P9-ASI-831

The Human
Nervous System

MURRAY L. BARR, M.D., D.Sc., F.R.C.P.(C), F.R.S.

PROFESSOR, DEPARTMENT OF ANATOMY,
HEALTH SCIENCES CENTRE, UNIVERSITY OF WESTERN ONTARIO,
LONDON, ONTARIO, CANADA

COVER PHOTOGRAPH BY NEDZAD GLUHBEGOVIC, M.D., PH.D.,
UTRECHT, THE NETHERLANDS

The Human Nervous System

AN ANATOMIC VIEWPOINT

THIRD EDITION

Presented to:

HARPER & ROW, PUBLISHERS
HAGERSTOWN, MARYLAND
NEW YORK, SAN FRANCISCO, LONDON

The author and publisher have exerted every effort to ensure that drug selection and dosage set forth in this text are in accord with current recommendations and practice at the time of publication. However, in view of ongoing research, changes in government regulations, and the constant flow of information relating to drug therapy and drug reactions, the reader is urged to check the package insert for each drug for any change in indications and dosage and for added warnings and precautions. This is particularly important when the recommended agent is a new and/or infrequently employed drug.

79 80 81 82 83 84   10 9 8 7 6 5 4 3 2 1

The Human Nervous System: An Anatomic Viewpoint, Third Edition. Copyright © 1979 by Harper & Row, Publishers, Inc. All rights reserved. No part of this book may be used or reproduced in any manner whatsoever without written permission except in the case of brief quotations embodied in critical articles and reviews. Printed in the United States of America. For information address Medical Department, Harper & Row, Publishers, Inc., 2350 Virginia Avenue, Hagerstown, Maryland 21740.
Library of Congress Cataloging in Publication Data
Barr, Murray Llewellyn, 1908-
    The human nervous system.
    Includes bibliographies and index.
    1. Central nervous system.   2. Neuroanatomy.
I. Title.
QM455.B37   1979   611'.8   79-430
ISBN 0-06-140312-1

Contents

BLOOD SUPPLY AND THE MENINGES

APPENDICES

INDEX   **327**

Preface to the Third Edition

The teaching of neuroanatomy varies so widely according to university and program that the preparation of a textbook of general suitability is an impossible goal. However, the acceptance of this book indicates that it approximates the requirements of many students in acquiring a basic understanding of the functional anatomy of the human central nervous system. This acceptance provided the encouragement to prepare an improved Third Edition.

The extensive revision of the text includes factual changes, as well as others designed to improve clarity and readability. The terminology conforms more closely with the recommendations of *Nomina Anatomica,* while not abandoning entirely synonyms of long standing which students are likely to encounter. References to clinical aspects of various topics have been retained as a bridge, small though it may be, between the basic neurosciences and clinical neurology. There are a few new illustrations and others have been revised.

The welcome letters from colleagues suggesting improvements were uniformly helpful. I am especially indebted to Dr. John A. Kiernan, Department of Anatomy, The University of Western Ontario, for his valued assistance throughout the preparation of this edition. I am indebted as well to Mrs. Aileen Densham for her efficient secretarial work, and to the staff of Harper & Row for their continued collaboration and encouragement.

M. L. B.

Preface to the First Edition

Because of the intricacies of neuronal connections and the necessity of being able to visualize structures three-dimensionally, the anatomy of the central nervous system offers a particular challenge to the student. It is only through an adequate understanding of the structure of the brain and spinal cord that concurrent studies along physiologic and clinical lines can progress. In particular, the interpretation of neurologic signs and symptoms must rest on a sound basis of neurologic anatomy. It is hoped that this textbook will provide such a basis for students in the health sciences and others studying the central nervous system of man. The book is written for those approaching the neurosciences for the first time; several excellent larger books on neurologic anatomy are available to the advanced student.

The material has been arranged in four sections. The first section deals mainly with neurohistology. The second and largest section is concerned with the regional anatomy of the central nervous system, beginning with the spinal cord and the progressing to the highest levels of the brain. Although the sensory and motor systems are discussed regionally, experience in teaching has shown the necessity of reviewing these clinically important systems in their entirety, and this is done in the third section. The fourth section deals with the blood supply of the central nervous system, its meningeal coverings, and the cerebrospinal fluid.

Eponyms are used freely in neurology, in spite of attempts to eliminate them; they frequently offer welcome alternatives to the more formal, and sometimes formidable, anatomic terms. Some facts concerning individuals whose names are attached to structures are provided at the end of the book for students who are curious about the source of the eponyms. In addition, since many neurologic terms are derived from Greek and Latin, a glossary is included for those students who have not received instruction in the classics.

It is a pleasure to acknowledge the valued assistance of several persons. A special note of appreciation goes to Mrs. Margaret Corrin for the preparation of the drawings, all of which are her own work. Illustrations of this type are of particular importance in a textbook of neurologic anatomy. I also wish to thank Mrs. Aileen Densham, who carried out the secretarial work most efficiently. I am greatly indebted to Mr. J. E. Walker for the technical preparation of anatomic specimens for reproduction, to Mr. C. E. Jarvis for the photomicrographs, and to the staff of the Art Service Department of this Health Services Centre for their fine photography.

Several colleagues have given of their time to read drafts of all chapters and make valuable suggestions. They are Dr. H. W. K. Barr, of the Department of Clinical Neurological Sciences, and Drs. R. C. Buck, M. J. Hollenberg, and D. G. Montemurro, of the Department of Anatomy. I am also grateful for the many helpful discussions on specific topics with Dr. J. P. Girvin, of the Departments of Clinical Neurological Sciences and Physiology, and with Dr. A. Kertesz, of the Department of Clinical Neurological Sciences. Finally, I wish to express my appreciation to the staff of Harper & Row for their patience, advice, and assistance.

M. L. B.

The Human Nervous System

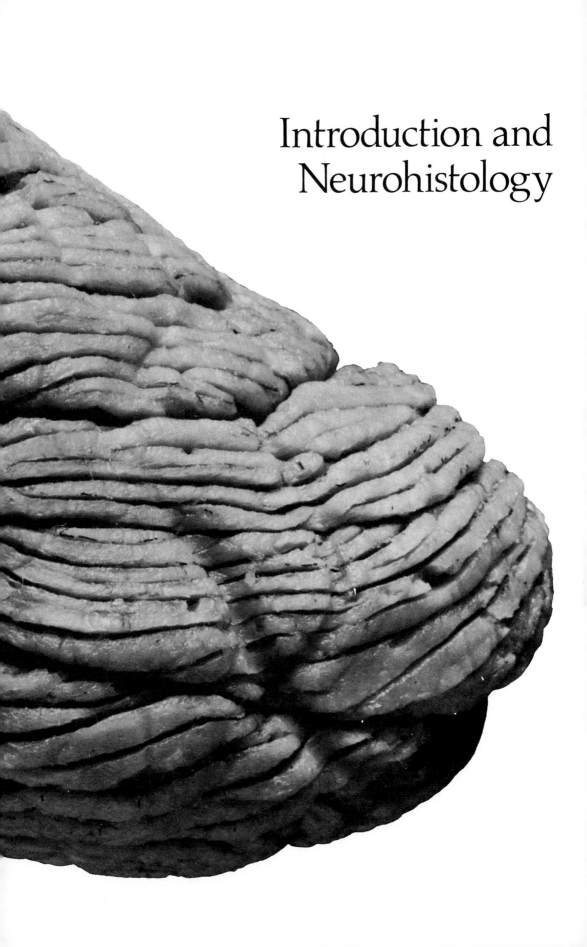

Introduction and Neurohistology

1

Origin of the Central Nervous System and Composition of Its Major Divisions

The nervous system regulates and integrates the systems of the body, and it provides for the behavior and intellectual attainments of man. The **central nervous system** consists of the brain and spinal cord, whereas the cranial and spinal nerves comprise the **peripheral nervous system.** There is also an **autonomic nervous system** which innervates the smooth muscle and glands of viscera, together with cardiac muscle. It is situated partly in the central and partly in the peripheral nervous system, and it is closely related functionally with the afferent or sensory supply of viscera. The peripheral and autonomic nervous systems are described in textbooks of gross anatomy. In this book, which deals mainly with the central nervous system, general features of the peripheral nervous system are discussed in Chapter 3, and a survey of visceral innervation is presented in Chapter 24. The details of neuroembryology are more appropriate for textbooks of embryology. However, it is helpful to refer briefly to early stages of development, in which the major divisions of the mature brain are established and receive their names.

The nervous system develops from the dorsal ectoderm of the early embryo. Nerve cells, together with most of the neuroglial or interstitial cells, are therefore derived from the outer, ectodermal layer, like the cells of the epidermis covering the body surface. The first indication of the future nervous system is the neuroectoderm comprising the **neural plate,** which appears in the dorsal midline of

the embryo at the 16th day of development. The neural plate changes 2 days later into a **neural groove** with a **neural fold** along each side; by the end of the 3rd week the neural folds have begun to fuse with one another, thereby converting the neural groove into a **neural tube** (Fig. 1–1). The transformation proceeds rostrally and caudally, and the openings at each end (the rostral and caudal neuropores) close at about the 24th and 26th days, respectively. The neural tube is the forerunner of the brain and spinal cord. Neuroectodermal cells not incorporated in the neural tube form **neural crests** running dorsolaterally along each side of the neural tube. From the neural crests are derived the dorsal root ganglia of spinal nerves, comparable ganglia on cranial nerves, autonomic ganglia, and secretory cells of the adrenal medulla.

Growth and differentiation are greatest in the rostral portion of the neural tube, from which the large and complex brain develops, and the remainder of the neural tube becomes the spinal cord. As described conventionally, three **primary brain vesicles** appear at the end of the 4th week: the **prosencephalon** (forebrain), **mesencephalon** (midbrain), and **rhombencephalon** (hindbrain) (Fig. 1–2A). During the 5th week each of the first and third vesicles changes into two swellings, so that there are five **secondary brain vesicles: telencephalon, diencephalon, mesencephalon, metencephalon,** and **myelencephalon** (Fig. 1–2B). As cellular proliferation and

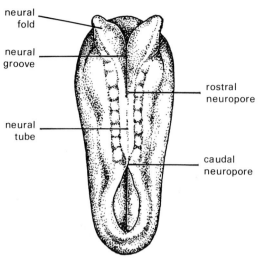

neural fold

neural groove

neural tube

rostral neuropore

caudal neuropore

FIG. 1–1. Dorsal view of embryo at about 22 days.

differentiation proceed in the spinal cord, a longitudinal groove called the **sulcus limitans** appears along the inner aspect of each lateral wall. The sulcus demarcates a dorsal **alar plate** from a ventral **basal plate;** they acquire afferent and efferent connections, respectively, and continue forward as far as the rostral end of the mesencephalon. The neural canal within the neural tube becomes the ventricles of the brain and the central canal of the spinal cord.

Congenital malformations of the central nervous system include those which result from failure of the neural folds to fuse normally. In anencephaly the folds do not fuse at the rostral end of the developing neural tube, so that forebrain derivatives are lacking and the concurrent absence of a cranial vault exposes the rudiment of the brain to the exterior. Anencephaly occurs once in about 1000 births and is incompatible with sustained life. As a rarer condition the neural folds fail to meet and fuse in the lumbar region. This error results in an especially severe form of spina bifida, known as spina bifida with myeloschisis (cleft spinal cord).

DERIVATIVES OF THE BRAIN VESICLES

The regions of the brain which develop from the secondary brain vesicles acquire a distinctive structure, and some of the formal embryologic names are replaced by others for common usage (Table 1–1 and Fig. 1–3). The myelencephalon becomes the medulla oblongata, and the metencephalon develops into the pons and cerebellum. The mesencephalon of the mature brain is usually called the midbrain. The names diencephalon and telencephalon are retained because of the diverse nature of their derivatives. A large mass of gray matter, the thalamus, develops in the diencephalon. Adjacent regions are known as the epithalamus, hypothalamus, and subthalamus, each with distinctive structural and functional characteristics. The telencephalon undergoes the greatest development in the human brain, in respect both to other regions and to the telencephalon of other animals. It includes the olfactory system, the corpus striatum (a mass of gray matter with motor functions), an extensive surface layer of gray matter known as the cortex or pallium, and a medullary center of white matter.

The medulla, pons, and midbrain together make up the brain stem, to which the cere-

TABLE 1–1. DEVELOPMENT OF THE MATURE BRAIN FROM THE BRAIN VESICLES

PRIMARY BRAIN VESICLES	SECONDARY BRAIN VESICLES	MATURE BRAIN
Rhombencephalon	Myelencephalon	Medulla oblongata
	Metencephalon	Pons and cerebellum
Mesencephalon	Mesencephalon	Midbrain
Prosencephalon	Diencephalon	Thalamus, epithalamus, hypothalamus, and subthalamus
	Telencephalon	Cerebral hemispheres, consisting of the olfactory system, corpus striatum, cortex, and medullary center

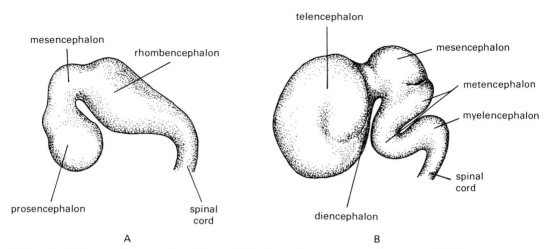

FIG. 1–2. **A.** Primary brain vesicles (5th week). **B.** Secondary brain vesicles (7th week). The diencephalon is partly hidden by the expanding telencephalon, which develops into the cerebral hemispheres.

FIG. 1–3. Regions of the mature central nervous system, as seen in sagittal section. (× ⅝)

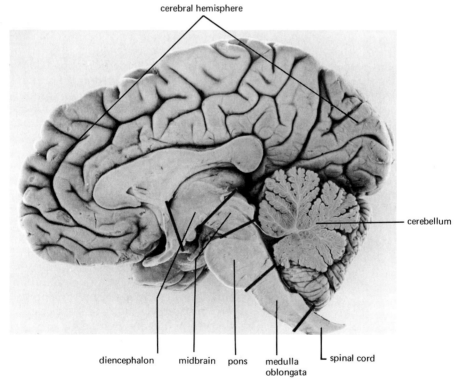

bellum is attached by three pairs of peduncles. The diencephalon and telencephalon constitute the cerebrum, of which the telencephalon is represented by the massive cerebral hemispheres. The lumen of the neural tube is converted into a lateral ventricle in each cerebral hemisphere, a third ventricle in the diencephalon, and a fourth ventricle bounded by the medulla, pons, and cerebellum. The third and fourth ventricles are connected by a narrow channel or aqueduct through the midbrain.

SUMMARY OF MAIN REGIONS OF THE NERVOUS SYSTEM

Certain features of the main regions are noted in the following summary, by way of introduction and to provide a first acquaintance with some neurologic terms.

SPINAL CORD

The **spinal cord** is the least differentiated component of the central nervous system. The segmental nature of the spinal cord is reflected in a series of paired spinal nerves, each of which is attached to the cord by a dorsal sensory root and ventral motor root. The central gray matter, in which nerve cell bodies are located, has a roughly H-shaped outline in transverse section. White matter, which consists of nerve fibers running longitudinally, occupies the periphery of the cord. The spinal cord includes neuronal connections which provide for important spinal reflexes. There are also pathways conveying sensory data to the brain and other pathways conducting impulses from the brain to motor neurons in the spinal cord.

MEDULLA OBLONGATA

The fiber tracts of the spinal cord are continued in the **medulla,** which also contains clusters of nerve cells called nuclei. The most prominent of these, the inferior olivary nuclei, send fibers to the cerebellum through the inferior cerebellar peduncles, which attach the cerebellum to the medulla oblongata. Of the smaller nuclei, some are components of the following cranial nerves: hypoglossal (CN12), accessory (CN11), vagus (CN10), glossopharyngeal (CN9), and vestibulocochlear (CN8).

PONS

The **pons** consists of two distinct parts. The dorsal portion has features shared with the rest of the brain stem. It therefore includes sensory and motor tracts, together with nuclei of the facial (CN7), abducens (CN6), and trigeminal (CN5) nerves. (Trigeminal nuclei are also present in the medulla and midbrain.) The basal (ventral) portion of the pons is special to this part of the brain stem. Its function is to provide for extensive connections between the cortex of a cerebral hemisphere and that of the contralateral cerebellar hemisphere. These connections are important for maximal efficiency of motor activities. A pair of middle cerebellar peduncles attaches the cerebellum to the pons.

MIDBRAIN

Like other parts of the brain stem, the **midbrain** contains sensory and motor pathways, together with nuclei for two cranial nerves, the trochlear (CN4) and the oculomotor (CN3). There is a dorsal region, the roof or tectum, which is concerned principally with the visual and auditory systems. The midbrain also includes two important motor nuclei, the red nucleus and the substantia nigra. The cerebellum is attached to the midbrain by the superior cerebellar peduncles.

CEREBELLUM

The **cerebellum** is especially large in the human brain. Receiving data from most of the sensory systems and the cerebral cortex, the cerebellum eventually influences motor neurons supplying the skeletal musculature. The function of the cerebellum is to influence muscle tonus in relation to equilibrium, locomotion and posture, and nonstereotyped movements based on individual experience. The cerebellum operates behind the scenes at a subconscious level.

DIENCEPHALON

The **diencephalon** forms the central core of the cerebrum. The largest component of the diencephalon, the **thalamus,** receives data from all sensory systems except the olfactory and projects to sensory areas of the cerebral cortex. Part of the thalamus is involved in reverberating circuits with nonspecific cortical areas that are concerned with complex mental processes. Other regions of the thalamus participate in neural circuits related to emotions, and certain thalamic nuclei are incorporated in pathways from the cerebellum and corpus striatum to motor areas of the cerebral cortex. The **epithalamus** includes small tracts and a nucleus, together with the pineal gland, an endocrine organ. The **hypothalamus** is the principal autonomic center of the brain and as such has an important controlling influence over the sympathetic and parasympathetic systems. In addition neurosecretory cells in the hypothalamus synthesize hormones which reach the blood stream by way of the neurohypophysis or influence the hormonal output of the adenohypophysis through a special portal system of blood vessels. The **subthalamus** includes sensory tracts proceeding to the thalamus, nerve fibers originating in the cerebellum and corpus striatum, and the subthalamic nucleus (a motor nucleus). The retina is a derivative of the diencephalon; the optic nerve (CN2) and the visual system are therefore intimately related to this part of the brain.

TELENCEPHALON
(Cerebral Hemispheres)

Within the **telencephalon,** the corpus striatum is a large mass of gray matter with motor functions, situated near the base of each hemisphere. The corpus striatum consists of caudate and lenticular (lentiform) nuclei, the latter being subdivided into a putamen and a globus pallidus. The medullary center of the hemisphere consists of 1) fibers connecting cortical areas of the same hemisphere, 2) fibers crossing the midline in a large commissure known as the corpus callosum to connect cortical areas of the two hemispheres, and 3) fibers passing in both directions between cortex and subcortical centers. Fibers of the last category converge to form a compact internal capsule in the region of the thalamus and corpus striatum.

Small areas of cerebral cortex have an ancient lineage (paleocortex); they are olfactory in function, receiving data from the olfactory nerves (CNI) and forming part of the rhinencephalon or nosebrain, which dominates the cerebrum of lower vertebrates. Certain areas of cortex were once part of the rhinencephalon but acquired other roles in the evolution of the mammalian brain. These areas are referred to as archicortex; they are included in the limbic system, which is involved with emotions and the influence of emotions on visceral function through the autonomic nervous system. The development of cortex still further removed from olfactory influence (neocortex) was a most significant event, and the presence of substantial amounts of neocortex is a mammalian characteristic. Its extent and volume have increased during mammalian evolution, and the human brain is notable for having much more neocortex than the brain of any other animal. Nine-tenths of the cortex of the human cerebral hemispheres is neocortex, which includes areas for all modalities of sensation, exclusive of smell, and special motor areas. There are also extensive areas of association cortex in which the highest levels of neural function take place, including those inherent in intellectual activity. The unique place of the human species is an endowment conferred by an expanse of neocortex that is possessed by no other animal.

The weight of the mature brain varies according to age and body stature. The normal range in the adult male is 1100–1700 g (average 1360 g). The lower figures for the adult female (1050–1550 g, average 1275 g) reflect the smaller body stature of females in general, compared with males. There is no evidence of a relation between brain weight, within the normal limits, and a person's level of intelligence.

SUGGESTED READING

Lemire RJ, Loeser JD, Leech RW, Alvord EC Jr: Normal and Abnormal Development of the Nervous System. Hagerstown, Harper & Row, 1975

Moore KL: The Developing Human; Clinically Oriented Embryology, 2nd ed. Philadelphia, Saunders, 1977

2

Cells of the Central Nervous System

There are two classes of cells in the central nervous system aside from the usual cells found in walls of blood vessels. **Nerve cells** or **neurons** are specialized for excitation (or inhibition) and nerve impulse conduction, and are therefore responsible for most of the functional characteristics of nervous tissue. **Neuroglial cells,** also known as interstitial cells, have important ancillary functions. There are four types of neuroglial cell, namely, astrocytes, oligodendrocytes, microglial cells, and ependymal cells.

The central nervous system consists of gray matter and white matter. **Gray matter** contains the cell bodies of neurons, each with a nucleus, embedded in a **neuropil** made up predominantly of delicate neuronal processes. **White matter,** on the other hand, consists mainly of long processes of neurons, the majority being surrounded by myelin sheaths, and nerve cell bodies are lacking. Both the gray and the white matter contain large numbers of neuroglial cells and a network of blood capillaries. In some parts of the central nervous system, notably the brain stem (medulla, pons, and midbrain), there are regions which contain both nerve cell bodies and numerous myelinated fibers. These regions are therefore an admixture of gray matter and white matter.

The cytology of the nervous system is described in some detail in textbooks of histology. However, a subject so basic to the neurologic sciences can hardly be omitted from a student's textbook of neurologic anatomy. An account of the cellular components of the brain and spinal cord is therefore introduced at this point.

THE NEURON

Neurons have special features for reception of nerve impulses from other neurons, the effect of which may be either excitation or inhibition, and conduction of nerve impulses. The part of the cell that includes the nucleus is called the **cell body** or **perikaryon. Dendrites** are typically short, branching processes which form a major part of the receptor area of the cell. Most neurons of the central nervous system have several dendrites and are therefore multipolar in shape. By reaching out in various directions, these processes improve the capacity of a neuron to receive nerve impulses from diverse sources. Each cell has a single **axon.** This process, which varies greatly in length from one type of neuron to another, conducts impulses away from the cell body, usually to other neurons in the central nervous system. Axons of efferent neurons in the spinal cord and brain stem are included in spinal and cranial nerves; they end on striated muscle fibers or on nerve cells of sympathetic or parasympathetic ganglia in the case of neurons belonging to the autonomic system.

Each neuron is a structural and functional unit. This statement is implicit in the Neuron Theory, which is an extension of the Cell Theory to include nerve cells. The Neuron Theory, as opposed to the view that nerve cells form a continuous reticulum, was advanced by His on the basis of embryologic studies, by Forel on the basis of the response of nerve cells to injury, and by Ramón y Cajal from his observations with silver staining methods. The Neuron Theory was given wide distribution in a general review of the whole subject of the individuality of nerve cells by Waldeyer. Because of the special relationship between neurons at synapses, wholly convincing evidence in support of the Neuron Theory had to await the introduction of electron microscopy. It is now clear that plasma membranes of two neurons are in fact separated by a narrow interval known as a synaptic cleft.

VARIATIONS AMONG NEURONS

Although all nerve cells conform to the general principles outlined above, there is a wide range of structural diversity. The size of the perikaryon varies from 5μ for the smallest cells in complex circuits to 135μ for large motor neurons. Dendritic morphology, in particular the pattern of branching, varies greatly and is distinctive for neurons composing a specific cell group or nucleus. The axon of minute neurons is a fraction of a millimeter in length, exceedingly fine, and devoid of a myelin covering. The axon of large neurons, on the other hand, is several feet long in extreme cases, has a substantial diameter, and is typically enclosed in a sheath of myelin. Large and small neurons are known as Golgi type I and Golgi type II neurons, respectively. Intermediate grades, difficult to assign to type I and type II, occur in special locations. The following examples will serve to illustrate the range of variability among neurons of the central nervous system.

Examples of Large Neurons

Large pyramidal cells of the cerebral cortex, Purkinje cells of the cerebellar cortex, and motor cells of the spinal cord are familiar examples of Golgi type I neurons. These cells and examples of small neurons are illustrated in Figure 2-1 as they might appear in sections stained by the Golgi bichromate–silver or bichromate–osmium method, or one of the many modifications of the Golgi technique.

The **pyramidal cell** derives its name from the shape of the cell body. An apical dendrite extends toward the surface of the cortex, and there are several basal or horizontal dendrites. The dendrites branch extensively, and the smaller branches are beset with minute protuberances (dendritic spines or gemmules), with which axons of other neurons make synaptic contact. The axon of a pyramidal cell arises from the base of the perikaryon or occasionally from the root of a basal dendrite. It leaves the cortex and may continue for a considerable distance, even to lower levels of the spinal cord. The axon gives off collateral branches and these, together with the terminal branches, make synaptic contact with other neurons.

The cell bodies of **Purkinje cells** constitute a single layer of cells throughout the extensive cerebellar cortex. The cell body is flask shaped, tapering into one or two dendrites which extend toward the cortical surface. The dendritic branching, which is exceptionally profuse, occurs in a plane at right angles to the cortical fold or folium. The branches bear many thousands of dendritic spines, and these provide for unusually abundant synaptic contacts with axons of other cortical cells which relay data they receive from outside the cerebellum. The axon arises from the base of the cell body, gives off collateral branches, and then traverses the white matter of the cerebellum to end in its central nuclei.

Lower motor neurons are found in the ventral gray horns of the spinal cord and motor nuclei of cranial nerves. They are "lower motor neurons" in the sense that they come under the influence of "upper motor neurons" whose cell bodies are at higher levels, including the cerebral cortex. These large multipolar cells give off several dendrites which branch in the vicinity of the cell body. Large numbers of axon terminals (up to 2000 in the case of spinal motor neurons) establish synaptic contact with the dendrites and the cell body. The axon leaves the central nervous system in a spinal or cranial nerve and terminates in motor end plates on striated muscle fibers.

Examples of Small Neurons

Although Golgi type I neurons are impressive because of their large size, they are vastly outnumbered by Golgi type II cells. The latter are variously called intercalary, intercalated, or internuncial neurons (or simply interneurons) because they are typically interposed between other neurons to establish circuits which may be of great com-

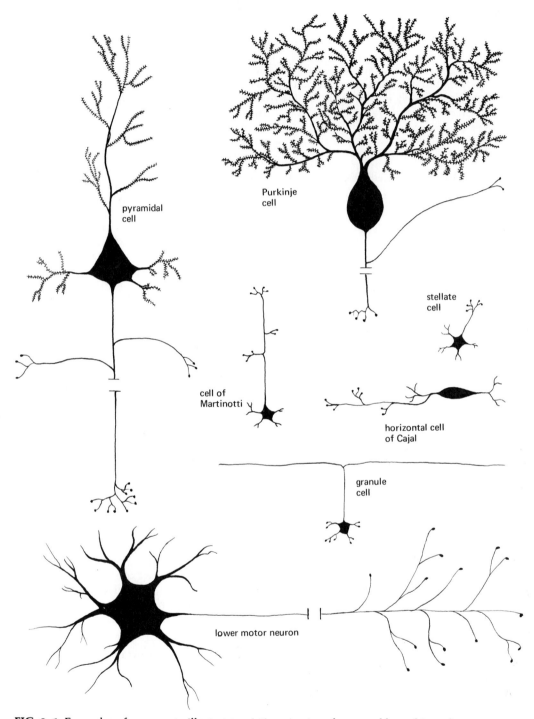

FIG. 2–1. Examples of neurons to illustrate variations in size, shape, and branching of processes. The axon of the lower motor neuron traverses cranial or spinal nerves and branches terminally within a muscle. The other neurons shown are confined to the central nervous system.

plexity. Such circuits are basic to the most complex neural functions, including the intellectual capabilities of man. These small cells are especially numerous in the cerebral cortex.

In the cerebral cortex and at certain other sites many of the Golgi type II neurons take the form of **stellate cells,** so-called because their multipolar form gives a star-shaped profile (Fig. 2–1). Several short dendrites branch close to the cell body and establish contact with axon terminals. The thin axon, which is unmyelinated in most Golgi type II cells, ends on one or more nerve cells in the immediate vicinity. **Cells of Martinotti** and **horizontal cells of Cajal** are additional examples of interneurons in the cerebral cortex. The cell of Martinotti is like a stellate cell, except that the axon is longer and directed toward the surface of the cortex. The horizontal cell of Cajal lies in the outer cortex with its long axis parallel to the cortical surface.

The **granule cell** of the cerebellar cortex is another example of a Golgi type II neuron. The small cell bodies of granule cells are closely packed in the deepest of the three cortical layers. Several short dendrites establish contact with axons conveying impulses from outside the cerebellum. The axon is directed toward the surface of the cortex, bifurcates on reaching the outer layer containing Purkinje cell dendrites, and establishes synaptic contact with many Purkinje cells by running parallel with the cortical fold or folium.

The examples just given will serve to illustrate the morphologic diversity of nerve cells within the broad limits of a common pattern. In addition to size differences, there are variations in the number of dendrites, the pattern of dendritic branching, and other morphologic characteristics, according to the specific role of the neuron. It follows that the neurons of different cell aggregates or nuclei tend to be structurally similar within a nucleus.

CYTOLOGY OF THE NEURON

The intrinsic structure of the neuron, although basically like that of other cells, has some specialized characteristics. Knowledge of neurocytology has accumulated over many decades through the application of an assortment of staining methods for light microscopy and more recently through the use of electron microscopy. Hematoxylin and eosin stain, which is so widely used for most tissues, has less to offer with respect to nervous tissue, mainly because the processes of neurons and neuroglial cells are not revealed. Many staining methods have been devised to demonstrate the processes of these cells and specialized components or organelles of the cytoplasm. Because of chemical and physical differences between the various organelles, each requires a specific staining method. In order to visualize the nerve cell in its entirety, it is necessary to combine the results of several staining methods conceptually. This is true of most cell types, but the situation is made more difficult in the case of neurons by the cell processes, synaptic contacts, and myelin covering of axons.

Electron microscopy has the distinct advantage of showing the components of a cell without differential staining, depending instead on variations in scattering of electrons as they pass through the cell. The necessity of using ultrathin sections makes it difficult, although not impossible, to reconstruct the neuron three-dimensionally. In the end, a combination of light and electron microscopy gives a comprehensive view of neuronal structure. Figure 2–2 does not pretend to represent a typical neuron, because the diversity among nerve cells makes the "typical neuron" an abstraction. The figure is intended to represent, in simplified and semidiagrammatic form, a large nerve cell as conceived by combining the results of several staining techniques. The drawing also forms a basis for comments on the ultrastructure of the cellular components as shown with the electron microscope. It is assumed that most users of this book have become acquainted with cell ultrastructure through courses in biology or histology. Where this is not so, standard texts in those subjects may be consulted.

Cell Surface

The surface or limiting membrane of the neuron assumes special importance because of its role in the initiation and transmission of nerve impulses. There is a plasma membrane composed of lipid and protein molecules, whose arrangement is a subject of cur-

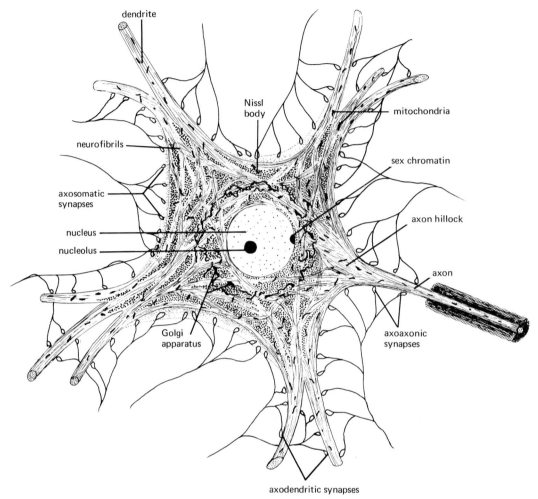

FIG. 2–2. Semidiagrammatic representation of the constituents of a nerve cell.

rent research, together with an external "cell coat" consisting of glycoproteins containing sialic acids. Briefly stated, the participation of the cell surface with respect to the nerve impulse is as follows.

The cell membrane, considering the plasma membrane and the cell coat as a unit, is semipermeable in that it allows diffusion of some ions through it, but restricts others. In the resting state, the membrane is disproportionately permeable to K^+ ions. The latter diffuse from the cytoplasm, in which they are in high concentration, to the outer surface of the cell membrane. In this way the outer surface acquires a positive resting potential of about 80 mV (millivolts). During excitation, when the membrane potential has been re-

duced by about 10–15 mV to threshold value, there is a sudden functional alteration in the membrane, characterized by a selective increase in permeability to Na^+ ions. These surge locally from the outer to the inner surface, the concentration of Na^+ ions being relatively high externally, causing a reversal of charge and creating an **action potential.** Once generated the action potential is self-propagated along the membrane by local circuits of electrical current. This is the **nerve impulse,** which can be recorded electrically from the outer surface of a nerve fiber as a wave of negative potential. The resting and active membrane potentials of excitable cells are dependent upon the semipermeable nature of the membrane and its ionic polarization, which is maintained by active metabolic processes.

Nucleus

The spherical nucleus is usually situated centrally in the cell body; it is vesicular in large neurons, *i.e.,* the chromatin is finely dispersed, whereas in small neurons the chromatin is likely to be in coarse clumps. There are a few binucleate nerve cells in sympathetic ganglia. The **nuclear membrane** or **envelope** has the usual double-layered ultrastructure with numerous small pores. Although the pores are closed by thin diaphragms, they enhance the permeability of the nuclear membrane for passage of certain chemicals from the nucleoplasm to the cytoplasm or in the reverse direction. There is usually a single prominent **nucleolus.** The large size of the nucleolus is related to its role in the synthesis of ribonucleic acid (RNA) and the transfer of RNA to the cytoplasm. The further role of RNA in protein synthesis has a special significance in nerve cells, particularly Golgi type I neurons, because an unusually large volume of proteins must be maintained in the long cell processes. In females one of the two X chromosomes of the interphase nucleus is compact (heterochromatic), rather than elongated (euchromatic) like the remaining 45 chromosomes of the complement. The compact X chromosome is evident as a mass of **sex chromatin,** which is usually situated at the inner surface of the nuclear membrane. A small, spherical intranuclear structure of unknown significance, called the **accessory body of Cajal,** is seen in sections stained by silver methods (Fig. 4–5).

Cytoplasmic Organelles

NEUROFIBRILS, NEUROFILAMENTS, AND MICROTUBULES. When certain silver stains are used the cytoplasm is seen by light microscopy to contain neurofibrils, sometimes grouped into bundles, running through the perikaryon and into the cell processes. In electron micrographs of nerve cells, the cytoplasm contains neurofilaments of the order of 75–100A in thickness (A= one ten-thousandth of a micron). The neurofilaments are probably responsible for the neurofibrils of light microscopy, although this is uncertain. Electron microscopy also shows microtubules about 200–300A in external diameter, similar

to those of other types of cell. These appear to be involved in the rapid transport of essential metabolites from the perinuclear zone throughout the neuron. The neurofilaments and microtubules consist of helically organized protein threads.

NISSL MATERIAL. When nervous tissue is stained with basic dyes such as cresyl violet or thionine, clumps of basophilic material are seen in most nerve cells. These are known as Nissl bodies, after Franz Nissl (1860–1919), a Heidelberg neurologist. The amount of Nissl material increases with the size of the neuron, and its arrangement varies from one type of nerve cell to another. For example the clumps are coarse in motor neurons (Fig. 2–3), whereas the basophilic material is more finely distributed in sensory neurons. The Nissl substance extends into dendritic processes, but is lacking in both the axon hillock, *i.e.,* the peripheral zone of the perikaryon where the axon emerges, and the axon itself. Nissl material is the same as the basophilic substance, sometimes called ergastoplasm or chromidial substance, in the cytoplasm of cells such as those composing the pancreatic acini.

The nature of the Nissl substance was made apparent by electron microscopy. Virtually all cells of the body contain an ultrastructural cytoplasmic constituent, known as **granular endoplasmic reticulum,** in amounts ranging from scanty to abundant. This consists of a system of flattened cisternae or vesicles bearing ribosomal particles on their outer surfaces, and often with free ribosomes in the adjacent cytoplasmic matrix. The ribosomes contain RNA, and the granular or rough-surfaced endoplasmic reticulum is therefore basophilic. The clumps of Nissl substance consist of orderly arrays of granular endoplasmic reticulum with many free ribosomes (Fig. 2–4). The ribosomes participate in the synthesis of structural and enzymatic proteins, accounting for the abundance of Nissl material in large neurons having considerable cytoplasm to maintain in long processes. To be more specific it has been shown by several methods, including autoradiography following the administration of labeled amino acids, that the proteins of nerve cells are synthesized predominantly in the perikaryon, then flow along the neuronal

FIG. 2–3. Motor neuron in the spinal cord. (Cresyl violet stain, × 1000)

processes, notably the axon, at a rate of about 1 mm a day. The axoplasmic flow away from the perikaryon replaces proteins that are degraded during cellular activity. This aspect of cell metabolism is important as well as in the growth of neurons and regeneration of peripheral nerve fibers. Axoplasmic flow is of cardinal significance in the phenomenon of neurosecretion by certain cells in the hypothalamus.

MITOCHONDRIA. These cytoplasmic organelles are scattered through the perikaryon, dendrites, and axon. They are spherical, rod-shaped, or filamentous, measuring from 0.2–1.0μ in their greatest dimension and about 0.2μ in diameter. With electron microscopy, the mitochondria of nerve cells show the surface double membrane and internal folds or cristae that are present in mitochondria of cells generally. Mitochondria are the repository of enzymes, which are involved in several aspects of cell metabolism, including the respiratory and phosphorylating enzymes of the Krebs citric acid cycle. They are therefore important in nerve cells, as in all cells, in the energy-producing reactions of cellular physiology.

GOLGI APPARATUS. The Golgi apparatus (complex) is a universal cytoplasmic organelle with special historic interest in relation to nerve cells, having been first demonstrated in these cells by the Italian histologist Camillo Golgi (1843–1926). With a silver-osmium staining method for light microscopy, the Golgi apparatus appears as a dark, irregular network, which is often disposed around the nuclear envelope, midway between the latter and the cell surface. The Golgi apparatus appears in electron micrographs as clusters of closely apposed, flattened cisternae, arranged in stacks and surrounded by many small vesicles. This membranous system is continuous with agranular or smooth-surfaced endoplasmic reticulum, and the latter is continuous with granular endoplasmic reticulum. The three membranous systems are in a sense regional differentiations of a single, extensive cytoplasmic organelle. The function of the Golgi complex is imperfectly understood. In secretory cells there is good evidence that the secretory products are "packaged" in the Golgi area, including incorporation of the carbohydrate moiety of the secretory product. In cells generally, the Golgi apparatus appears to be in dynamic relationship with vacuoles and other membranous components of the cytoplasm.

FIG. 2-4. Electron micrograph of a portion of a neuron in the preoptic nucleus of the rabbit's hypothalamus. The series of membranous profiles, together with the free ribosomes (polysomes) between the profiles, constitute the Nissl material of light microscopy. **M.** Mitochondria. **Memb.** Membranes of endoplasmic reticulum. **N.** Nucleus. **PM.** Plasma membrane. (× 36,000) (Courtesy of Dr. R. Clattenburg)

CENTROSOME. This cell organelle, which includes a pair of centrioles, has an important role in the dynamics of mitosis. A centrosome is present in the precursors of mature neurons during the developmental period, as is to be expected, and has been seen in neurons in cell cultures. A centrosome is lacking, or poorly developed at best, in mature neurons. It is generally believed that there is little increase in the neuronal population after birth, although some increment in the number of small internuncial neurons during infancy is a distinct possibility. The size of the brain increases most during the later part of fetal life. The increase in size of the brain and spinal cord during the postnatal growth period is caused by a number of factors. These include further development of existing neurons, especially branching of dendrites and growth of axons, and completion of myelination of certain fiber systems.

Pigment Material

The perikaryon may contain nonliving material or cytoplasmic inclusions, of which the most important are pigment granules. **Lipofuscin** (lipochrome) pigment occurs as clumps of yellowish-brown granules. Traces of this pigment appear in neurons of the spinal cord and medulla at about the 8th year of life, and in cells of spinal and sympathetic ganglia at about the same time. The amount of the pigment increases with age. The significance of lipofuscin is unknown, except that it is related to the aging process and is found at other sites, including cardiac muscle fibers. Some types of neuron, of which Purkinje cells are an example, do not accumulate lipofuscin, even in old age.

The presence of dark **melanin** pigment in the cytoplasm is restricted to a few cell groups, the largest being the substantia nigra, a motor nucleus in the midbrain. The significance of melanin at this site is not known with certainty, although it may be a by-product of a series of chemical reactions in which tyrosine and dihydroxyphenylalanine (dopa) figure prominently. The pigment appears at the end of the first year, increases until puberty, and remains relatively constant thereafter. Fine, iron-containing granules are present in some nerve cells of the substantia nigra and in the globus pallidus, a component of the corpus striatum. The amount of this material is not age dependent.

Processes of the Nerve Cell

Dendrites taper from the perikaryon and branch at acute angles in the environs of the cell body. The branching may be exceedingly profuse and intricate, the Purkinje cell of cerebellar cortex being outstanding in this respect. In some neurons, the smaller branches bear large numbers of minute projections, called dendritic **spines** or **gemmules,** which participate in synapses. The surface of the perikaryon may be included in the receptive area or "dendritic field" of the neuron. In motor neurons of the spinal cord,

for example, large numbers of axonal endings are in synaptic relationship with the cell body, as well as with the dendrites.

The single **axon** of a nerve cell tends to have a uniform diameter throughout its length. It is a short delicate process in the case of Golgi type II cells, branching terminally to establish synaptic contact with one or more adjacent neurons. In Golgi type I cells, the diameter of the axon increases in proportion to its length. Collateral branches may be given off at right angles to the axon. The terminal branches are known as telodendria; they end typically as swellings or synaptic end bulbs. The cytoplasm of the axon is called **axoplasm** and the surface membrane is known as the **axolemma.** The axoplasm includes neurofilaments and microtubules, scattered mitochondria, and patches of smooth-surfaced or agranular endoplasmic reticulum.

Axons of Golgi type I neurons are surrounded as a rule by a myelin sheath, which begins near the origin of the axon and ends short of its terminal branching. Within the central nervous system the myelin is laid down by oligodendrocytes and consists essentially of closely apposed layers of their plasma membranes. The sheath therefore has a lipoprotein composition, and interruptions called nodes of Ranvier indicate where regions formed by different oligodendrocytes adjoin. The thickness of the myelin sheath tends to be directly proportional to the diameter and length of the axon. The greater the diameter of the nerve fiber, the faster is the conduction of the nerve impulse. (A nerve "fiber" in the central nervous system consists of the axon and the surrounding myelin sheath, or of the axon only in the case of unmyelinated fibers.) The formation and structure of the myelin sheath are discussed in the following chapter in the context of peripheral nerve fibers, in which these aspects of the myelin have been studied in greater detail.

Synapses

A neuron brings its influence to bear on other neurons at junctional points or synapses. "Synapse," meaning a conjunction or connection, was introduced by Sherrington in 1897. A nerve impulse can be propagated in any direction on the surface of a nerve cell. However, the direction followed under physiologic conditions is determined by a consis-

FIG. 2-5. Model of a nerve cell in the spinal cord, prepared from sections stained by Cajal's silver nitrate method. (From Haggar RA, Barr ML: J Comp Neurol 93:17–36, 1950)

tent polarity at the synapse, where transmission is from the axon of one neuron to the cell surface of another neuron.

Synapses assume a variety of forms, ranging from a simple apposition of axon and dendrite to rather complicated arrangements. In most instances, a synapse consists of an expansion of the end of an axonal branch in close apposition to the cell surface of another neuron (Fig. 2-5). The terminals are variously called **synaptic end bulbs, end bulbs of Held-Auerbach,** or **boutons terminaux.** Synaptic endings are always present on dendrites of cells in the central nervous system, the role of dendritic processes being to receive stimuli.

Depending on the type of neuron, there may also be synaptic terminals on the cell body, on the proximal portion of an axon before the myelin sheath begins, or even synaptic association between end bulbs derived from different neurons. On the foregoing basis, synapses are said to be **axodendritic, axosomatic,** or **axoaxonic.** Depending on the pathway or circuit in which a synapse is included, the particular neurotransmitter substance at the synapse, and perhaps other factors, the influence of an end bulb on the succeeding neuron is one of either excitation or inhibition.

When examined in electron micrographs (Figs. 2-6 and 2-7), the end bulb usually contains a number of mitochondria; bundles of neurofilaments continue into some end bulbs but not into others. The most characteristic constituent consists of large numbers of **synaptic vesicles,** which tend to accumulate near the synaptic surface. The vesicles vary from 200 to 800A in diameter, the majority being about 500A. They are of two types, clear or granular, the former having clear centers and the latter containing a dense particle; an end bulb usually contains either clear or granular vesicles, but both types are present occasionally in the same end bulb. The vesicles contain the chemical mediator at the synapse, which is released when nerve impulses reach the end bulb. Acetylcholine is known to be the mediator at synapses between preganglionic and postganglionic neurons of the autonomic system, at terminals of postganglionic parasympathetic fibers, and at motor end plates on striated muscle fibers. Norepinephrine (noradrenalin) is the transmitter agent at the terminals of postganglionic sympathetic fibers. Some synapses can therefore be classified as cholinergic or adrenergic. Establishing specific sites within the central nervous system at which acetylcholine, norepinephrine, or other substances act as neurotransmitters is an important aspect of current research.

The apposed surfaces of the end bulb and the neuron on which it terminates are called the **presynaptic** and **postsynaptic membranes,** respectively. They are separated by a 200A-wide **synaptic cleft.** The pre- and postsynaptic membranes are thickened in places, and there is an increase in the density of the cytoplasm beneath the thickened areas,

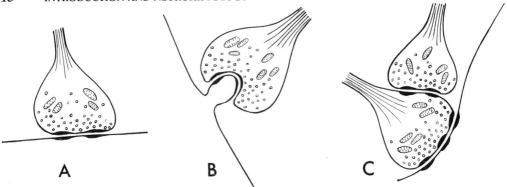

FIG. 2-6. Ultrastructure of synapses. **A.** Axodendritic or axosomatic synapse. **B.** Axodendritic synapse, in which an end bulb is in synaptic relation with a dendritic spine. **C.** Axoaxonic synapse of the end bulb to end bulb type. See text for details.

FIG. 2-7. Electron micrograph of a synapse in the suprachiasmatic nucleus of the rabbit's hypothalamus. **D.** Dendrite. **M.** Mitochondria. **Pre.** Presynaptic membrane. **Post.** Postsynaptic membrane. **SV.** Synaptic vesicles in the end bulb of an axon. (× 82,000) (Courtesy of Dr. R. Clattenburg)

especially of the postsynaptic membrane. The cell coat, consisting of glycoproteins containing sialic acids, continues through the synaptic cleft and binds the two membranes together. If the synapse is excitatory, the chemical mediator released from the synaptic vesicles by a nerve impulse produces a functional alteration in the postsynaptic membrane, which may result in an action potential, as described above. If the synapse is inhibitory, release of the transmitter substance stabilizes the postsynaptic membrane and lessens the likelihood of an action potential originating in the vicinity of the synapse.

Ultrastructural variations among synapses include differences in the size and shape of the synaptic vesicles and whether they are clear or granular. The pre- and postsynaptic membranes may be symmetrical or asymmetrical, depending mainly on the amount of increase in cytoplasmic density beneath the postsynaptic membrane. Considerable evidence has accumulated which indicates that synaptic morphology may be related to a particular chemical mediator and to either an excitatory or an inhibitory role. For example end bulbs containing clear vesicles have become associated with acetylcholine as the neurotransmitter substance, whereas end bulbs containing granular vesicles have become associated with norepinephrine and other catecholamines. The relevant studies are complicated by the range of structural diversity and possible neurotransmitter substances, as well as by technical difficulties, and further correlated studies are needed in order to establish relationships between synaptic structure and function.

Electrical synapses, as opposed to the chemical synapses already described, are common in invertebrates and lower vertebrates, and they have been observed at a few sites in the mammalian nervous system. They consist essentially of a close apposition of pre- and postsynaptic membranes, the interval between them being only 20A. Electrical synapses offer a low-resistance pathway between neurons, and there is a minimal delay in synaptic transmission because a chemical mediator is not involved. Unlike chemical synapses electrical synapses are not polarized, and the direction of transmission is determined by the interrelations of the neurons in a pathway.

NEUROGLIAL CELLS

Although neuroglial cells are not involved in the first instance with excitation, inhibition, and propagation of the nerve impulse, they have their own essential roles. It has also become evident that certain of these cells have an intimate relationship with nerve cells, leading to a high degree of interdependence. As noted previously neuroglial cells are classified as astrocytes, oligodendrocytes, microglial cells, and ependymal cells (Fig. 2–8). The first two mentioned are sometimes combined under the heading of **macroglia.** All but the microglia differentiate from neuroectodermal cells of the embryo, whereas microglial cells are derived from the mesoderm.

ASTROCYTES (Astroglia)

Astrocytes are present in profusion throughout the gray and the white matter of the brain and spinal cord. Cytoplasmic processes reach out in all directions, and the name of these cells is derived from the conventional representation of a star. The nucleus is round or oval in profile, often indented, and in general larger than the nuclei of other neuroglial cells. The nucleus is moderately vesicular and the nucleolus is small, if visible at all. It is difficult to distinguish nuclei of astrocytes from those of small neurons in sections stained with basic dyes. The cytoplasm contains granules (gliosomes), which are resolved by electron microscopy into clumps of mitochondria or of lysosomes. The latter are membrane-bound vesicles, containing enzymes that digest macromolecular material, not only taken up by the cell, but also worn-out protoplasm (autophagia). Electron micrographs also show numerous gliofilaments 75–100A in thickness; they are similar to the neurofilaments of nerve cells and the microfilaments of other cell types. Endoplasmic reticulum is scanty, but free ribosomes may be present.

Special staining methods, such as the gold-sublimate method of Cajal, are necessary to show the processes of astrocytes in light microscopy. Many of the processes end on capillaries or vessels of larger caliber as foot plates or perivascular feet. Much of the capillary wall, perhaps 80% of its surface, is covered with astrocytic foot plates, which are attached to the basement membrane sur-

FIG. 2-8. Neuroglial cells of the central nervous system.

rounding the endothelial lining. The processes of astrocytes in the gray matter also end in close apposition to neurons at such intervals as are free of synapses. The processes of astrocytes near the surface of the brain and spinal cord are attached as foot plates to the pia mater, a thin meningeal layer which adheres to the surface, to form an **external limiting membrane.** The ventricles are lined by a single layer of ependymal cells giving off short processes from their deep aspect. There is a concentration of astrocytes beneath the ependyma, and their processes intertwine with those of ependymal cells to form an **internal limiting membrane.**

Astrocytes in the white matter tend to have rather coarse processes and contain bundles of gliofilaments visible as fibrils with the light microscope. This type of cell is called a **fibrous astrocyte.** The **protoplasmic astrocytes** found in gray matter have more delicately branching processes, and the gliofilaments are not sufficiently numerous to be seen as fibrils with light microscopy. There are intermediate grades between typical fibrous and protoplasmic astrocytes, especially in transitional zones between white matter and gray matter.

The conventional view is that astrocytes, by virtue of the attachment of processes to blood vessels, constitute a structural and supporting framework for nerve cells and capillaries. However, they no doubt have additional, more dynamic, roles. For example it now seems likely that the transport of chemicals essential for the metabolic reactions of nerve cells occurs partly within astrocytes, some astrocytic processes being adherent to capillaries and others being adjacent to the surfaces of neurons. This is a corollary of the narrow intercellular spaces of nervous tissue, which are of the order of 200A in width.

OLIGODENDROCYTES (Oligodendroglia)

The **oligodendrocytes** have, until comparatively recent years, been the most underrated cells among the neuroglia because no satisfactory stain for their study by light microscopy had been developed. They could be seen only as cells rather smaller than astrocytes with spherical nuclei, scanty cytoplasm, and a few short processes (accounting for their name). They are situated adjacent to nerve cells in gray matter and in larger numbers among the nerve fibers of white matter.

As in certain other aspects of neurocytology, the morphology of oligodendrocytes has been placed on a sound basis by ultrastructural studies. This is especially true of the **interfascicular oligodendrocytes** of white matter, where they make up some 75% of neuroglial cells. The cytoplasm contains a considerable amount of endoplasmic reticulum and many ribosomes. But the most striking revelation is that the oligodendrocytes are responsible for the formation of myelin sheaths, in the same way as neurolemmal or Schwann cells form the myelin sheaths of peripheral nerve fibers. The lipoprotein plasma membrane of an oligodendrocyte is wrapped around the axon in numbers of layers that determine the thickness of the myelin sheath. The intervals between the territories of oligodendrocytes are identified as nodes of Ranvier. One oligodendrocyte forms internodal myelin for from 3 to 50 fibers, depending in part on the caliber of the fibers. A single oligodendrocyte also surrounds numerous axons when the fibers are unmyelinated, but the plasma membrane is not wrapped around the axons in layers to form myelin sheaths.

Other oligodendrocytes lie close to the cell bodies and dendritic processes of nerve cells. These **perineuronal oligodendrocytes** seem to have a symbiotic relationship with nerve cells in the central nervous system, similar to that of the satellite cells surrounding nerve cell bodies in peripheral ganglia. The close relationship between neurons and neuroglia is demonstrated in cultures of nervous tissue, in which neurons do not thrive and grow unless they are accompanied by neuroglial cells.

EPENDYMA

The **ependymal epithelium** lining the ventricles of the brain and the central canal of the spinal cord is included among the neuroglia. The cells of this epithelium are arranged as a single layer in the adult and they are flattened endothelial-like to cuboidal-columnar in shape. Throughout most of the ventricular surface, the epithelium is characterized by a carpet of cilia projecting into the ventricle (Fig. 2-9). In other areas ciliated ependymal cells are interspersed among nonciliated

FIG. 2–9. Scanning electron micrograph showing the surface of the third ventricle in the rabbit. This illustration represents an area in which the ependymal lining is heavily ciliated. (× 2,880) (Courtesy of Dr. J. E. Bruni and Dr. D. G. Montemurro)

cells. The deep surface of some ependymal cells gives off processes that intertwine with those of astrocytes to form an internal limiting membrane. Suitable staining methods show intracellular fibrils similar to those of fibrous astrocytes.

MICROGLIAL CELLS (Microglia)

There remain the **microglial cells,** which are scattered through the gray and the white matter in fewer numbers than the macroglial cells. Microglial cells can be stained by the silver-carbonate method of Rio Hortega. As was mentioned, these are the only neuroglial components that are not of ectodermal origin. Instead they are derived rather late in intrauterine life from mesenchymal cells which invade the central nervous system from its surface, and they are therefore known alternatively as **mesoglial cells.**

Microglial cells are small and have an ir-

regular-shaped nucleus; the cytoplasm is scanty and there are several short, branching processes. No special function has been attributed to them under normal conditions. However, when nervous tissue is damaged from any cause, microglial cells become rounded and enlarged, and display ameboid and phagocytic properties. Under these circumstances, the cells ingest and digest tissue debris. In view of their mesodermal origin and role as scavenger cells, the microglial elements are regarded as belonging to the reticuloendothelial system of the body, with properties similar to those of histiocytes in connective tissue.

DEVELOPMENT OF NEURONS AND NEUROGLIAL CELLS

Neurons and neuroglial cells (except the microglia) differentiate from the neuroepithelial cells which constitute the neural tube at an early state of its maturation. Some of these cells change into **neuroblasts,** which are capable of cell division, and neuroblasts become neurons with the appearance of cytoplasmic processes (dendrites and an axon). The number of neurons is largely stabilized by the time of birth, although there are probably additions to the pools of small interneurons during the 1st year or so postnatally. Cells known as **glioblasts** (spongioblasts) appear a little later than the neuroblasts. Glioblasts differentiate into **astroblasts** and **oligodendroblasts,** which multiply and differentiate into astrocytes and oligodendrocytes. The ependymal cells lining the ventricles of the brain and the central canal of the spinal cord are likewise derived from the neuroepithelial cells of the neural tube.

SUGGESTED READING

Barr ML: The significance of the sex chromatin. Int Rev Cytol 19:35–95, 1966

Bodian D: Synaptic types on spinal motoneurons: an electron microscopic study. Johns Hopkins Med J 119:16–45, 1966

Bourne GH (ed): The Structure and Function of Nervous Tissue, Vol 1. New York, Academic Press, 1968

Bunge RP: Glial cells and the central myelin sheath. Physiol Rev 48:197–251, 1968

Droz B, Leblond CP: Axonal migration of proteins in the central nervous system and peripheral nerves as shown by radioautography. J Comp Neurol 121:325–346, 1963

Francoeur J, Olszewski J: Axonal reaction and axoplasmic flow as studied by radioautography. Neurology (Minneap) 18:178–184, 1968

Gray EG, Guillery RW: Synaptic morphology in the normal and degenerating nervous system. Int Rev Cytol 19:111–182, 1966

Haggar RA, Barr ML: Quantitative data on the size of synaptic end-bulbs in the cat's spinal cord. With a note on the preparation of cell models. J Comp Neurol 93:17–35, 1950

Hydén H (ed): The Neuron. Amsterdam, Elsevier, 1967

Krnjević K: Chemical nature of synaptic transmission in vertebrates. Physiol Rev 54:418–540, 1974

Luse SA: Electron microscopic observations on the central nervous system. J Biophys Biochem Cytol 2:531–542, 1956

Mori S, Leblond CP: Identification of microglia in light and electron microscopy. J Comp Neurol 135:57–79, 1969

Mori S, Leblond CP: Electron microscopic features and proliferation of astrocytes in the corpus callosum of the rat. J Comp Neurol 137:197–225, 1969

Mori S, Leblond CP: Electron microscopic identification of three classes of oligodendrocytes and a preliminary study of their proliferative activity in the corpus callosum of young rats. J Comp Neurol 139:1–29, 1970

Palay SL, Palade GE: The fine structure of neurons. J Biophys Biochem Cytol 1:69–88, 1955

Peters A, Palay SL, Webster HdeF: The Fine Structure of the Nervous System: The Neurons and Supporting Cells. Philadelphia, Saunders, 1976

Siekevitz P: The organization of biologic membranes. N Engl J Med 283:1035–1041, 1970

Uchizono K: Characteristics of excitatory and inhibitory synapses in the central nervous system of the cat. Nature 207:642–643, 1965

Windle WF (ed): Biology of Neuroglia. Springfield, IL, Thomas, 1958

Worthington WC Jr, Cathcart RS: Ependymal cilia: distribution and activity in the adult human brain. Science 139:221–222, 1963

Wuerker RB, Palay SL: Neurofilaments and microtubules in anterior horn cells of the rat. Tissue Cell 1:387–402, 1969

3

Peripheral Nervous System

Certain aspects of the peripheral nervous system are especially pertinent to a study of the brain and spinal cord. These include the general sensory receptors, the motor endings, the histology of peripheral nerves, and the structure of ganglia. The following introductory comments refer to all spinal nerves and to those cranial nerves which are not restricted to the special senses. The structures discussed in this chapter are shown in Figure 3–1; this figure represents a spinal nerve in the thoracic and upper lumbar region in which neurons for visceral innervation are included.

The general sensory endings are scattered profusely throughout the body. They are biologic transducers, in which physical or chemical stimuli create action potentials in nerve endings. The resulting nerve impulses, on reaching the central nervous system, give rise to reflex responses, awareness of the stimuli, or both. Sensory endings which are superficially located, such as those in the skin, are called **exteroceptors;** they respond to stimuli for pain, temperature, touch, and pressure. **Proprioceptors** in muscles, tendons, and joints provide data for reflex adjustments of muscle action and for awareness of position and movement.

Nerve impulses from exteroceptors and proprioceptors are conducted centrally by primary sensory neurons, whose cell bodies are located in dorsal root ganglia (or a cranial nerve ganglion). On entering the spinal cord, the dorsal root fibers divide into ascending and descending branches; these are distributed as necessary for reflex responses and for transmission of sensory data to the brain.

There is a third class of sensory endings, known as **interoceptors,** in the viscera. Central conduction is through primary sensory neurons like those already noted, except that the peripheral process follows a different route. The fiber reaches the sympathetic trunk through a white communicating ramus and continues to a viscus in a nerve arising from the sympathetic trunk. The spinal connections of these neurons are those required for visceral reflex responses and for transmission of data of visceral origin to the brain. There are therefore two broad categories of sensory endings and afferent neurons, namely, **somatic afferents** for the body (soma) generally and **visceral afferents.**

There are also two categories of efferent or motor neurons. The cell bodies of **somatic efferent** neurons are situated in the ventral gray horns of the spinal cord and motor nuclei of cranial nerves. The axons of ventral horn cells traverse the ventral roots and spinal nerves, and terminate in motor end plates on skeletal muscle fibers. The **visceral efferent** or autonomic system has a special feature in that two neurons take part in transmission from the central nervous system to the viscera. In the sympathetic division of the autonomic system, for example, the cell bodies of preganglionic neurons are located in the thoracic and upper lumbar segments of the spinal cord. The axons traverse the corresponding ventral roots and white communicating rami, ending either in ganglia of the sympathetic trunk or in prevertebral ganglia such as those found in the celiac and superior mesenteric plexuses of the abdomen. Axons of postganglionic neurons in these locations proceed to smooth muscle and secretory cells of viscera and to the heart. Axons from some of the cells in ganglia of the sympathetic trunk enter spinal nerves through gray com-

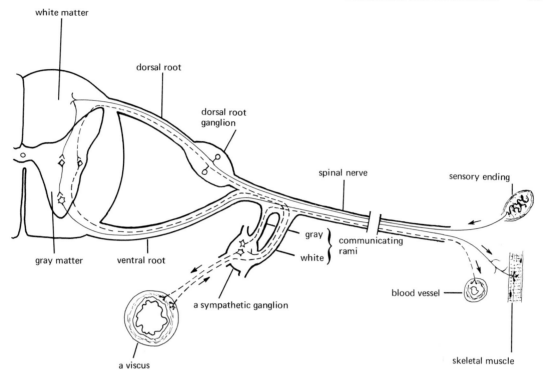

white matter

dorsal root

dorsal root ganglion

spinal nerve

sensory ending

gray

communicating rami

white

gray matter

ventral root

blood vessel

a sympathetic ganglion

a viscus

skeletal muscle

FIG. 3-1. Components of a spinal nerve between the first thoracic and the second or third lumbar segments.

municating rami for distribution to blood vessels, sweat glands, and arrector pili muscles of hairs.

SENSORY ENDINGS

The sensory endings are supplied by nerve fibers differing in size and other characteristics. This is a matter of some importance because there is a correlation between fiber diameter and the rate of conduction of the nerve impulse and because different sensory endings tend to be supplied by fibers of specific sizes.

A commonly used classification of peripheral nerve fibers is given in Table 3-1, which includes the sensory modalities and efferent neurons associated with the three main categories. (The table does not include a population of unmyelinated fibers that has been described in certain ventral roots, and for which a definite function has yet to be assigned.) The diameters of group A and group B fibers

include the myelin sheaths. Group A is further subdivided into alpha, beta, gamma, and delta fibers in decreasing order of size. There is some overlapping of the diameters of the A, B, and C groups because physiologic properties, especially the form of the spike potential and after potential, are taken into consideration when defining the groups. In brief the smallest fibers (group C) are unmyelinated and have the slowest conduction rate, whereas the myelinated fibers of group B and group A exhibit rates of conduction which increase progressively with increasing size of the fibers.

A second classification of nerve fibers applies specifically to somatic afferent fibers of the dorsal roots. Table 3-2 lists the receptors from which impulses traverse each of the four categories in the numerical system, together with the equivalents in the alternative classification.

It is customary to recognize two classes of sensory endings on a structural basis. **Nonencapsulated** endings are simple, undifferentiated terminal arborizations of the nerve fibers; they have a long phylogenetic history

TABLE 3–1. CLASSIFICATION OF FIBERS IN PERIPHERAL NERVES

	GROUP	DIAMETER (μ)	SPEED OF IMPULSE CONDUCTION (METERS/SEC)	FUNCTION
Myelinated	A ($\alpha, \beta, \gamma, \delta$)	1–20	5–120	Afferent fibers for proprioception, vibration, touch, pressure, pain, and temperature; somatic efferent fibers
Myelinated	B	1–3	3–15	Visceral afferent fibers; preganglionic visceral efferent fibers
Unmyelinated	C	0.5–1.5	0.6–2.0	Afferent fibers for pain and temperature; postganglionic visceral efferent fibers

and respond to various forms of stimuli that are identified by the general senses. **Encapsulated** endings are more specialized and of more recent phylogenetic origin.

NONENCAPSULATED ENDINGS

Sensory nerve terminals of the nonencapsulated type are widely distributed throughout the body. They are present in epithelia, serous membranes, connective tissue, muscles, tendons, joints, periosteum, and viscera, as well as in special locations such as the cornea, tympanic membrane, and dental pulp.

Simple nerve endings in the skin may be taken as the first example (Fig. 3–2A). Smaller fibers of group A and group C fibers form a plexus in the dermis and continue into

TABLE 3–2. CLASSIFICATION OF SOMATIC DORSAL ROOT FIBERS

NUMBER	RECEPTORS	LETTER EQUIVALENT
I.a.	Annulospiral ending of neuromuscular spindle	Aα
b.	Neurotendinous spindle	
II.	Flower spray ending of neuromuscular spindle; touch and pressure receptors	Aβ and γ
III.	Pain and temperature receptors	Aδ
IV.	Pain and temperature receptors	C

the epidermis as unmyelinated fibers. They then divide into terminal branches, which run between the cells of the deep epidermal layers. These are endings for pain, among other senses, responding to stimuli that are damaging or potentially damaging to the skin. Endings such as these function in relation to pain in many tissues, including mucous membranes, joint capsules, dental pulp, and other sites known through experience to react painfully to trauma or disease. Reliable observations on the nature of sensory endings for temperature are scanty. Endings similar to those responding to painful stimuli are probably sensitive to changes of temperature, although more complex endings may also function in temperature sensibility. Sensations of pain and temperature have protective functions; they give warning of real or potential injury and are hence known as **nociceptive** senses (*noceo*, to injure). As such they are phylogenetically old sensory modalities, and information concerning both pain and temperature reaches the brain through a common pathway in the spinal cord. Simple endings also respond to touch, as shown by the cornea, in which the sensory endings are all of this type.

Modifications of this simple type of nerve ending are sensitive to touch. In the first example group A fibers of medium caliber pass from the dermal plexus into the epidermis and terminate as leaf-like, meniscal expansions, known as **Merkel's disks,** in contact with epidermal cells (Fig. 3–2B). There may

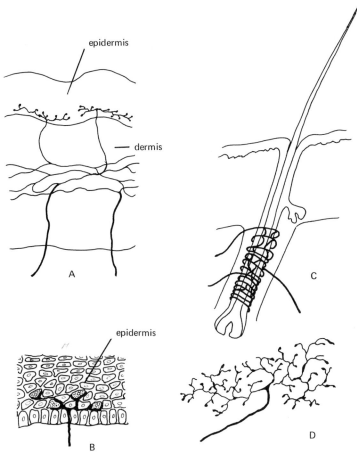

FIG. 3–2. Main types of nonencapsulated sensory endings. **A.** Dermal plexus and simple endings in the epidermis. **B.** Merkel's disks in the epidermis. **C.** Hair follicle plexus. **D.** Undifferentiated ending in deep somatic tissues or in viscera.

be as many as 50 Merkel's disks for a single nerve fiber, and they are confined to the deeper layers of the epidermis. The cells with which disks make contact are stained more darkly than neighboring epidermal cells because of an accumulation of glycoprotein granules in the cytoplasm. Merkel's disks are most numerous in the skin of the palm, sole, and nipple, but are also present at other sites, including the borders of the tongue.

The **hair follicle plexuses** (Fig. 3–2C), also known as peritrichial endings, are the second example of modified nonencapsulated endings for the sense of touch. Hairs are present on most of the body surface and their role in man is that of touch receptors, aside from a cosmetic value in the head area. Depending on the size of the hair, from 2 to 20 fibers in the medium group A range approach a hair follicle deep to the sebaceous gland from various directions. The unmyelinated terminals wind around the follicle in its connective tissue sheath, giving off collateral branches to form a basket-like network. The hair is exquisitely sensitive to touch, acting as a lever in which slight changes in position produce an action potential in the nerve plexus.

Rather complicated terminal ramifications of sensory fibers occur in the ligaments of joints, and in periosteum, tendons, and fascia (Fig. 3–2D). These endings of group A fibers, especially those associated with joints, give precise information concerning the position and movements of parts of the body (proprioception). Nonencapsulated nerve terminals in the periosteum respond to vibration. Similar terminals of group B fibers are numerous in the viscera. These are sensory

gamma motor endings

nuclear bag fiber

nuclear chain fiber

annulospiral endings

gamma
motor
fiber

flower spray endings

A

B

C

D

E

FIG. 3–3. Main types of encapsulated sensory endings. **A.** Meissner's corpuscle in a dermal papilla. **B.** Pacinian corpuscle. **C.** Neuromuscular spindle. **D.** Neurotendinous spindle. **E.** Sensory end bulb.

endings for visceral reflexes and for the sensation of fullness of the stomach, bladder, and rectum, together with general feelings of well-being or malaise.

In summary, the undifferentiated, nonencapsulated sensory endings have a long evolutionary history and serve several modalities of sensation. Receptors for pain are entirely of this category. The simple endings also make important contributions to the senses of touch, proprioception, and vibration, probably to the sense of temperature, and to the visceral afferent system. These conclu-

sions, and in particular the foregoing description of nonencapsulated sensory endings, are based mainly on light microscopic studies and the use of staining techniques which may not reveal fully the morphology of the fine terminal portions of nerve fibers. The interpretation of these sensory endings, especially cutaneous endings, will probably be modified as investigations proceed using electron microscopy and physiologic techniques.

ENCAPSULATED ENDINGS

Meissner's Corpuscles

These sensors of touch are mainly in the skin, where they occur in the dermal papillae projecting into the epidermis (Fig. 3–3A). Meissner's corpuscles are most numerous and best developed on the palmar surface of the hand (especially the fingers), the plantar surface of the foot, and around the mouth. They are present in smaller numbers in the volar surface of the forearm, tip of the tongue, margin of the eyelid, nipple, and external genitalia. The corpuscle is usually ovoid in shape and of the order of 50 by 100μ in size; a thin capsule encloses epithelioid cells, which tend to be arranged transversely. From one to four group A fibers, usually of large diameter, enter the deep pole of the corpuscle, give up their myelin sheaths, and pursue an irregular course among the epithelioid cells.

Meissner's corpuscles are exquisitely sensitive tactile endings which appeared rather late in evolution. They enable a person to detect that two points on the skin are touched, even though separated by millimeters (two-point discrimination). Among other properties, this delicate form of touch discrimination permits recognition of slight differences in the texture of surfaces.

Pacinian Corpuscles

Pacinian corpuscles, also called corpuscles of Vater–Pacini, are widely distributed. They are present (among other sites) in subcutaneous connective tissue and connective tissue in the vicinity of tendons, ligaments and joints, the nipple and mammary gland, external genitalia, serous membranes and mesenteries, and some viscera. The corpuscles are typically ellipsoidal in shape and from 1–4 mm long. They are therefore visible to the unaided eye; for this and other reasons the physiologic properties of pacinian corpuscles have been studied in considerable detail.

With light microscopy a pacinian corpuscle is seen to consist of a cylindrical core surrounded by numerous lamellae (Fig. 3–3B). A large group A nerve fiber enters the corpuscle at one pole, at which point the myelin sheath terminates, and continues along the central axis. In electron micrographs the cylindrical core consists of about 60 closely packed lamellae formed by much-flattened cells, and the nerve fiber occupying the core is notable for containing an unusual concentration of mitochondria. In the imma-

ture corpuscle the core is surrounded by an intermediate growth zone containing numerous nuclei, but this is no longer a feature when full development has been reached. The peripheral zone making up the bulk of the corpuscle consists of 30 or more concentric lamellae, each consisting of flattened cells with greatly attenuated cytoplasm. The lamellae are bounded sparsely by collagen fibers and separated by spaces containing fluid. A few of the outer lamellae are close together and underlie a condensation of connective tissue which constitutes the capsule of the corpuscle.

Pacinian corpuscles are sensitive to pressure exerted on them; they serve several functions, depending on their location and the central connections of afferent neurons. Those in subcutaneous tissues respond to pressure on the skin. Pacinian corpuscles adjacent to joints are proprioceptors; through excitation of these endings and nonencapsulated endings in the capsules of joints, there is accurate awareness of the position and movement of body parts (kinesthetic sense). Pacinian corpuscles close to bone respond to vibration. These corpuscles in viscera and mesenteries contribute to sensations of fullness of hollow organs as well as to the more generalized feelings of well-being or malaise.

Neuromuscular Spindles

The neuromuscular spindles (Fig. 3–3C) are the most complex of the receptors, both structurally and functionally. They provide sensory data for spinal reflex adjustments of muscle tonus, for the contribution of the cerebellum to motor functions, and for sensorimotor integration at the cerebral cortical level. In addition to functioning as a sensory receptor, the neuromuscular spindle has a significant motor role because it is a component of the gamma reflex loop.

These slender spindles are a fraction of a millimeter wide and up to about 6 mm long. They are inserted in considerable numbers parallel with the fibers of voluntary muscles, being most numerous toward the tendinous insertion of a muscle. Each spindle consists of a fusiform-shaped capsule of connective tissue and from two to ten intrafusal muscle fibers. The latter differ in several respects from the main or extrafusal fibers of the muscle. Intrafusal fibers are considerably smaller than the extrafusal, the middle zone lacks cross-striations, and this region contains numerous nuclei which are not in the subsarcolemmal position characteristic of mature striated muscle. In some intrafusal fibers the midregion is expanded, and in others it is not; they are known as **nuclear bag fibers** and **nuclear chain fibers,** respectively.

Each neuromuscular spindle is supplied by two afferent nerve fibers. One of these is a large member of the A group; the myelin covering ends as the fiber pierces the capsule, and the terminal portion of the fiber winds spirally around the midportion of the intrafusal muscle fibers in the form of an **annulospiral ending.** The second, slightly smaller, afferent fiber branches terminally and ends as varicosities on the intrafusal muscle fibers some distance from the midregion. The latter terminals are called **flower spray endings.** The annulospiral and flower spray terminals are also known as primary and secondary sensory endings of the spindle. The neuromuscular spindles are unique sensory endings in several respects, most significantly in having an efferent or motor innervation. The extrafusal fibers comprising the main mass of a muscle are innervated by large motor cells (alpha motor neurons), whose axons are of alpha size in the A group. Smaller motor cells (gamma motor neurons), with axons of gamma size in the A group, supply the intrafusal muscle fibers of the spindle. There are motor end plates on both sides of the specialized midregion of the intrafusal muscle fibers.

Neuromuscular spindles contribute to muscular function in several ways, the simplest role being that of a receptor for the stretch or extensor reflex. Slight stretching of a muscle includes the intrafusal muscle fibers; the sensory endings are stimulated and nerve impulses pass to alpha motor neurons supplying the main mass of the muscle. The latter thereupon contracts, in response to stretch, through a two-neuron reflex arc. Stimulation of the spindles ceases when the muscle contracts, because the spindle fibers are in parallel with the other muscle fibers. The stretch reflex is in almost constant use in the adjustment of muscle tonus. It also forms the basis of tests for tendon reflexes, such as the knee jerk test or extension at the knee on tapping the patellar tendon, which are standard items in a clinical examination.

The spindles also have an important role in muscle action resulting from neurologic processes in the brain. A considerable proportion of the motor fibers originating in the brain and descending in the white matter of the spinal cord synapse with gamma motor neurons in the ventral gray horns. Contraction of the intrafusal muscle fibers in response to stimulation by gamma motor neurons causes augmented firing of the sensory nerve terminals, partly through increasing the sensitivity of the spindle to stretch. This results in contraction of the regular muscle fibers through reflex stimulation of alpha motor neurons. The **gamma reflex loop** consists of the gamma motor neuron, neuromuscular spindle, afferent or sensory neuron, and the alpha motor neuron supplying extrafusal muscle fibers. It is an important adjunct to the more direct control of muscular activity by means of descending fibers from the brain which synapse with alpha motor neurons.

Neurotendinous Spindles

Neurotendinous spindles, also known as Golgi tendon organs or simply tendon spindles, are most numerous near the attachment of tendons to muscles. These receptors consist only of a thin capsule of connective tissue enclosing a few collagenous fibers of the tendon on which a nerve fiber ends (Fig. 3–3D). It is a large group A fiber (there may be more than one), which enters the spindle and breaks up into branches ending as varicosities on the intrafusal tendon fibers. These sensory endings are stimulated by tension on the tendon, greater tension being required than for excitation of neuromuscular spindles by stretch. The afferent impulses reach intercalated neurons in the spinal cord. These have an inhibitory effect on alpha motor neurons, causing relaxation of the muscle to which the particular tendon is attached. The opposing functions of the neuromuscular spindles (excitatory) and the neurotendinous spindles (inhibitory) are in balance in the total integration of spinal reflex activity. By acting as constant monitors of tension, the inhibitory role of neurotendinous spindles also provides protection against damage to muscle or tendon because of excessive tension.

Four types of ending which serve as proprioceptors have now been discussed. They are the nonencapsulated endings and pacinian corpuscles related to joints (both of which function elsewhere in other modalities of sensation), neuromuscular spindles, and Golgi tendon organs. All of them provide data for motor responses of a reflex or automatic nature through pathways of varying degrees of complexity—from the simplest in the spinal cord to the more complicated connections inherent in circuits in the cerebellar and cerebral cortices. In addition, all of the receptors contribute to proprioception at the conscious level, *i.e.*, to awareness of position and movement of body parts. However, the nonencapsulated endings and pacinian corpuscles associated with joints appear to be of special significance in this respect.

Sensory End Bulbs

There is a group of sensory endings, known collectively as end bulbs, which are difficult to appraise because their structural variations and physiologic properties are poorly understood. The end bulbs consist of a thin capsule enclosing poorly organized cellular and fibrous material (Fig. 3-3E). A group A fiber of small to medium caliber pierces the capsule, and the unmyelinated terminal forms an irregular pattern with numerous branches. The end bulbs vary in size (many are of the order of $50-100\mu$ in diameter) and they are spherical, elongated, or irregular in shape. They also differ in the configuration of the intrinsic nerve fiber. The wide distribution of end bulbs includes the dermis and subcutaneous connective tissue, mucous membranes and mucocutaneous junctions, glans of the clitoris and penis, conjunctiva, serous membranes, and joint capsules. Various types of end bulb have been identified on a histologic basis. They were given names derived from their location or the person who described them initially—names such as mucocutaneous endings, genital corpuscles, and end bulbs of Krause and Ruffini. However, it is doubtful that all the types of end bulb so described can be identified with confidence because there are intermediate gradations.

With regard to functions it was thought at one time that end bulbs of Krause were receptors for coolness and that end bulbs of Ruffini were for warmth, but the evidence that they are special temperature sensors is no longer regarded as conclusive. As a group these general sensory receptors are obviously in need of further study. Although they appear to participate in touch, pressure, temperature, and proprioception, definite correlations between such modalities of sensation and specific end bulbs have yet to be firmly established.

MOTOR ENDINGS

The **motor end plates** or **myoneural junctions** on extrafusal and intrafusal fibers of voluntary muscles are synapselike structures with two components: the ending of a motor nerve fiber and the subjacent part of the muscle fiber. In regard specifically to the extrafusal fibers, the axon of an alpha motor neuron divides terminally to supply variable numbers of muscle fibers. A **motor unit** consists of a motor neuron and the muscle fibers innervated by the neuron. The number of muscle fibers in a motor unit varies from one to several hundred, depending on the size and function of the muscle. A large motor unit, in which a single neuron supplies many muscle fibers, is adequate for the functions of such muscles as those of the trunk and proximal portions of the limbs. However, in small muscles such as the extraocular and intrinsic hand muscles, which must function with precision, the motor units include only a few muscle fibers. Such an anatomic arrangement provides for intricate control of muscle action.

Each branch of the nerve fiber gives up its myelin sheath on approaching a muscle fiber and ends in the form of bulbous expansions which constitute the neural component of the end plate (Fig. 3-4). The end plate is typically $40-60\mu$ in diameter and is usually located midway along the length of the muscle fiber. Each peripheral nerve fiber is surrounded by two sheaths external to the myelin sheath. The neurolemmal sheath consists of the nucleated cytoplasmic portion of Schwann cells, whose cell membrane wraps around the axon or axis cylinder to form the myelin sheath. The neurolemmal sheath continues around the terminal branches of the motor

FIG. 3-4. Motor end plates. (Gold chloride stain, × 500) (Courtesy of Dr. R. Mitchell and Dr. A. S. Wilson)

fiber after the Schwann cells cease to form a myelin sheath but does not intervene between the nerve ending and the muscle fiber. The nerve fiber is surrounded outside the neurolemma by a delicate endoneurial sheath of connective tissue. The endoneurium is continuous at the motor end plate with the thin endomysium or connective tissue sheath of the muscle fiber, forming a "tent" over the myoneural junction.

The ultrastructure of the axonal expansions within the end plate is like that of a synaptic end bulb, in that they contain synaptic vesicles and mitochondria. The surface of the muscle fiber is slightly elevated at the myoneural junction. The accumulation of sarcoplasm at this site constitutes the sole plate, in which there are nuclei of the muscle fiber and mitochondria. Each neural expansion occupies a groove or trough on the surface of the sole plate; there is an interval of 200–500A, constituting a synaptic cleft between the surface of the nerve terminal and that of the muscle fiber. The plasma membrane or sarcolemma of the muscle fiber has a wavy outline where it apposes the nerve terminal, the irregularities being known as junctional folds. The synaptic cleft contains glycoprotein material which is continuous with the boundary layer that invests the sarcolemma elsewhere.

Acetylcholine released from the synaptic vesicles by nerve impulses traveling along the axon reduces the membrane potential of the sarcolemma, as in postsynaptic neuronal membranes. The resulting action potential is self-propagated along the sarcolemma and carried into the muscle fiber to the contractile myofibrils by means of an ultramicroscopic membrane system in the form of tubules (transverse tubular system).

The characteristic feature of myasthenia gravis is an abnormal fatiguability of muscles due to progressive failure of neuromuscular transmission, and oculomotor, facial, pharyngeal, and laryngeal muscles are likely to be affected first. The disorder is caused by an autoimmune mechanism in which antibodies formed in the thymus have a deleterious effect on the postsynaptic portion of myoneural junctions. The ultrastructural changes, notably degeneration of the junctional folds and widening of the synaptic cleft, are accompanied by decreased responsiveness of the postsynaptic region to acetylcholine.

Postganglionic autonomic endings on smooth muscle and secretory cells are also similar to synapses. The fine axons make contact with the effector cell, and there is often a swelling along the course of the axon or at its end, which fits into a depression on the surface of the muscle or gland cell. The nerve fiber contains an accumulation of mitochondria at these sites, together with synaptic vesicles from which either norepinephrine or acetylcholine is released, according to whether the neuron is sympathetic or parasympathetic.

GANGLIA

The **spinal ganglia** are swellings on the dorsal roots of spinal nerves. They are situated in the intervertebral foramina, just proximal to the union of dorsal and ventral roots to form the spinal nerves. These ganglia contain the cell bodies of primary sensory neurons, mainly in a large peripheral zone. The center of the ganglion is occupied by nerve fibers, which are the proximal portions of peripheral and central processes of the nerve cells. Dorsal root ganglia and ganglia of cranial nerves involved with general sensation have the same histologic structure.

These sensory neurons develop from the embryonal neural crests, which consist of neuroectodermal cells and lie along the dorsolateral borders of the neural tube. The cells are bipolar at first, but the two processes soon unite to form the single process of this unipolar type of neuron. The processes arising from the smaller cell bodies are short and straight, whereas those given off by larger cells often wind at first around the parent cell body. In either case the fiber divides into peripheral and central branches or processes; the former terminates in a sensory ending, and the latter enters the spinal cord through a dorsal root. The nerve impulse passes directly from the peripheral to the central process, thereby bypassing the cell body. Both processes have the structural characteristics of axons, although the peripheral one is a dendrite in the sense of conduction toward the cell body. Alternatively the terminal part of the peripheral branch in the sensory ending may be considered as the dendrite. The major portion of the peripheral process and the central process then constitute a long axon, to which the cell body forms a necessary appendage with genetic and metabolic functions.

The spherical cell bodies vary from 20–100μ in diameter; their processes are similarly of graded size, ranging from small unmyelinated fibers of the C group to the largest myelinated fibers in the A group. The large neurons are for proprioception and discriminative touch; those of intermediate size are concerned with light touch, pressure, pain, and temperature; the smallest neurons transmit impulses for pain and temperature. Each cell body is closely invested by a capsule consisting of two types of cells. An inner layer of satellite cells is continuous with the neurolemmal sheath surrounding the processes. External to this, there are cells supported by connective tissue fibers, forming a layer of the capsule that is continuous with the endoneurial sheath of the processes. One of the most common disorders involving spinal or cranial nerve ganglia is herpes zoster (shingles), in which a viral infection of the ganglion causes pain and other sensory disturbances in the cutaneous area of distribution of the affected nerve.

Autonomic ganglia include those of the sympathetic trunks along the sides of the vertebral bodies, collateral or prevertebral ganglia in plexuses of the thorax and abdomen (*e.g.*, the cardiac, celiac, and mesenteric plexuses), and terminal ganglia in or near the viscera. The multipolar nerve cells of autonomic ganglia are 20–45μ in diameter. The nucleus is often eccentric, and binucleate cells are encountered occasionally. The cell body is surrounded by satellite cells similar to those which constitute the inner capsular layer around the nerve cells of spinal ganglia. The dendrites, of which there are several, branch externally to the capsule and are in synaptic contact with terminals of preganglionic fibers. The thin unmyelinated axon (group C fiber) takes the most convenient route to smooth muscle and gland cells in the viscera, to the heart, to blood vessels throughout the body, and to sweat glands and arrector pili muscles in the skin.

PERIPHERAL NERVES

The constituent fibers of all but the smallest peripheral nerves are arranged in bundles or fasciculi, and three connective tissue sheaths are recognized. The entire nerve is surrounded by an **epineurium;** the sheath enclosing a bundle of fibers is known as the **perineurium;** and individual nerve fibers have a delicate covering of connective tissue constituting the **endoneurium** or sheath of Henle.

NERVE FIBERS

A **nerve fiber** consists of the axon or axis cylinder, the myelin sheath in the case of fibers belonging to groups A and B, and the neurolemmal sheath (of Schwann). The **axis cylin-**

der has no features that are not shared with long axons in the central nervous system. Its cytoplasm **(axoplasm)** contains neurofilaments, microtubules, patches of smooth–surfaced endoplasmic reticulum, and mitochondria. The plasma membrane is called the **axolemma.**

Neurolemma and Myelin Sheath

The neurolemma (also spelled neurilemma) and the myelin sheath have several points of interest, centering around the fact that both are components of Schwann cells. The myelin has no significant intrinsic structure at the level of light microscopy (Fig. 3–5A). That it contains lipids has been obvious because the myelin is dissolved by lipid solvents and stained black by osmic acid, which is known to react with lipids. Proteins were also known to be present in myelin; they remain as fibrillar material after the lipids have been dissolved.

The myelin sheath is interrupted at intervals by **nodes of Ranvier;** the length of an internode varies from 100μ to about 1 mm, depending on the length and thickness of the fiber. Funnel-shaped clefts, called the **incisures of Schmidt-Lanterman,** are clearly visible in the myelin sheath in longitudinal sections of a nerve stained with osmic acid. (These incisures have not been seen in the central nervous system.) With light microscopy the neurolemmal sheath is seen as a series of **Schwann cells,** one for each internode. Most of the cytoplasm is in the region of the ellipsoidal nucleus, but traces of cytoplasm and the plasma membrane closely surround the myelin sheath from one node of Ranvier to the next.

Observations on the growth of nerve fibers in cell cultures and on regeneration of fibers following trauma to a peripheral nerve have established that Schwann cells are responsible for laying down the myelin sheath around the axis cylinder. X-ray diffraction studies have shown that the myelin consists of alternating protein and lipid layers, and the lipids have been identified chemically as cholesterol, phospholipids, and cerebrosides. More recently the technique of electron microscopy has established that the myelin is not only formed by the Schwann cell but in fact consists of its plasma membrane wrapped around the axis cylinder. The term neurolemmal sheath or sheath of Schwann is used to distinguish the nucleated cytoplasmic layer from the layer of myelin. In fact, the Schwann cell is included in both sheaths, the cytoplasmic portion forming the neurolemma and an extensive proliferation of the plasma membrane constituting the myelin. The Schwann cells are continuous with satellite cells surrounding nerve cell bodies in cerebrospinal and autonomic ganglia. The cellular layer that is in such intimate relationship with all nerve fibers and ganglion cells of the peripheral nervous system originates mainly from cells of the embryonal neural crest, with the addition of some cells which migrate from the neural tube along with growing motor fibers. Oligodendrocytes are the comparable cells in the central nervous system, the transition between oligodendrocytes and Schwann cells occurring at the junction of the nerve roots and spinal cord (or brain stem). Other oligodendrocytes lie close to neuronal cell bodies without forming a continuous layer like the satellite cells of peripheral ganglia.

Myelin sheaths are laid down during the later part of fetal development and during the first year postnatally, in the manner shown diagrammatically in Figure 3–5B, C, and D. The ultrastructure of the myelin sheath is seen in Figure 3–6. In order to explain the alternating layers of electron dense and less dense material, it is necessary to show the plasma membrane as a double line, representing outer and inner protein layers separated by an interval composed of lipids. Whether this trilaminar structure applies to the membrane of the Schwann cell generally, or only the extension of the membrane which constitutes the myelin sheath, is an open question.

The axis cylinder is first surrounded by the Schwann cell; the external plasma membrane is continuous with the membrane immediately around the axon through a **mesaxon.** Subsequent events could be explained by rotation of the Schwann cell around the axon, but the precise mechanism is not yet clear. The direction of the spiral is clockwise in some internodes and anticlockwise in others. In any event the cytoplasm between the layers of cell membrane gradually disappears, except for surface cytoplasm which is most abundant in the region of the nucleus. The myelin sheath comes to consist of from a

FIG. 3-5. A. The myelin sheath and neurolemmal sheath, as seen with light microscopy. B, C, D. Successive stages in the development of the myelin sheath from the plasma membrane of a Schwann cell. E. Ultrastructure of a node of Ranvier. F. Relation of a Schwann cell to several unmyelinated fibers.

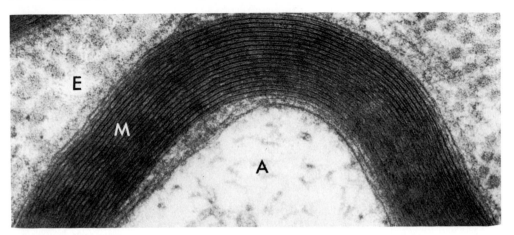

FIG. 3-6. Ultrastructure of the myelin sheath **M** consisting of alternating dense and less dense layers; the latter includes a thin intraperiod line. **A.** Axoplasm. **E.** Collagen fibers of the endoneurium. (× 107,500) (Courtesy of Dr. R. C. Buck)

few to 50 turns of membrane, depending on the diameter and length of the axis cylinder. The major dense line, 25A in thickness, consists of two inner protein layers of the plasma membrane, which fuse along a line indicated by the arrow in Figure 3-5D. The less dense layer, about 100A wide, consists of a double thickness of the lipid layer of the cell membrane. The fused outer protein layers of the membrane become exceedingly thin, forming an inconspicuous intraperiod line in the middle of the lighter lipid layer (Fig. 3-6).

The node of Ranvier is the interval between the plasma membrane systems of two Schwann cells (Fig. 3-5E). The neurolemmal sheath portion of the adjoining Schwann cells has an irregular edge at the node, and there is a space between the Schwann cells through which the axolemma at the node is bathed by tissue fluid. The action potential skips electronically from node to node, and the transmission of a nerve impulse along a myelinated fiber is called saltatory conduction (*saltare*, to jump). The length of internodes has therefore a bearing on the conduction rate of the nerve impulse and the internodes are longer, up to a maximum of about 1 mm, the thicker and longer the nerve fiber. The Schmidt–Lanterman incisures, which are of unknown functional significance, are formed by a loosening of the plasma membrane layers of the sheath with retention of cytoplasm between the membranes.

With respect to unmyelinated fibers a Schwann cell envelops several (up to 15) thin axons, as shown in Figure 3-5F. The axon is surrounded by a single layer of the Schwann cell's plasma membrane; it is therefore unmyelinated and there are no nodes of Ranvier. The nerve impulse is a self-propagating action potential along the axolemma, without the accelerating factor of node-to-node or saltatory conduction. This accounts for the slow rate of conduction which is characteristic of unmyelinated fibers.

DISORDERS

The peripheral nervous system is subject to various disorders. Peripheral neuropathy (neuritis) is the most common of these and consists of degenerative changes in peripheral nerves, causing sensory loss and motor weakness. Distal portions of nerves are affected first, with symptoms in the hands and feet. There are multiple causes of peripheral neuropathy, including nutritional deficiencies, toxins of various kinds, and metabolic disorders such as diabetes.

Damage to a peripheral nerve by a penetrating wound may result in an incapacitating disorder known as causalgia. There is severe pain in the affected limb, together with tropic changes in the skin. A nerve may be pressed upon where it passes through a restricted aperture; for example, the ulnar nerve is subject to pressure at the elbow and the median nerve in the carpal tunnel at the wrist. The resulting "entrapment syndrome" includes motor and sensory disturbances in the area of distribution of the nerve. The major plexuses, especially the brachial plexus, may be involved in a traumatic lesion, or there may be compression of major bundles of a plexus (as in crutch palsy). The nerve roots are involved in a variety of disorders (radiculopathy), causing motor and sensory disturbances. The latter may include pain in cutaneous areas and in muscles supplied by the affected nerve roots.

SUGGESTED READING

Bodian D: The generalized vertebrate neuron. Science 137:323–326, 1962

Boyd IA: The structure and innervation of the nuclear bag muscle fibre system and the nuclear chain muscle fibre system in mammalian muscle spindles. Philos Trans R Soc Lond [Biol] 245:81–136, 1962

Bridgman CF: Comparisons in structure of tendon organs in the rat, cat and man. J Comp Neurol 138:369–372, 1970

Causey G: The Cell of Schwann. Edinburgh, Livingstone, 1960

Coggeshall RE, Emery DG, Ito H, Maynard CW: Unmyelinated and small myelinated axons in rat ventral roots. J Comp Neurol 173:175–184, 1977

Davis H: Some principles of sensory receptor action. Physiol Rev 41:391–416, 1961

Eames RA, Gamble HJ: Schwann cell relationships in normal human cutaneous nerves. J Anat 106:417–435, 1970

Geren BB: Structural studies of the formation of the myelin sheath in peripheral nerve fibers. In Rudnick D (ed): Cellular Mechanisms in Differentiation and Growth. Princeton, Princeton University Press, 1956, pp 213–220

Keller JH, Moffett BC Jr: Nerve endings in the temporomandibular joint of the Rhesus macaque. Anat Rec 160:587–594, 1968

Kennedy WR: Innervation of normal human muscle spindles. Neurology (Minneap) 20:463–475, 1970

Landon DN (ed): The Peripheral Nerve. New York, Wiley, 1976

Munger BL: Neural-epithelial interactions in sensory receptors. J Invest Dermatol 69:27–40, 1977

Nishi K, Oura C, Pallie W: Fine structure of Pacinian corpuscles in the mesentery of the cat. J Cell Biol 43:539–552, 1969

Pease DC, Quilliam TA: Electron microscopy of the Pacinian corpuscle. J Biophys Biochem Cytol 3:331–350, 1957

Robertson JD: The ultrastructure of adult vertebrate peripheral myelinated nerve fibers in relation to myelinogenesis. J Biophys Biochem Cytol 1:271–278, 1955

Sinclair DC: Cutaneous Sensation. London, Oxford University Press, 1967

Straile WE: Encapsulated nerve end-organs in the rabbit, mouse, sheep and man. J Comp Neurol 136:317–335, 1969

Thaemert JC: Ultrastructural interrelationships of nerve processes and smooth muscle cells in three dimensions. J Cell Biol 28:37–49, 1966

Winkelmann RK: Nerve Endings in Normal and Pathological Skin. Springfield, IL, Thomas, 1960

Response of Nerve Cells to Injury; Nerve Fiber Regeneration; Neuroanatomic Methods

There are usually changes in the parent cell body following damage to an axon, and there are always degenerative changes in the nerve fiber distal to the injury. The effect on the cell body is called **axon reaction,** and the peripheral changes are known as **wallerian degeneration.** Axon reaction consists of a similar sequence of events whether the traumatized fiber is in the central nervous system or in a peripheral nerve. However, there are significant differences in what happens in the distal portion of the severed fiber, more specifically with respect to regeneration, depending on whether the fiber is centrally or peripherally located. Nerve fibers in the central nervous system may be damaged by natural causes. Fibers may be included, for example, in a region of infarction caused by vascular occlusion or in a region affected by one of the demyelinating diseases. Bundles of nerve fibers may also be interrupted by trauma, such as occurs in accidental injuries and neurosurgical procedures. Neurologic research may require the interruption of a fiber tract, under anesthesia, in an experimental animal. Fibers of a peripheral nerve may lose their continuity as a result of various forms of trauma to the nerve.

The sequelae of axon interruption, and regeneration of nerve fibers when this occurs, have important clinical implications. In addition advantage is taken of wallerian degeneration to trace specific fiber pathways in the central nervous system.

AXON REACTION

The changes in the proximal portion of the affected neuron vary according to the type of neuron and the species, among other variables. Cells in some locations undergo progressive degeneration and ultimately disappear. Conversely the proximal portion of the neuron may not be altered significantly by axon section. For example the cell bodies of cerebrospinal ganglia react to section of their peripheral, but not their central, processes. Species differences include absence of axon reaction in motor cells of the spinal cord of the rat and rabbit following peripheral nerve section, whereas a typical reaction occurs in the same motor cells in most animals, including man. The cytologic details of axon reaction are best seen in large neurons of motor type, which contain coarse clumps of Nissl material. The following account includes the more typical aspects of this fundamental response to injury in such cells.

The nerve fiber between the cell body and the lesion is not altered appreciably, except for traumatic degeneration immediately adjacent to the lesion. The cell body, in sections stained by a basic dye (the Nissl method), first shows signs of reaction 24–48 hours after interruption of the axon. The coarse clumps of Nissl material are changed to a finely granular dispersion; this change, which is known as **chromatolysis,** occurs first between the axon hillock and the nucleus, grad-

FIG. 4-1. Motor neuron undergoing axon reaction, 6 days after axon section. (Cresyl violet stain, × 800)

ually spreading through the perikaryon. The nucleus assumes an eccentric position, moving away from the axon hillock, and the cell body swells, giving it a rounded contour (Fig. 4-1). This aspect of the reaction reaches a maximum 10–20 days after axon injury, and it is more severe the closer the injury to the cell body. The total amount of cytoplasmic RNA, as determined by cytochemical measurements, is not altered appreciably. Electron microscopy shows that there is disruption of the orderly array of granular endoplasmic reticulum, with some loss of ribosomes from the outer surfaces of the cisternae and an increase in the number of free ribosomes in the cytoplasmic matrix. This early phase of reaction appears to be partly in the nature of cellular edema, which is a well-known response of cells in general when affected by a harmful agent.

There are signs of recovery from the early effects of trauma to the axon, even while the changes just mentioned are in progress. The nucleolus enlarges and dense basophilic caps are often seen on the cytoplasmic side of the nuclear membrane. Both the nucleolar enlargement and the nuclear caps are evidence of accelerated RNA and protein synthesis, which would favor regeneration of the axon when conditions make regeneration possible. The recovery period is long, often several months. The cell may pass through a phase

during which the RNA and protein contents are in excess of normal; normal levels are then gradually restored, together with the usual Nissl pattern for the type of cell. The cell body is eventually smaller than normal if the axon does not regenerate. Histochemical studies show that there are quantitative changes in cytoplasmic enzymes, including oxidative and hydrolytic enzymes, throughout the period of morphologic alteration of the cell.

Reacting cells can be identified with little difficulty, thus providing a method of determining the location of parent cell bodies of interrupted fibers. The method has been valuable in establishing the source of numerous fasciculi in the brain and spinal cord, together with the cells of origin of fibers in cerebrospinal nerves. In view of the limitation of the method to large neurons, most of the information that can be obtained from its use is now available.

WALLERIAN DEGENERATION IN A PERIPHERAL NERVE

The nucleus is essential for the synthesis of cytoplasmic proteins, which are carried distally by axoplasmic flow, replacing proteins that have been degraded as part of the metabolic activity of the cell. The axon therefore does not long survive when separated from the cell body. Simultaneously throughout its length, that part of the axon distal to the lesion becomes slightly swollen and irregular within the 1st day and breaks up into fragments by the 3rd–5th day. Muscular contraction on electrical stimulation of a degenerating motor nerve ceases abruptly 2–3 days after the nerve is interrupted. The degeneration includes the neural component of sensory and motor endings, although they remain intact otherwise for a considerable time and are reinnervated under favourable conditions.

The myelin sheath, which becomes converted into short ellipsoidal segments during the first few days after interruption of the fiber, gradually undergoes complete disintegration and the particles of degenerating myelin disappear over a period of several weeks. While the axis cylinder and myelin sheath are degenerating, or the axon only in the case of unmyelinated fibers, the Schwann cells become much altered. Each cell loses the extensive membrane system that constitutes the myelin sheath, leaving only the part of the cell forming the neurolemmal sheath. The cells multiply by mitosis and fill the slightly contracted endoneurial sheath. This sheath and the altered cells of Schwann occupying its lumen compose the **band fiber** or **band of von Büngner**. It has been assumed that the fragments of axon and myelin are ingested by tissue macrophages and others of hematogenous origin. However, there is evidence that the Schwann cells take on phagocytic properties and assist in removal of myelin by autodigestion of the membrane systems that envelop the axis cylinders.

REGENERATION OF PERIPHERAL NERVE FIBERS

If a nerve has been severed, regeneration of fibers requires close apposition of the cut ends by placing sutures through the outer connective tissue sheaths. Assuming that this condition has been met, the following sequence of events takes place.

REGENERATION OF AXONS

During the first few days, proliferating Schwann cells fill the interval between the apposed nerve ends. Regenerating fibers begin to invade the region by about the fourth day, each fiber dividing into numerous branches with bulbous tips which grow along the clefts between Schwann cells. The rate of growth is slow at first; 2–3 weeks may elapse before the fibers have traversed the region of the lesion. The fine branches may then find their way into endoneurial tubes of the distal segment, these tubes now being the band fibers of von Büngner. Several filaments enter each tube, and the invasion of a particular endoneurial tube leading to a specific type of end organ appears to be determined by chance alone. Many filaments fail to enter an endoneurial tube and grow into adjacent tissue. This is the fate of all regenerating axons if the severed ends are too widely separated or if connective tissue or extraneous material intervenes. Such fibers tend to form complicated whorls (spirals of Perroncito), producing a swelling or neuroma which may be a source of spontaneous pain. At the other extreme is the almost perfect regeneration of the nerve through the growth of each fiber along its original endoneurial tube. Such regeneration may occur if the nerve is crushed just enough to interrupt axis cylinders without disruption of the connective tissue sheaths.

Having crossed the region of the lesion, the filaments grow distally among the Schwann cells in the endoneurial tube. The regenerating fibers eventually reach motor and sensory endings; the proportion of endings that are reinnervated depends on conditions at the site of the original injury. The rate of growth is approximately 2–4 mm daily. The number of days that will elapse between nerve suture and the beginning of functional return may be estimated on the basis of a regeneration rate of 1.5 mm daily. This value allows for the time required for the fibers to traverse the lesion and for reinnervation of the peripheral endings.

RECONSTITUTION OF NERVE FIBERS

Changes occur meanwhile along the course of the fibers. A myelin sheath is laid down by Schwann cells if the growing axon extends from a myelinated fiber in the proximal segment. Myelination begins near the lesion and proceeds in a proximodistal direction, the mechanism being like that described in the preceding chapter for myelination of fibers in the first instance. Of the several axons growing in an endoneurial tube, only one matures fully; the others gradually regress and disappear. The branching of axons as they begin to regenerate, the entry of branches from a single axon into a number of endoneurial tubes, and the presence of branches from several neurons in an individual endoneurial tube all improve a neuron's chance of becoming reconnected with a suitable sensory or motor ending. The appropriate fiber for the ending persists, whereas others in the endoneurial tube regress. A regenerated fiber tends to have a diameter, internodal length, and conduction velocity that are about 80% of the corresponding values for the original fiber. The motor unit for a regenerated fiber is larger, compared with the preexisting motor unit, *i.e.*, the axon supplies more muscle fibers than formerly. This contributes to less precise function of a reinnervated muscle. When all things are considered it is understandable that there are limitations to functional recovery after peripheral nerve injuries.

The cut ends of a nerve can be placed in fairly accurate apposition by fine sutures inserted at intervals through the epineurium and including some subjacent perineurium. It may be desirable to postpone suturing for 2–3 weeks after the nerve is interrupted, but the delay should not extend much beyond 1 month. Later there is atrophy of muscle fibers and end organs and excessive shrinkage of endoneurial tubes. Delay beyond 6 months is likely to jeopardize seriously the chances of obtaining useful restoration of motor and sensory functions.

DEGENERATION AND REGENERATION IN THE CENTRAL NERVOUS SYSTEM

Following destruction of cell bodies or interruption of nerve fibers, degeneration of axis cylinders and myelin sheaths follows as in peripheral nerves. The presence of degenerative material serves as a stimulus to microglial cells, which then reveal their potentiality as macrophages and remove the debris by phagocytosis. Although severed axons regenerate in the central nervous system of adult urodele amphibia, regeneration is minimal at best in mammals. Instead, the affected region or fasciculus is converted into a special form of scar tissue by astroglial proliferation.

The histologic, functional, and clinical events subsequent to wallerian degeneration in the brain and spinal cord are a consequence of the ineffectiveness of nerve fiber regeneration. Much of the research on this important problem has involved section of white matter in the mammalian spinal cord in experimental animals. The findings are in agreement that there is sprouting of axons and that a few regenerating fibers traverse the cut and even grow beyond it for some distance. However, most of those that do so degenerate again 2–3 weeks after the transection, and there is no convincing evidence of clinically significant regeneration of nerve fibers when they are severed by trauma to the human spinal cord. Several possible explanations have been offered. They include the imposition of a barrier at the site of injury by astroglial proliferation, the necessity of endoneurial tubes for guidance of regenerating fibers, and the lack on the part of oligodendrocytes of properties possessed by Schwann cells which favor regeneration. Another possibility is that for effective regeneration the growing tips of axons must be bathed by extracellular fluid containing proteins derived from the blood plasma, a requirement which is made possible by the vascular permeability in peripheral nerves but not in the central nervous system.

The disability resulting from such injuries as compression of the spinal cord by a spinal fracture is so serious that any possibility of stimulating nerve fiber regeneration is of the first importance. Several chemicals have been investigated in the hope of reducing the glial reaction. They have been shown to improve the growth of axons through and beyond a cut made in the spinal cord of experimental animals, the effect being greater in young than in mature animals. Some improvement in axonal regeneration also accompanies the administration of thyroid hormones, which stimulate protein synthesis in the perikarya of affected neurons. The discovery of a "nerve growth factor" which can be extracted from mouse salivary glands and other sources has stimulated interest in future possibilities. The active substance, which consists of proteins, has the property of stimulating RNA and protein synthesis in sympathetic ganglion cells and cells of cerebrospinal ganglia *in vitro.* The cells increase in size and there is remarkable proliferation of their processes. An antiserum has been prepared by injecting the nerve growth factor into rabbits; cells of sympathetic and sensory ganglia are destroyed selectively when the antiserum is administered to young mice.

NEUROANATOMIC METHODS BASED ON WALLERIAN DEGENERATION

Advantage is taken of the structural and chemical changes in fibers undergoing wallerian degeneration to establish the position of fasciculi in the central nervous system and to trace the distribution of their constituent fibers. Of the two methods described the first is applicable to myelinated fibers only, whereas the second method can be used to trace unmyelinated axons and the fine terminal branches of myelinated axons.

MARCHI TECHNIQUE

The **Marchi technique** (Fig. 4–2) for staining degenerating myelin sheaths has contributed a great deal to our understanding of the organization of the nervous system, and its usefulness is not yet exhausted. A fasciculus of myelinated fibers can be traced to the point where myelin sheaths cease, *i.e.,* almost to the cells with which the fibers synapse. The principles of the technique are as follows.

As has been mentioned, in the interval between 1–3 weeks of fiber degeneration the myelin is in the form of droplets. The physical change is accompanied by chemical degradation, the complex lipids being broken down into simpler compounds and ultimately fatty acids. Lipids are stained black by osmium tetroxide whether they are those of normal myelin or the chemically altered lipids of degenerating myelin. However, if the tissue is treated with osmium tetroxide and potassium chlorate simultaneously, only the hydrophobic cholesterol esters of unsaturated fatty acids in the degenerating myelin are stained. The degenerating fibers appear as black particles against a lighter background; their course can be followed with considerable precision by mapping the Marchi particles in sections taken at appropriate intervals.

SILVER STAINING METHODS

The use of solutions of silver nitrate forms the basis of most of the methods for staining degenerating unmyelinated fibers or the terminal branches of myelinated fibers. For example the **Nauta** and **Fink–Heimer techniques** act by suppressing the argyrophilia of normal axons but not of those undergoing degeneration (Fig. 4–3). With these techniques, therefore, degenerating fibers have a beaded or fragmented appearance and are stained more darkly than normal fibers in the interval of 5–7 days following separation from the parent cell bodies. The degenerating fibers can be traced to the synaptic terminals with the Cajal method using formalin fixation (see Methods for Normal Cytology and Histology) because the end bulbs are first swollen and then fragmented, accompanied by an increase in affinity for silver nitrate. Degenerating synaptic terminals can also be recognized in electron micrographs. These procedures are capable of yielding precise information, and they are therefore especially useful for the study of connections in the complex brain stem and diencephalon.

METHODS FOR NORMAL CYTOLOGY AND HISTOLOGY

The **Nissl method** employs basic aniline dyes, such as cresyl violet, toluidine blue, and thionine. Basophilic components of nerve cells are stained, *i.e.,* parts of the cell containing nucleic acids (DNA and RNA). The Nissl method therefore stains the nucleus, nucleolus, and the granular endoplasmic reticulum or Nissl substance (Fig. 2–3). In addition to its use to show intrinsic cellular detail the Nissl stain is used to establish the spatial pattern of nerve cells and to demonstrate functional groups of cells. Only the nuclei of neuroglial cells are stained by the Nissl method. These cells require special staining procedures, such as Cajal's gold chloride method for astrocytes and the silver carbonate staining method of Rio Hortega for microglia and, less usefully, for oligodendrocytes.

In spite of its usefulness, the Nissl method has the drawback of leaving the nerve cell processes unstained. Of several techniques

FIG. 4-2. Section of human spinal cord at the level of the third cervical segment. The patient succumbed 9 days after a traumatic lesion involved the dorsal roots of the second, third, and fourth cervical nerves on the right side, together with the dorsal portion of the lateral white column in the second cervical segment. There are the following areas of Marchi degeneration: **A.** Entering fibers of the third cervical dorsal root. **B.** Ascending branches of fibers that entered the spinal cord in the third and fourth cervical dorsal roots (branches of these fibers are seen entering the gray matter). **C.** Descending corticospinal fibers in the lateral white column. (Marchi preparation, × 10)

FIG. 4-3. Degenerating nerve fibers in the cerebral cortex, stained by a modification of the Nauta method. (× 320) (Courtesy of Dr. Elizabeth Hall)

FIG. 4-4. Pyramidal cell in the cerebral cortex. (Golgi technique, × 90) (Courtesy of Dr. E. G. Bertram)

that have been devised to overcome this deficiency, the Golgi and Cajal methods are best known. In the **Golgi method,** small pieces of nervous tissue are fixed in potassium dichromate, then treated in a silver nitrate solution, following which sections are prepared. The nerve cells, including the finest branches of their dendrites, stand out as brownish-black silhouettes (Fig. 4–4). Only a proportion of the cells react to the Golgi process. This is a distinct advantage because the section would be too densely stained to be useful if all the nerve cells were blackened by the silver.

In the **Cajal method,** blocks of tissue are fixed in any one of a variety of solutions (*e.g.,* alcohol, formalin, pyridine, or chloral hydrate), immersed for several days in a solution of silver nitrate, treated with a photographic reducing agent such as hydroquinone, and sectioned. The nerve cells are stained a golden-yellow color, the details varying according to the method of fixation. In general the Cajal technique is useful for staining neurofibrils, the neuropil or complex mesh of fibers between cell bodies (Fig. 4–5), and synaptic end bulbs (Fig. 4–6). Other silver methods accomplish similar purposes. Examples are the Bielschowsky method, in which an ammoniacal silver solution is used, and Bodian's method, which employs protargol, an organic silver compound.

The **Weigert method** is a stain for myelin sheaths and therefore for fiber bundles and white matter generally. The method is particularly useful in studying the intrinsic structure of the brain stem (Figs. 7–2 through 7–15). There are several modifications, but in the classic technique rather large blocks of nervous tissue are treated in a solution of potassium dichromate, embedded in celloidin, and sections about 30μ in thickness are stained with hematoxylin. The white matter takes on a bluish-black color. Luxol-fast-blue dyes for myelin are a useful alternative to the Weigert method. These dyes stain the protein-bound phospholipids of myelin; they are used for paraffin sections and these can be counterstained by the Nissl method for nerve cells. Page's iron alum-solochrome technique is commonly used for the same purpose in neuropathology.

Perfection of the **electron microscope** for biologic use made possible important advances in neurocytology and contributed to an integration of structure, function, and chemistry. A few examples will serve as illustrations. Electron microscopy has confirmed the Neuron Theory by demonstrating the synaptic cleft and has shown the synaptic vesicles which contain a chemical mediator for synaptic transmission. The myelin sheath is now known to consist of the Schwann cell membrane, wrapped in layers around the axis cylinder. Electron micrographs provide information concerning the volume of the extracellular space in the central nervous system. In view of the complexity of nervous tissue, a great deal of research at the ultrastructural level remains to be done.

ADDITIONAL METHODS OF VALUE IN NEUROANATOMY

The following lines of research have made valuable contributions to our understanding of the structure of the nervous system.

Developmental studies have made a distinct contribution, in part because different fiber tracts of the brain and spinal cord are myelinated at different times. Certain pathways can therefore be traced in myelinstained sections of the nervous system at appropriate stages of development (the method of Flechsig). Once a cell group or fiber system has been acquired in the course of evolution, the structure persists, even though relegated to a minor role on being superseded by newer parts of the brain. For this reason comparative neuroanatomy has been helpful in clarifying the significance of certain components of the human brain.

Procedures that originate in biochemistry, physiology, and pharmacology are complementary to those of morphology. Histochemical techniques help to identify the chemical constituents of the neuron and give useful information concerning monoamine neurotransmitter substances. Autoradiography after administration of radioactive isotopes supplies information concerning metabolic processes in the cells of nervous tissue. A method recently introduced consists of making a tritiated amino acid available to perikarya of neurons and tracing the intraaxonal transport of the radioactive amino acid to axon terminals by autoradiography. Another new method involves the injection of a tracer protein (usually horseradish peroxidase) into a region containing synaptic bou-

FIG. 4–5. A nerve cell surrounded by the neuropil. In addition to the nucleolus, the small accessory body of Cajal is seen in the nucleus. (Cajal silver nitrate method, chloral hydrate fixation, × 1200)

FIG. 4–6. A nerve cell surrounded by the neuropil; numerous synaptic end bulbs are stained. (Cajal silver nitrate method, formalin fixation, × 1000)

tons. The protein is imbibed by the nerve endings and transported retrogradely to the perikarya, where it can be detected by a simple histochemical method.

Nicotine has been used to block synapses and thus to establish their location, especially in autonomic ganglia. Anatomic studies of neuronal pathways are supplemented by stimulation of neurons and observing the destination of nerve impulses by recording the "evoked potentials" elsewhere. Accurate measurement of elapsed time between stimulation and recording gives information which may aid in determining the number of neurons, or synaptic delays, that are included in the pathway. This procedure is called "physiologic neuronography."

It is the hope of neurologists that there will be an increasing convergence of structural, functional, biochemical, and pharmacologic approaches resulting in a unified basic neurologic science with close ties to clinical aspects of neurology.

SUGGESTED READING

Angeletti PU, Gandini-Attardi D, Toschi G, Salvi ML, Levi-Montalcini R: Metabolic aspects of the effect of nerve growth factor on sympathetic and sensory ganglia: protein and ribonucleic acid synthesis. Biochim Biophys Acta 95:111–120, 1965

Bignami A, Ralston HJ III: The cellular reaction to Wallerian degeneration in the central nervous system of the cat. Brain Res 13:444–461, 1969

Clemente CD: Regeneration in the vertebrate central nervous system. Int Rev Neurobiol 6:257–301, 1964

Edwards SB: The ascending and descending projections of the red nucleus in the cat: an experimental study using an autoradiographic tracing method. Brain Res 48:45–63, 1972

Guth L: Regeneration in the mammalian peripheral nervous system. Physiol Rev 36:441–478, 1956

Heimer L: Silver impregnation of terminal degeneration in some forebrain fiber systems: a comparative evaluation of current methods. Brain Res 5:86–108, 1967

Heinicke E: Influence of exogenous triiodothyronine on axonal regeneration and wound healing in the brain of the rat. J Neurol Sci 31:293–305, 1977

Johnstone G, Bowsher D: A new method for the selective impregnation of degenerating axon terminals. Brain Res 12:47–53, 1969

Kiernan JA: An explanation of axonal regeneration in peripheral nerves and its failure in the central nervous system. Med Hypotheses 4:15–26, 1978

Levi-Montalcini R, Angeletti PU: Growth control of the sympathetic system by a specific protein factor. Q Rev Biol 36:99–108, 1961

Matthews MR, Cowan WM, Powell TPS: Transneuronal cell degeneration in the lateral geniculate nucleus of the macaque monkey. J Anat 94:145–169, 1960

McIsaac G, Kiernan JA: Accelerated recovery from peripheral nerve injury in experimental hyperthyroidism. Exp Neurol 48: 88–94, 1975

Nandy K: Histochemical study on chromatolytic neurons. Arch Neurol 18:425–434, 1968

Nauta WJH, Gygax PA: Silver impregnation of degenerating axons in the central nervous system: a modified technic. Stain Technol 29:91–93, 1954

Olsson Y, Sjöstrand J: Origin of macrophages in Wallerian degeneration of peripheral nerves demonstrated autoradiographically. Exp Neurol 23:102–112, 1969

Parent A: Distribution of monoamine-containing nerve terminals in the brain of the Painted Turtle, *Chrysemys picta.* J Comp Neurol 148:153–165, 1973

Puchala E, Windle WF: The possibility of structural and functional restitution after spinal cord injury. A review. Exp Neurol 55:1–42, 1977

Ramón y Cajal S: Degeneration and Regeneration of the Nervous System. London, Oxford University Press, 1928

Sunderland S: Nerves and Nerve Injuries. Edinburgh, Livingstone, 1968

Torvik A: Central chromatolysis and the axon reaction. A reappraisal. Neuropathol Appl Neurobiol 2:423–432, 1976

Windle WF (ed): Regeneration in the Central Nervous System. Springfield, IL, Thomas, 1955

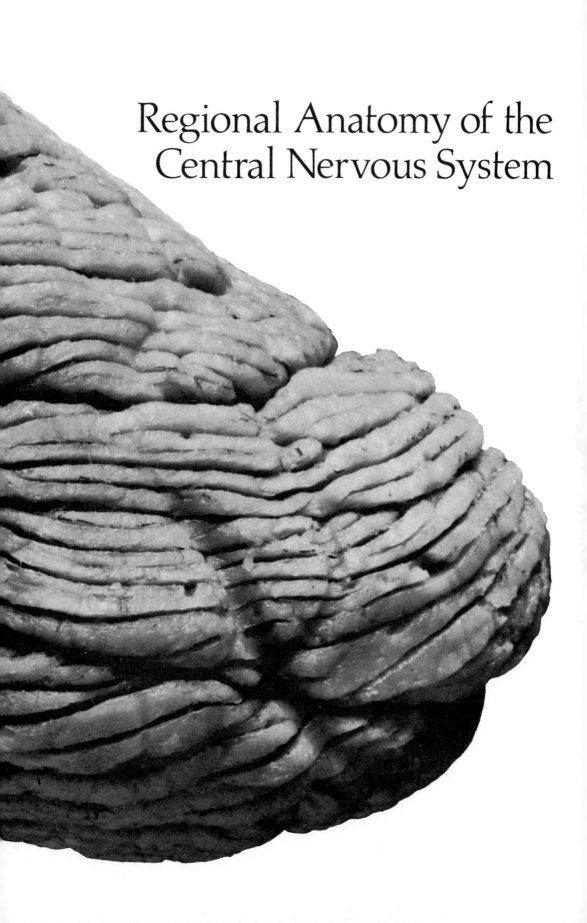

Regional Anatomy of the
Central Nervous System

Spinal Cord

The spinal cord and dorsal root ganglia are directly responsible for innervation of the body, exclusive of most of the head. Afferent or sensory fibers enter the spinal cord through the dorsal roots of spinal nerves, and efferent or motor fibers leave by way of the ventral roots (the Bell–Magendie Law). In addition to initiating spinal reflex responses, data originating in sensory endings are relayed to the brain stem and cerebellum, where they are utilized in various circuits, including those that influence motor performance. Sensory information is also transmitted to the thalamus and then the cerebral cortex where it becomes part of conscious experience, with the possibility of immediate or delayed behavioral responses. Motor neurons in the spinal cord are excited or inhibited by impulses originating at various levels of the brain from the medulla to the cerebral cortex. The spinal cord has therefore a complex internal structure.

As the fiber tracts of the spinal cord are identified, there will be references to components of the brain that are discussed in subsequent chapters. When the central nervous system is described by regions, it is necessary to probe ahead of the region under immediate consideration. An appreciation of the major systems is thus acquired step by step. The general sensory and motor systems are reviewed in Chapters 19 and 23, respectively.

GROSS FEATURES OF THE SPINAL CORD AND NERVE ROOTS

The spinal cord is a cylindrical structure, slightly flattened dorsoventrally, in the spinal canal of the vertebral column. Protection to the cord is provided not only by the vertebrae and their ligaments, but also by the meninges and a cushion of cerebrospinal fluid. The innermost meningeal layer of pia mater adheres to the surface of the spinal cord. The outermost layer of thick dura mater forms a tube extending from the level of the second sacral vertebra to the foramen magnum at the base of the skull, where it is continuous with the dura mater around the brain. The delicate arachnoid lies against the inner surface of the dura mater, forming the outer boundary of the fluid-filled subarachnoid space. The spinal cord is suspended in the dural sheath by a **denticulate ligament** on each side. This ligament takes the form of a ribbon or shelf, which is attached along the lateral surface of the cord midway between the dorsal and ventral roots (Fig. 5–1A). The lateral edge of the denticulate ligament is serrated. Twenty-one points or processes are attached to the dural sheath at intervals between the foramen magnum and the level at which the dura mater is pierced by the roots of the first lumbar spinal nerve. An epidural space, filled with fatty tissue containing a venous plexus, occupies the interval between the dural sheath and the wall of the spinal canal.

The segmented nature of the spinal cord is demonstrated by the presence of 31 pairs of spinal nerves, but there is little indication of segmentation in its internal structure. Each dorsal root breaks up into a series of rootlets, which are attached to the cord along the corresponding segment (Fig. 5–1). The ventral root arises similarly as a series of rootlets. The spinal nerves are distributed as follows: cervical, 8; thoracic, 12; lumbar, 5; sacral, 5; coccygeal, 1. The first cervical nerves lack dorsal roots in 50% of individuals, and the coccygeal nerves may be absent.

Segments of the neural tube (neuromeres) correspond in position with segments of the

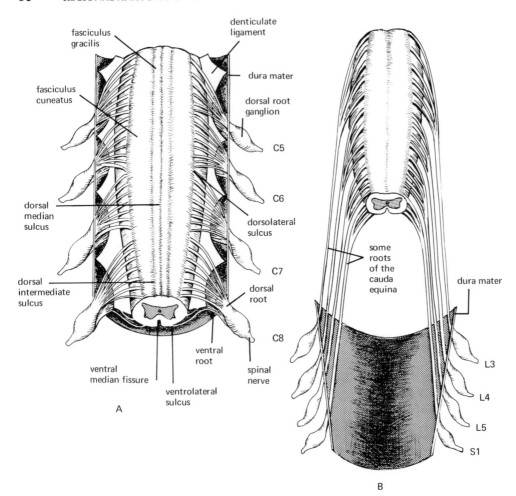

FIG. 5–1. Dorsal views of **(A)** cervical enlargement and **(B)** lumbosacral enlargement of the spinal cord and the corresponding roots of spinal nerves. In **(B)** the dorsal and ventral roots **(S1)** appear to join one another close to the spinal cord. In fact the dorsal and ventral roots of all spinal nerves unite just distal to the dorsal root ganglia to form the spinal nerves.

vertebral column (scleromeres) until the 3rd month of fetal development. The vertebral column elongates more rapidly than the spinal cord during the remainder of fetal life. The cord, which is fixed at its rostral end, gradually advances; by the time of birth the caudal end is opposite the disk between the second and third lumbar vertebrae. A slight difference in growth rate continues during childhood, bringing the caudal end of the cord in the adult opposite the disk between the first and second lumbar vetebrae (Fig. 5–2). This is an average level because the

length of the spinal cord varies less from one individual to another than the length of the vertebral column. The caudal end of the cord may be as high as the twelfth thoracic vertebral body or as low as the third lumbar vertebra. In any event, the spinal cord occupies about the upper two-thirds of the spinal canal; the cord is approximately 45 cm long in the adult male and 42 cm in the adult female.

The rostral shift of the cord during development determines the direction of spinal nerve roots in the subarachnoid space. As shown in Figure 5–2, spinal nerves from C1 through C7 leave the spinal canal through the intervertebral foramina above the corresponding vertebra. (The first and second cervical nerves lie on the vertebral arches of the atlas and axis, respectively.) The eighth cervical nerve passes through the foramen

cervical
nerves
1-8

thoracic
nerves
1-12

sacral 1-5
coccygeal 1

lumbar
nerves
1-5

sacral
nerves
1-5

coccygeal
nerve

FIG. 5–2. Relation of segments of the spinal cord and the spinal nerves to the vertebral column.

between the seventh cervical and first thoracic vertebrae, because there are eight cervical cord segments and seven cervical vertebrae. From that point caudally, the spinal nerves leave the canal through foramina immediately below the corresponding vertebrae. To be more precise, the nerves exit from the spinal canal by passing immediately inferior to the pedicles of the vertebrae and therefore slightly above the levels of the intervertebral disks.

The dorsal and ventral roots traverse the subarachnoid space and pierce the arachnoid and dura mater, at which point these meninges become continuous with the epineurium. After a short course in the epidural space, the roots reach the intervertebral foramina, where the dorsal root ganglia are located. The dorsal and ventral roots join immediately distal to a ganglion, forming the spinal nerve. The length and obliquity of the roots increase progressively in a rostrocaudal direction, because of the increasing distance between cord segments and corresponding vertebral segments (Figs. 5–1 and 5–2). The lumbosacral roots are of necessity the longest and constitute the **cauda equina** in the lower part of the subarachnoid space. The cord tapers into a slender filament called the **filum terminale,** which lies in the midst of the cauda equina and has a distinctive bluishwhite color. The filum terminale picks up a dural investment opposite the second segment of the sacrum and finally attaches to the dorsum of the coccyx. The filum terminale consists of pia mater and neuroglial elements; it has no functional significance.

Insertion of a needle into the subarachnoid space may be required to obtain a sample of cerebrospinal fluid for analysis or for other reasons. A spinal lumbar puncture is the method of choice, and the needle is inserted between the arches of the third and fourth lumbar vertebrae in order to avoid any damage to the spinal cord. It is helpful when examining a patient with a possible lesion involving the spinal cord or nerve roots to determine the location of segments of the cord in relation to vertebral spines or bodies. These relations are shown for reference in Figure 5–2.

The spinal cord is enlarged in two regions for innervation of the limbs. The cervical enlargement extends from C4 through T1 segments, most of the corresponding spinal nerves forming the brachial plexuses for the nerve supply of the upper limbs. Segments L2 through S3 are included in the lumbosacral enlargement, and the corresponding nerves constitute most of the lumbosacral plexuses for innervation of the lower limbs. Individual segments are longest in the thoracic region and shortest in the lower lumbar and sacral regions. The caudal end of the cord tapers rather abruptly, forming the **conus medullaris** from which the filum terminale arises.

The surface of the spinal cord is marked off into dorsal, lateral, and ventral areas by longitudinal furrows. The deep **ventral median fissure** contains connective tissue of the pia mater and branches of the anterior spinal artery. The **dorsal median sulcus** is a shallow midline furrow. The **ventrolateral sulcus** is indistinct, but its position is indicated by the zone of attachment of the ventral roots. The **dorsolateral sulcus** marks the line of attachment of the dorsal roots. The dorsal area on each side is divided above the midthoracic level into a medial part containing the **fasciculus gracilis** and a lateral part containing the **fasciculus cuneatus.** The intervening groove is called the **dorsal intermediate sulcus** (Fig. 5-1).

GRAY MATTER AND WHITE MATTER

As seen in transverse section, the gray matter has a roughly H-shaped or butterfly outline (Figs. 5-3 through 5-5). The small central canal is lined by ependymal epithelium and the lumen may be obliterated in places. Thin **dorsal** and **ventral gray commissures** surround the central canal. The gray matter on each side consists of **dorsal** and **ventral horns** and an **intermediate zone.** A small **lateral horn,** containing sympathetic efferent neurons, is added in the thoracic and upper lumbar segments.

There are three main categories of neuron in the spinal gray matter. The smallest cells may be classified broadly as **internuncial neurons;** although they are most prevalent in the dorsal horn and intermediate zone, there are many such cells in the ventral horn. Internuncial neurons receive afferents mainly from dorsal root fibers and fibers in descending fasciculi of the white matter. Their axons terminate for the most part on motor cells and tract cells. **Motor cells** of the ventral horn supply the skeletal musculature and

consist of alpha and gamma motor neurons. The cells of the lateral horn and the sacral autonomic nucleus are preganglionic neurons of the sympathetic and parasympathetic divisions of the autonomic system, respectively. The cell bodies of **tract cells,** whose axons constitute the ascending fasciculi of the lateral and ventral white columns, are located mainly in the dorsal horn and the intermediate zone of gray matter.

The white matter consists of three columns or funiculi (Figs. 5-3 through 5-5). The **dorsal column** is bounded by the median septum and the dorsal gray horn. As was noted, this column consists of a medial **fasciculus gracilis** and a lateral **fasciculus cuneatus** above the midthoracic level, the former corresponding with the entire dorsal column caudal to the midthoracic region. The two fasciculi are separated by a thin **dorsal intermediate septum.** The remainder of the white matter consists of **lateral** and **ventral columns,** between which there is no anatomic demarcation; they are sometimes combined under the heading of the ventrolateral white column. Nerve fibers decussate in the **ventral white commissure.** The **dorsolateral fasciculus** or **zone of Lissauer** occupies the interval between the apex of the dorsal horn and the surface of the cord. The white matter consists of partially overlapping fiber bundles (tracts or fasciculi), as will be described presently.

Although the general pattern of gray matter and white matter is the same throughout the spinal cord, regional differences are apparent in the photographs of transverse sections (Figs. 5-3 through 5-8). For example the amount of white matter increases in a caudal-to-rostral direction because fibers are added to ascending tracts and fibers leave descending tracts to terminate in the gray matter. The main variation in the gray matter is its increased volume in the cervical and lumbosacral enlargements for innervation of the limbs. The small lateral horn of gray matter is characteristic of the thoracic and upper lumbar segments.

CELL COLUMNS (NUCLEI) OF THE GRAY MATTER

Four cell columns are clearly delineated; these are the substantia gelatinosa and the nucleus dorsalis (thoracicus) in the dorsal horn, the somatic motor cells of the ventral

FIG. 5-3. Seventh cervical segment. (Weigert stain, ×7)

FIG. 5-4. Second thoracic segment. (Weigert stain, ×7)

FIG. 5–5. First sacral segment. (Weigert stain, × 7)

horn, and the visceral efferent cell column of the lateral horn. The remainder of the gray matter consists of a complex mixture of tract cells and internuncial neurons.

DORSAL HORN

The receptive or sensory part of the gray matter is in the dorsal horn and intermediate zone, in which most of the dorsal root fibers terminate. The following nuclei are recognized on the basis of cytoarchitecture and neuronal connections (Figs. 5–6 through 5–8).

Substantia Gelatinosa

The substantia gelatinosa (of Rolando) occupies the dorsal portion of the dorsal horn throughout the length of the spinal cord. The constituent cells are chiefly small neurons of the Golgi type II variety whose axons terminate within the nucleus, often after traveling a distance of one or two segments in the dorsolateral fasciculus (Lissauer's zone). Dendrites of neurons in the subjacent gray matter branch freely within the nucleus. Dorsal root fibers for pain and temperature in the dorsolateral fasciculus terminate in the substantia gelatinosa, where they synapse with invading dendrites, or with the intrinsic cells which in turn synapse with these dendrites. In this manner conduction for pain and temperature

is transferred to intercalated neurons on spinal reflex pathways and to tract cells for transmission to the brain. The cell bodies of second order neurons lie principally in the main part of the dorsal horn and the intermediate zone of gray matter.

Data for pain and temperature received by the substantia gelatinosa through primary sensory neurons may be modified when transferred to secondary sensory neurons or tract cells. The nucleus also receives afferents from the dorsal white column, and by means of this input transmission with respect to pain and temperature is perhaps modified by other modalities of general sensation. Further, fibers originating in the cerebral cortex enter the substantia gelatinosa from the lateral white column, and this input may modify synaptic transmission by inhibition or excitation of intrinsic neuronal elements. The nucleus appears to have a complex function, therefore, which may include the modification or "editing" of pain and temperature data by concurrent stimulation of various types of general sensory receptors and by activity at any given moment in the cerebral cortex. This is a difficult area of research, which is currently under investigation.

Nucleus Dorsalis

The nucleus dorsalis (nucleus thoracicus or Clarke's column) is a slender yet well-defined column of cells in the ventromedial part of the dorsal horn. The nucleus extends from C8 through L2 or L3 segments and is largest in the twelfth thoracic and first lumbar segments. The cells are unusual in having an eccentric nucleus and diffuse Nissl material, giving the erroneous appearance of cells undergoing axon reaction. Impulses impinging on cells of Clarke's column originate in proprioceptive endings, with a lesser contribution from touch and pressure receptors. The afferents to the nucleus are mainly collaterals of ascending and descending branches of dorsal column axons that entered the cord in the dorsal roots of spinal nerves. Fibers conveying data from the lower limb reach the nucleus through ascending branches; this may account for the larger size of the caudal part of Clarke's column. The nucleus dorsalis has no input from the upper four cervical spinal nerves, but descending branches of dorsal root fibers entering segments C5 through C7 transmit data to the upper part of Clarke's column. Axons from this nucleus enter the lateral white column of the same side, where they form the dorsal spinocerebellar tract. It is therefore an important nucleus through which proprioceptive data, and to a lesser extent information derived from touch and pressure receptors, are sent on to the cerebellum.

Nucleus Proprius

Almost all of the dorsal horn not accounted for by the substantia gelatinosa and nucleus dorsalis constitutes the nucleus proprius, also called the chief nucleus of the dorsal horn. This nucleus includes many internuncial neurons, together with tract cells whose axons contribute to ascending fasciculi in the white matter. Fibers enter the nucleus proprius from the dorsal white column, these being branches of dorsal root fibers for sensory modalities other than pain and temperature. Connections are thereby established for spinal reflexes and for transmission of sensory data to the brain. Many fibers of the lateral corticospinal tract, a large motor tract of the cord originating in the cerebral cortex, terminate on small neurons of the nucleus proprius. The latter cells in turn make synaptic contact with motor neurons of the ventral horn. The intermediate zone of gray matter between the dorsal and

ventral horns is similar to the nucleus proprius with respect to constituent nerve cells and their connections.

Visceral Afferent Nucleus

Certain cells in the base of the dorsal horn make up a poorly defined visceral afferent nucleus, which receives impulses by way of visceral afferent fibers in the dorsal roots. The nucleus is present in the thoracic and upper lumbar segments, and in the second to fourth sacral segments, because visceral afferents are restricted to segments that give rise to autonomic efferent fibers. The visceral afferent nucleus projects to visceral efferent cells of the spinal cord and to centers in the brain.

VENTRAL HORN

The efferent or motor part of the gray matter is included in the ventral horn, in which the large motor neurons are conspicuous. These are "lower motor neurons," in contrast to "upper motor neurons" whose cell bodies are in various gray areas of the brain. Dorsal root fibers and fibers of motor pathways from the brain excite or inhibit lower motor neurons, intercalated cells usually intervening, through synaptic end bulbs numbering in the thousands for each motor cell. The motor neuron in the ventral horn constitutes a "final common pathway" (Sherrington), through which impulses received from diverse sources are balanced one against the other, thereby determining the fluctuating activity of muscle fibers included in a motor unit. The large cells of the ventral horn are cell bodies of alpha motor neurons for the main mass of muscle fibers. Inconspicuous but functionally important cells giving rise to gamma efferents for intrafusal fibers of neuromuscular spindles are scattered among the larger alpha cells.

Somatic Motor Cell Columns

Several columns of motor cells have been identified in the ventral horn, as will be summarized (Figs. 5–6 through 5–8). In addition to motor neurons, the ventral horn contains a few tract cells, together with numerous small cells similar to those of the dorsal horn and intermediate gray matter. Many of these

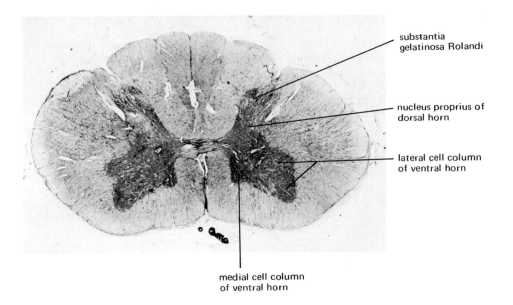

substantia
gelatinosa Rolandi

nucleus proprius of
dorsal horn

lateral cell column
of ventral horn

medial cell column
of ventral horn

FIG. 5–7. Third thoracic segment. (Cresyl violet stain, × 7)

nucleus dorsalis
(Clarke's column)

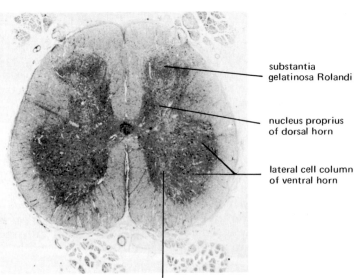

substantia
gelatinosa Rolandi

nucleus proprius of
dorsal horn

intermediolateral
cell column

medial motor
cell column

FIG. 5–8. Third sacral segment. (Cresyl violet stain, × 7)

substantia
gelatinosa Rolandi

nucleus proprius
of dorsal horn

lateral cell column
of ventral horn

medial cell column
of ventral horn

FIG. 5-6. Sixth cervical segment. (Cresyl violet
← stain, × 7)

---

small cells are interposed between fibers of
descending motor tracts and the motor
neurons.

A **medial cell column** is present throughout the spinal cord for innervation of the
muscles of the neck and truck, *i.e.*, muscles
attached to the axial skeleton together with
intercostal and abdominal muscles. A **lateral
cell column** innervates the muscles of the
limbs and is therefore present in the cervical
and lumbosacral enlargements. The lateral
column is subdivided according to parts of
the limbs innervated. The **ventrolateral nucleus** in segments C4 through C8 supplies
muscles of the shoulder and upper arm, and
in segments L2 to S2 this nucleus supplies
muscles of the hip and thigh. The **dorsolateral nucleus,** which is present in segments
C4 through T1 and L2 through S3, supplies
the muscles of the forearm and hand and the
leg and foot. There is a short **retrodorsolat-
eral nucleus** in segments C8 and T1, and also
in segments S1 through S3, for certain intrinsic muscles of the hand and foot. A **central
group** of motor cells has been described in
segments L2 through S2, but the distribution
of axons from these cells is not known.

Special Golgi type II neurons, called **Renshaw cells,** have been identified by physiologic methods; they are located in the medial
part of the ventral horn. These small nerve
cells receive collateral branches of axons of
alpha motor neurons; each Renshaw cell has
a short axon which terminates on the particular motor cell from which the axon collateral
arose or on a nearby alpha motor neuron.
This feedback circuit has an inhibitory effect
on alpha motor neurons.

Phrenic and Spinal Accessory Nuclei

There are two additional motor nuclei in the
cervical cord, one for the phrenic nerve and
the other for the spinal root of the accessory
nerve. The diaphragm develops from cervical
myotomes and, although it migrates caudally
during embryonic development, the origin of
the diaphragm is reflected in its nerve supply.
The phrenic nucleus is responsible for an enlargement of the medial group of ventral

horn cells in segments C3 through C5, most
prominently in C4. This nucleus receives afferents from higher motor centers, including
the cerebral cortex, and from respiratory centers in the brain stem, for voluntary and automatic movements of the diaphragm,
respectively.

The spinal accessory nucleus consists of
motor cells in the lateral region of the ventral
horn in segments C1 through C6. The axons
emerge in a series of rootlets along the lateral
aspect of the spinal cord, just behind the
denticulate ligament. The rootlets converge
to form the spinal root of the accessory
nerve, which ascends along the side of the
cord in the subarachnoid space and enters
the posterior cranial fossa through the foramen magnum. The spinal root joins the cranial (medullary) root along the side of the
medulla; the accessory nerve then leaves the
posterior cranial fossa through the jugular foramen, and the spinal component supplies the sternocleidomastoid and trapezius
muscles.

LATERAL HORN

An **intermediolateral cell column** forms the
small lateral horn of gray matter extending
from segment T1 through L2 or L3. Consisting of motor-type cells smaller than the alpha
cells of the ventral horn, the column gives
rise to preganglionic sympathetic fibers.
Stimuli are received from visceral afferents of
the dorsal roots and from autonomic centers
in the brain by way of fibers in the lateral
white column. Similar cells in the base of the
ventral horn in segments S2 through S4 constitute the **sacral autonomic nucleus,** from
which arise the preganglionic fibers of the
sacral portion of the parasympathetic system.

Certain data concerning the cell columns
are summarized in Table 5-1.

LAMINAE OF REXED

Studies of the architecture of neurons (cy-
toarchitectonics) provide the basis for
Rexed's laminar map of the spinal gray matter. This system of parceling the gray matter
is useful in experimental work, providing a
rather precise identification of areas in which
there is terminal fiber degeneration following
section of dorsal roots or descending fasciculi
of the white matter. Briefly described, the ten

TABLE 5-1. SUMMARY OF THE CHARACTERISTICS OF THE CELL COLUMNS

CELL COLUMN	EXTENT IN CORD	FUNCTION
Substantia gelatinosa Rolandi	Entire cord	Relay nucleus for pain and temperature, with modification of transmission of sensory input
Nucleus dorsalis (nucleus thoracicus or Clarke's column)	C8 through L2 or L3	Origin of dorsal spinocerebellar tract
Nucleus proprius of dorsal horn	Entire cord	Contains internuncial neurons, together with tract cells for ascending fasciculi of lateral and ventral white columns
Visceral afferent nucleus	T1 through L2 or L3; S2 through S4	Relay nucleus for visceral afferent impulses
Spinal cervical nucleus	C1 and C2	Termination of spinocervical tract
Medial motor cell column	Entire cord	Supplies muscles of neck and trunk
Lateral motor cell column	C4 through T1; L2 through S3	Supplies muscles of limbs
Phrenic nucleus	C3 through C5	Motor innervation of diaphragm
Spinal accessory nucleus	C1 through C6	Origin of spinal root of accessory nerve
Intermediolateral cell column	T1 through L2 or L3	Source of preganglionic sympathetic fibers
Sacral parasympathetic nucleus	S2 through S4	Source of preganglionic parasympathetic fibers for pelvic viscera

FIG. 5-9. Laminae of Rexed in the cervical enlargement.

laminae are as follows (Fig. 5-9). The thin **lamina I,** consisting of medium-sized and large neurons, is superficial to the substantia gelatinosa. **Lamina II** corresponds with the substantia gelatinosa Rolandi. The chief nucleus of the dorsal horn is divided into **laminae III, IV, V,** and **VI. Lamina VII** includes most of the intermediate zone, together with the intervals between motor nuclei in the lateral part of the ventral horn. Similarly **la-**mina VIII consists of areas in the medial part of the ventral horn, in which motor neurons are few or absent. **Lamina IX** is made up of the motor nuclei of the ventral horn. Finally, **lamina X** consists mainly of neuroglial cells surrounding the central canal.

COURSE OF DORSAL ROOT FIBERS WITHIN THE SPINAL CORD

Fibers of various calibers for the different modalities of general sensation are intermingled in the dorsal root. Just before reaching the spinal cord, unmyelinated and thinly myelinated fibers form a **lateral division** that enters the dorsolateral fasciculus or zone of Lissauer, whereas more heavily myelinated fibers form a **medial division** that continues into the dorsal white column. Fibers of the lateral division are concerned with conduction for pain and temperature, and those of the medial division transmit impulses for touch (simple and discriminative), pressure, proprioception, and vibration.

DORSOLATERAL FASCICULUS

Unmyelinated and thinly myelinated fibers comprising the lateral division of dorsal roots divide into short ascending and descending

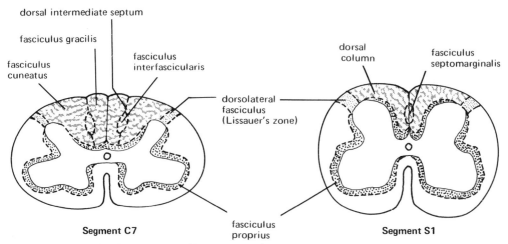

FIG. 5-10. Dorsal column, zone of Lissauer, and fasciculus proprius.

branches in the dorsolateral fasciculus or zone of Lissauer (Fig. 5-10). Each branch gives off numerous collaterals, and the entire fiber terminates in the substantia gelatinosa within the segment of entry or in the next rostral or caudal segment. As has been described, the substantia gelatinosa provides connections for spinal reflex responses and transmission of data for pain and temperature to the thalamus. The cell bodies of the tract cells concerned are located in the nucleus proprius and intermediate gray matter, their dendrites extending into the substantia gelatinosa. The axons of these cells cross to the opposite side of the cord, where they form the lateral spinothalamic tract. This tract traverses the brain stem and terminates in the general sensory nucleus of the thalamus. It is important to note that impulses for pain and temperature, in their passage from peripheral endings to the thalamus, cross to the opposite side in, or close to, the segment of entry into the spinal cord.

DORSAL COLUMN

The **dorsal white column** is constituted as follows. Myelinated fibers comprising the medial division of dorsal roots bifurcate on entering the spinal cord just medial to Lissauer's zone. The ascending and descending branches run longitudinally on the lateral side of similar fibers that entered the cord in the segment just below. However, some of the descending fibers, which may be several

segments in length, accumulate in the **fasciculus septomarginalis** in the lower half of the cord, and in the **fasciculus interfascicularis** in the upper half of the cord (Fig. 5-10). The descending fibers, which give off many collateral branches, synapse with tract cells, internuncial neurons, and motor cells.

Many of the ascending fibers of the dorsal column also end in the spinal gray matter, both as terminal fibers and as collateral branches. Some of these fibers, which vary in length from a few to many segments, are concerned with conduction for light (simple) touch and pressure. Synaptic contacts are effected with internuncial neurons for spinal reflexes and with tract cells. Axons of the latter cells cross to the opposite side of the cord, where they form the ventral spinothalamic tract. The central pathway for light touch and pressure is therefore ipsilateral for a considerable distance, as well as contralateral through the crossed ventral spinothalamic tract. Tract cells receiving afferents for light touch and pressure contribute to additional ascending fasciculi, as will be noted presently.

Other ascending branches of dorsal root fibers, specifically those transmitting impulses from the various proprioceptive endings, also give off branches to the gray matter as they traverse variable numbers of segments. These nerve fibers make synaptic contact with motor neurons, internuncial neurons, and tract cells, mainly for spinal reflexes and transmission of proprioceptive data to the cerebellum.

Finally axons of many primary sensory neurons enter the medulla from the dorsal white column of the spinal cord. They travel in the fasciculus gracilis or the fasciculus cuneatus, depending on whether they entered the cord below or above the midthoracic level, and terminate in the nucleus gracilis or the nucleus cuneatus in the medulla. These long fibers transmit impulses from proprioceptors, tactile endings, and endings that respond to vibration. Fibers from the nuclei gracilis and cuneatus cross the midline in the medulla and continue rostrally as the medial lemniscus, which terminates in the general sensory nucleus of the thalamus (ventral posterior nucleus). The ascending pathway thus identified, which is completed by thalamocortical projections, is the main conduction pathway for detailed awareness of position and movement, discriminative touch, and vibration. The results of animal experiments and the study of effects of lesions restricted to the dorsal column in man suggest that these sensory modalities may also be transmitted to the thalamus, to some extent, through other ascending pathways.

There is a regular lamination of the dorsal white column according to segments in which the long ascending branches originate. At the level of the first cervical segment, for example, fibers that entered the cord in the lowest sacral segment are most medial; fibers from higher segments are progressively added in layers, and the newest upper cervical fibers are most lateral. Segments concerned with innervation of the limbs are well represented, whereas those for the trunk occupy a relatively small area adjacent to the dorsal intermediate septum. The size of the dorsal white column increased in comparison with other parts of the spinal cord in the course of vertebrate evolution, and the dorsal column is maximally represented in man.

FASCICULUS PROPRIUS

The fasciculus proprius (fasciculus spino-spinalis) surrounds the gray matter and is rather thinner in the dorsal columns than elsewhere (Fig. 5-10). This zone of white matter consists of ascending and descending association fibers connecting different segments. The connections thereby established are important in intersegmental spinal reflexes. The fasciculus proprius also forms a two-directional, polysynaptic pathway between the spinal cord and the brain stem, providing a communication between the two that is additional to the uninterrupted tracts in the remainder of the white matter.

EXAMPLES OF SPINAL REFLEXES

Certain neuronal connections in the spinal cord form the basis of important spinal reflexes. The stretch reflex, gamma reflex loop, and flexor reflex will serve as examples.

The **stretch reflex** is based on a two-neuron or monosynaptic reflex arc (Fig. 5-11). Slight stretching of a muscle stimulates the sensory endings in neuromuscular spindles, and the resultant excitation reaches the spinal cord by way of primary sensory neurons having large group A processes. Axons of these cells in the dorsal white column give off collateral branches that excite alpha motor neurons, causing the stretched muscle to contract. This is an important postural reflex. The afferent impulses originate as an asynchronous discharge from the neuromuscular spindles, which are delicate monitors of changes in the length of the muscle. The reflex alters tension in the muscle in such a way as to maintain a constant length. The stretch reflex forms the basis of the knee-jerk test and other tendon reflex tests that are used in a neurologic examination. A sharp tap on the patellar tendon causes synchronous discharges from the spindles in the quadriceps femoris muscle, with prompt reflex contraction of the muscle and extension of the leg at the knee.

The reflex arc just described forms part of the **gamma reflex loop,** through which muscle tension comes under the control of descending motor pathways (Fig. 5-12). Fibers of these pathways (*e.g.*, reticulospinal, vestibulospinal, and others) excite gamma motor neurons, causing contraction of intrafusal muscle fibers and an increase in the rate of firing from sensory endings in the neuromuscular spindles. The impulses are conveyed to alpha motor neurons supplying the main muscle mass through the monosynaptic reflex arc described above for the stretch reflex.

The **flexor reflex,** which is protective as in withdrawal of the hand in response to a painful stimulus, is based on a series of at least three neurons and is therefore polysynaptic (Fig. 5-13). The cutaneous receptors are

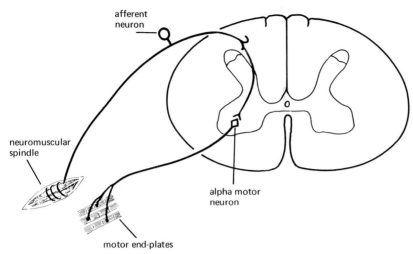

FIG. 5–11. Stretch reflex arc.

FIG. 5–12. Gamma reflex loop.

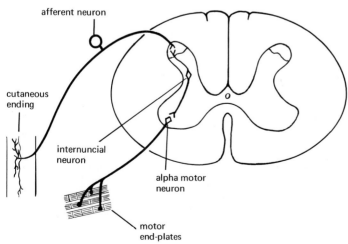

FIG. 5–13. Flexor reflex arc.

mainly nonencapsulated endings in the epidermis, and the afferent fibers synapse in the substantia gelatinosa with dendrites of internuncial neurons. The latter neurons end on alpha motor cells in several segments because a withdrawal response requires the action of groups of muscles.

The tension on a muscle is monitored by Golgi tendon spindles as well as neuromuscular spindles. When the tension reaches a certain level there is a distinct increase in the discharge from the tendon spindles. The resulting nerve impulses reach internuncial cells in the spinal gray matter, these cells inhibit alpha motor neurons, and relaxation of the muscle follows. This reflex therefore tends to prevent excessive tension on the muscle and tendon.

ASCENDING TRACTS OF THE LATERAL AND VENTRAL WHITE COLUMNS

The location of most of the pathways conducting sensory information to the brain is shown in Figure 5–14. Because of a degree of intermingling of fibers of adjacent tracts, both Figure 5–14 and Figure 5–15 indicate the sites in which fibers of a particular tract are concentrated. The cervical region of the cord is illustrated because not all tracts are present at lower levels.

The dorsal spinocerebellar tract originates in the distinctive nucleus dorsalis (thoracicus). Tract cells for the remaining ascending fasciculi are located primarily in the chief nucleus of the dorsal horn and the intermediate gray matter, with a few in the ventral gray horn.

SPINOTHALAMIC TRACTS

The **lateral spinothalamic tract** for pain and temperature is especially important clinically. The cells of origin receive afferents from the dorsolateral fasciculus or zone of Lissauer, small neurons of the substantia gelatinosa often intervening between the primary sensory neurons and the tract cells or second order sensory neurons. As has been noted, the dorsal root fibers for pain and temperature in Lissauer's zone do not extend longitudinally for more than a segment beyond the segment of entry. Axons of the tract

cells cross the midline in the ventral gray and white commissures, with a slight rostral inclination. The fibers then pass through the contralateral gray matter to reach the lateral spinothalamic tract. This fasciculus is present at all levels of the cord, fibers being added to its ventromedial aspect as they accumulate in a caudorostral direction. There is therefore a somatotopic arrangement of the constituent fibers. In the upper cervical region, for example, sacral segments are represented in the dorsolateral part of the tract, followed by fibers from lumbar and then thoracic segments, and fibers of cervical origin are in a ventromedial position. There is some indication that fibers for temperature are more dorsal than those for pain.

The lateral spinothalamic tract traverses the brain stem and ends in the general sensory nucleus of the thalamus. There is crude awareness of pain and temperature sensations, together with emotional responses, at the thalamic level. The somesthetic cortical area, to which the thalamic nucleus projects, adds discriminative qualities of localization and quantitative assessment. The lateral spinothalamic tract is the main central pathway for pain and temperature sensibilities. However, the study of patients following section of the tract (chordotomy) for relief of intractable pain suggests that there are additional routes for pain conduction to the thalamus; these may be provided by spinoreticular fibers, ascending visceral fibers, or the spinocervical tract (see Other Ascending Tracts).

The **ventral spinothalamic tract** is a crossed pathway for light touch and pressure, present at all levels of the cord. Some of the dorsal root fibers conveying data for these senses continue rostrally for considerable distances in the ipsilateral dorsal white column before synapsing with tract cells. The central pathway is therefore essentially bilateral; a unilateral cord lesion results in only slight and often undetectable impairment of light touch and pressure sensations. The ventral spinothalamic tract terminates in the thalamic nucleus for general sensation, which in turn projects to the somesthetic cortex where the information thus conveyed enters into conscious experience.

Figure 5–14 shows the lateral and ventral spinothalamic tracts as separated by the spinotectal and spinoolivary tracts. The latter

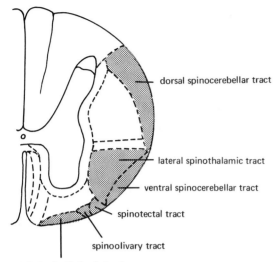

dorsal spinocerebellar tract

lateral spinothalamic tract

ventral spinocerebellar tract

spinotectal tract

spinoolivary tract

ventral spinothalamic tract

FIG. 5–14. Ascending tracts in the lateral and ventral white columns.

tracts are small and for the most part limited to the cervical region. There is also considerable overlapping of fibers of adjoining tracts, as already mentioned. For these reasons, the lateral and ventral spinothalamic tracts form virtually a single system for conduction of exteroceptive data from the periphery to the brain.

The major pathways in the spinal cord, through which information collected from general sensory endings is transmitted to the thalamus and the cerebral cortex, have now been noted. To recapitulate, the pathways are 1) the ipsilateral dorsal column for proprioception, discriminative touch, and vibration; 2) the crossed lateral spinothalamic tract for pain and temperature; and 3) the dorsal column of the same side and the ventral spinothalamic tract of the opposite side for light (simple) touch and pressure.

PATHWAYS TO THE CEREBELLUM

The **dorsal spinocerebellar tract** has its origin in the nucleus dorsalis (nucleus thoracicus or Clarke's column) of the same side and therefore begins in the upper lumbar segments. Afferents to the nucleus dorsalis come from the dorsal column of white matter, as described previously, the impulses originating mainly in proprioceptive endings, with an additional contribution from touch and

pressure receptors. The dorsal spinocerebellar tract continues through the medulla and enters the cerebellum by way of the inferior cerebellar peduncle.

The **ventral spinocerebellar tract** first appears in the lower lumbar region of the cord. This is a crossed tract, a large proportion of the fibers originating in the lumbosacral enlargement, where the cells of origin are located in the ventral horn. The ventral spinocerebellar tract traverses most of the brain stem and enters the cerebellum through the superior cerebellar peduncle in the region of the midbrain. The two spinocerebellar pathways differ in the location of their cells of origin, one is uncrossed and the other is crossed in the spinal cord, and they reach the cerebellum through different peduncles. However, they convey similar sensory data, which are mainly for proprioception, touch, and pressure, to the cerebellum. The part of the cerebellum receiving afferents from the spinal cord influences muscle tonus and maintains synergy among cooperating muscles, as appropriate in postural changes, locomotion, and other forms of movement.

The fibers of the **spinoolivary tract,** whose caudal extent is uncertain, originate in the contralateral gray matter of the spinal cord. The tract terminates in the inferior olivary complex in the medulla, which projects to the cerebellum.

OTHER ASCENDING TRACTS

The **spinocervical tract,** which is uncrossed and situated in the most dorsal part of the lateral white column, originates from cells of the nucleus proprius of the dorsal gray horn at all levels of the spinal cord. The tract terminates in the **lateral cervical nucleus,** which consists of a column of cells in the first two cervical segments of the spinal cord and continues for a short distance into the medulla. The axons of these cells cross the midline and traverse the brain stem to reach the general sensory nucleus of the thalamus. The sensory modalities conveyed by this pathway appear to include touch, pressure, pain, and temperature.

The **spinotectal tract** transmits general sensory data, originating principally in cutaneous receptors, to the roof (tectum) of the midbrain. This is a crossed tract, which has been identified most distinctly in the cervical region. The fibers end in a region of the tectum known as the superior colliculus, which also receives afferents from the visual and auditory systems. The superior colliculus serves as a midbrain center for reflex motor responses to various types of sensory stimuli.

Spinoreticular fibers are not well localized in the white matter and are therefore not shown in Figure 5–14. The reticular formation, which is discussed in Chapter 9, is a diffuse system of neurons in the brain stem. It has afferent and efferent connections with many parts of the central nervous system. Among other significant functions, the reticular formation is part of an "activating system," which has an important influence on levels of consciousness and one's alertness through projections to the diencephalon and cerebral cortex. The spinoreticular fibers convey data from general sensory receptors, both somatic and visceral, to the reticular formation. The pathway, which is for the most part uncrossed, consists of fibers scattered among the various tracts of the lateral and ventral white columns, together with spinospinalis relays.

An **ascending visceral system** of fibers is also poorly localized and is not entirely distinct from the spinoreticular system. The fibers, which are both crossed and uncrossed, originate in the visceral afferent nucleus and other parts of the dorsal gray horn. They run mainly in the deeper part of the lateral white column, and the system consists in part of chains of neurons (spinospinalis relays). This indefinite pathway transmits sensory data of visceral origin to the reticular formation of the brain stem and to the diencephalon. Conduction for visceral pain appears to be a significant role of the ascending visceral fibers.

DESCENDING TRACTS OF THE LATERAL AND VENTRAL WHITE COLUMNS

The descending or motor tracts originate in the cerebral cortex and in various centers in the brain stem. The position of most of the tracts in the cervical region of the spinal cord is shown in Figure 5–15.

CORTICOSPINAL TRACTS

The corticospinal tract runs through a region of the ventral medulla known as the pyramid, hence the alternative name of **pyramidal tract.** The term **pyramidal system** includes, in addition to the corticospinal tract, the corticobulbar tract, which bears the same relationship to motor neurons of cranial nerves as does the corticospinal tract to motor neurons of spinal nerves.

Parent cell bodies of about 40% of corticospinal fibers are located in the motor cortex of the frontal lobe, and the remainder are in other cortical areas of the frontal and parietal lobes. At the lower end of the medulla, about 85% of the fibers cross into the opposite side of the spinal cord through the pyramidal decussation. These crossed fibers constitute the **lateral corticospinal tract,** which extends throughout the cord. A few of the fibers synapse directly with alpha motor neurons, but the great majority (about 95%) terminate on internuncial neurons, which in turn synapse with alpha cells. The proportions of lateral corticospinal fibers terminating in the major regions of the cord are: cervical, 55%; thoracic, 20%; lumbosacral, 25%. The large proportion of fibers ending in the cervical cord reflects the role of the corticospinal tract with respect to nonstereotyped movements of the upper limbs, especially independent movements of the digits.

FIG. 5–15. Descending tracts in the lateral and ventral white columns.

A few of the fibers not included in the decussation of the pyramids continue into the lateral corticospinal tract of the same side. However, most of the uncrossed fibers constitute the **ventral corticospinal tract,** whose fibers terminate in either ventral horn (mostly contralateral) of cervical and upper thoracic segments. Myelination of corticospinal fibers begins at about the time of birth and is not fully completed until near the end of the second year of childhood.

TRACTS ORIGINATING IN THE BRAIN STEM

Motor tracts originating in brain stem nuclei convey impulses that impinge on gamma motor neurons as well as on alpha motor neurons, either directly or through internuncial cells. Stimulation of alpha motor neurons through the gamma reflex loop is therefore an important aspect of the control of movements through extrapyramidal motor pathways. The relative contributions of the pyramidal and extrapyramidal systems to motor functions are discussed in Chapter 23.

The **rubrospinal tract** originates in the contralateral red nucleus in the midbrain; its fibers terminate in all segments of the spinal cord, although mainly in the cervical region. The red nucleus is included in a pathway through which the cerebellum influences lower motor neurons. The nucleus also receives fibers from motor areas of the cerebral cortex; these, together with rubrospinal fibers, constitute one of the pathways of the extrapyramidal motor system. The **tecto-spinal tract** is also a crossed fasciculus, originating in the contralateral superior colliculus in the tectum of the midbrain. This tract, which is limited to the cervical cord, is part of a reflex pathway for turning the head and perhaps moving the arms in response to visual, acoustic, and cutaneous stimuli. The **interstitiospinal tract** originates in the interstitial nucleus of Cajal, a small nucleus in the rostral part of the midbrain. The constituent fibers, which are for the most part uncrossed, descend in the sulcomarginal fasciculus of the spinal cord, which is discussed later in this section. This minor tract appears to function in optic and vestibular reflexes.

The parent cell bodies of two descending tracts are in the vestibular nuclear complex, which is situated mainly in the medulla and receives afferents from the vestibular portion of the internal ear and the cerebellum. The complex, one on each side, consists of four nuclei: the lateral, superior, medial, and inferior vestibular nuclei (Chapter 22). The cells of origin of the large **vestibulospinal tract** are in the lateral vestibular (Deiters') nucleus of the same side. The tract extends the length of the cord, most of the fibers ending in the ventral gray horn of the cervical and lumbosacral enlargements. The tonus of muscles is altered according to the position of the head and in response to head movements; the vestibulospinal tract is therefore important in the maintenance of equilibrium.

The **sulcomarginal fasciculus** (of Marie) consists mainly of fibers whose cell bodies are located in the medial and inferior vestibular nuclei of both sides. These fibers make up the descending portion of a bundle in the brain stem known as the medial longitudinal fasciculus, of which the ascending component goes to cranial nerve nuclei that innervate the extraocular muscles. The descending fibers terminate in the ventral gray horn throughout the cervical cord, providing for changes in the tonus of neck muscles as required to support the head in various positions. The sulcomarginal fasciculus includes additional fibers with parent cell bodies in the reticular formation of the brain stem, as well as the interstitiospinal fibers already mentioned.

There remain two systems of descending fibers that are not sufficiently well localized to be shown in Figure 5-15. **Reticulospinal fibers** originate in the reticular formation of the brain stem and descend in the ventral and lateral white columns. Conduction is partly by means of long fibers and partly through polysynaptic relays in the fasciculus proprius. Among other functions, reticulospinal connections constitute an important part of the extrapyramidal system, through which motor areas of the cerebral cortex influence motor cells of the ventral horns. **Descending autonomic fibers** are not clearly marked off from reticulospinal fibers of the lateral white column. Most of the autonomic fibers originate in the reticular formation of the brain stem. They constitute a pathway through which the hypothalamus and visceral centers in the brain stem are brought into communication with the intermediolateral cell column (sympathetic) and the sacral parasympathetic nucleus. Other descending autonomic fibers originate in the nucleus of the tractus solitarius in the medulla and are said to comprise a **solitariospinal tract.** The cells of origin of this minor tract, which terminates in the intermediolateral cell column, receive impulses for taste by way of the facial, glossopharyngeal, and vagus nerves, as well as general sensory data from the viscera through the last two of these nerves.

SOME ANATOMIC AND CLINICAL CORRELATIONS

Lesions of the spinal cord result from trauma, degenerative and demyelinating disorders,

tumors, infections, and impairment of blood supply. Testing for impairment or loss of cutaneous sensation is an important part of the neurologic examination, being particularly useful in detecting the site of a lesion involving the spinal cord or nerve roots. The distribution of cutaneous areas (dermatomes) supplied by the spinal nerves is shown for reference in Figure 5–16. (Because different methods of investigation give different results, a dermatomal map receiving general acceptance in all details has yet to be devised.) Cutaneous areas supplied by adjacent spinal nerves overlap. For example, the upper half of the area supplied by T6 is also supplied by T5, and the lower half by T7. There is therefore little sensory loss, if any, following interruption of a single dorsal root of a spinal nerve.

FIG. 5–16. Cutaneous distribution of spinal nerves (dermatomes).

Reflex contraction of muscles is also used in testing for the integrity of segments of the cord and the spinal nerves. The segments involved in the more commonly tested stretch or tendon reflexes are as follows: biceps reflex, C5 and C6; triceps reflex, C6 through C8; quadriceps reflex, L2 through L4; gastrocnemius reflex, S1 and S2.

Before specific pathologic conditions are mentioned, it should be pointed out that a distinction is made between the effects of a lesion involving lower motor neurons as opposed to upper motor neurons. Destruction or atrophy of lower motor neurons (in the present context those of the ventral horn) results in 1) flaccid paralysis of the affected muscles, 2) diminished or absent tendon reflexes, and 3) progressive atrophy of the muscles deprived of motor fibers. The term "upper motor neuron lesion," although regularly used clinically, leaves much to be desired. The lesion may be in the cerebral cortex or another part of the cerebral hemisphere, in the brain stem, or in the spinal cord. Both pyramidal and extrapyramidal motor pathways are almost certain to be involved. In any event, the following signs are associated with an "upper motor neuron lesion" after the acute effects have worn off: 1) varying degrees of voluntary paralysis, which is most severe in the upper limb; 2) the sign of Babinski (up-turning of the great toe and spreading of the toes on stroking the sole); and 3) spasticity with exaggerated tendon reflexes. The voluntary paralysis is now considered to be a result of both pyramidal and extrapyramidal dysfunction, the former being reflected especially in impairment of the more delicate, nonstereotyped movements such as independent use of the fingers. The Babinski sign is attributed to interruption of the pyramidal or corticospinal tract. (A sign of Babinski is normal in infants prior to completion of myelination of the corticospinal tracts.) The muscle spasticity and hyperactive deep reflexes are thought to be caused by interruption of constituent fibers of extrapyramidal pathways. These fibers project from the cerebral cortex to the reticular formation and the red nucleus, which influence ventral horn cells through reticulospinal connections and the rubrospinal tract.

The following elementary notes on selected lesions will show the necessity of understanding the intrinsic anatomy of the spinal cord in order to interpret signs and symptoms.

The cord may be damaged by spinal fracture or dislocation, by penetrating wounds caused by projectile metal fragments, or by other traumatic events. Complete **transection** results in loss of all sensibility and voluntary movement below the lesion. The patient is quadriplegic (both arms and both legs paralyzed) if the upper cervical cord is transected, and paraplegic (both legs paralyzed) if the transection is between the cervical and lumbosacral enlargements. There is an initial period of spinal shock, lasting from a few days to several weeks, during which all somatic and visceral reflex activity is abolished. On return of reflex activity, there is spasticity of muscles and exaggerated tendon reflexes. Bladder and bowel functions are no longer under voluntary control.

The events following partial section of the spinal cord depend on the size and location of the lesion. **Hemisection,** although unusual in the literal sense, is an instructive lesion anatomically. The neurologic signs caudal to the hemisected region of the cord constitute the Brown–Séquard syndrome. Position sense, tactile discrimination, and the feeling of vibration are lost *on the side of the lesion* because of interruption of the dorsal funiculus. There is anesthesia for pain and temperature *on the opposite side* because of interruption of the lateral spinothalamic tract. Light touch is not affected prominently, because of essentially bilateral conduction in the dorsal column (uncrossed) and the ventral spinothalamic tract (crossed). The patient is hemiplegic if the lesion is in the upper cervical cord, whereas hemisection of the thoracic cord results in paralysis of the leg (monoplegia). The paralysis is *ipsilateral* to the lesion and is of the "upper motor neuron" type, as has been described. A patient with hemisection of the cervical cord has a sympathetic disturbance, known as Horner's syndrome, on the side of the lesion. This syndrome is a sequel to interruption of descending autonomic fibers in the lateral white column, with withdrawal of stimuli to cells of the intermediolateral cell column. Horner's syndrome consists of 1) pupillary constriction due to paralysis of the dilator pupillae muscle; 2) slight lowering of the upper eyelid (ptosis) because of paralysis of the smooth muscle component (tarsal muscle) of the levator palpebrae superioris muscle; 3) slight enophthalmos resulting from paralysis of Müller's orbital muscle; and 4) in some cases, vasodilation and absence of sweating on the face and neck.

The following degenerative diseases also illustrate the anatomic basis of neurologic signs. In **subacute combined degeneration** there is bilateral demyelination and loss of nerve fibers in the dorsal column and the dorsal part of the lateral column. The principal etiologic factor is vitamin B_{12} deficiency, and the disorder is usually encountered in association with pernicious anemia. The dorsal column lesion results in loss of the senses of position, discriminative touch, and vibration. The gait is ataxic (without coordination) because the patient is unaware of the position of the legs. However, the ataxia tends to be obscured by paraplegic signs caused by degeneration of the lateral corticospinal tracts and extrapyramidal pathways.

Friedreich's ataxia is a familial disease, usually beginning in childhood, in which the initial degenerative change affects Clarke's column and the dorsal spinocerebellar tract bilaterally. The dorsal white columns are involved to some extent, and the degenerative process spreads to the cerebellum and other parts of the brain. The characteristic sign of the disease is ataxia; disturbances of speech and other motor signs are added as the degeneration spreads, and there may be dementia late in the disease.

Amyotrophic lateral sclerosis is a bilateral degenerative disease that appears to be of viral origin. The degenerative process is restricted to the motor system, affecting the corticobulbar and corticospinal tracts along with motor nuclei of cranial nerves and ventral horn motor cells. The signs are therefore a combination of upper and lower motor neuron lesion effects.

Syringomyelia is a different disorder from those already mentioned in that neuronal degeneration is not the primary pathologic change. The condition is characterized by central cavitation of the spinal cord, usually beginning in the cervical region, with a glial reaction (gliosis) adjacent to the cavity. Decussating fibers for pain and temperature in the ventral gray and white commissures are interrupted early in the disease. The cavitation and gliosis spread into the gray matter and white matter, and also longitudinally, leading to variable signs and symptoms depending on the regions involved. The classic clinical picture is that of "yokelike" anesthesia for pain and temperature over the shoulders and upper limbs, accompanied by lower motor neuron weakness and wasting of the muscles of the upper limbs. Spread of the cavitation and glial reaction into the lateral white columns may result in voluntary paresis of the "upper motor neuron" type, affecting especially the lower limbs. The etiology of syringomyelia is not known, although there are hypotheses based on neuropathologic studies. It has been suggested, for example, that the pulsatile circulation through the choroid plexuses produces pressure waves in the cerebrospinal fluid, that these are carried into the central canal from the fourth ventricle, and that in rare instances the eventual result is cyst formation and surrounding gliosis in the region of the central canal. Another suggestion is that when the pressure of the cerebrospinal fluid in the spinal canal is increased for any reason, the pressure is transmitted into the central region of the cord through perivascular extensions of the spinal subarachnoid space.

SUGGESTED READING

Austin G: The Spinal Cord: Basic Aspects and Surgical Considerations. Springfield, IL, Thomas, 1961

Ball MJ, Dayan AD: Pathogenesis of syringomyelia. Lancet 2:799–801, 1972

Barson AJ: The vertebral level of termination of the spinal cord during normal and abnormal development. J Anat 106:489–497, 1970

Bryan RN, Coulter JD, Willis WD: Cells of origin of the spinocervical tract in the monkey. Exp Neurol 42:574–586, 1974

Calne DB, Pallis CA: Vibratory sense: a critical review. Brain 89:723–746, 1966

Eccles JC: Functional organization of the spinal cord. Anesthesiology 28:31–45, 1962

Gardner JW: Hydrodynamic mechanism of syringomyelia: its relation to myelocele. J Neurol Neurosurg Psychiatry 28:247–259, 1965

Grant FC, Wood FA: Experiences with cordotomy. Clin Neurosurg 5:38–65, 1958

Ha H, Liu CN: Cell origin of the ventral spinocerebellar tract. J Comp Neurol 133:185–205, 1968

Heimer L, Wall PD: The dorsal root distribution to the substantia gelatinosa of the rat with a note on the distribution in the cat. Exp Brain Res 6: 89–99, 1968

LaMotte C: Distribution of the tract of Lissauer and the dorsal root fibers in the primate spinal cord. J Comp Neurol 172:529–561, 1977

Nathan PW, Smith MC: Fasciculi proprii of the spinal cord in man: review of present knowledge. Brain 82:610–668, 1959

Oscarsson O: Functional organization of the spino- and cuneocerebellar tracts. Physiol Rev 45:495–522, 1965

Pearson AA: Role of gelatinous substance of spinal cord in conduction of pain. Arch Neurol Psychiatry 68:515–529, 1952

Poirer LJ, Bertrand C: Experimental and anatomical investigation of the lateral spino-thalamic and spinotectal tracts. J Comp Neurol 102:745–757, 1955

Renshaw B: Central effects of centripetal impulses in axons of spinal ventral roots. J Neurophysiol 9:191–204, 1946

Réthelyi M, Szentágothai J: The large synaptic complexes of the substantia gelatinosa. Exp Brain Res 7:258–274, 1969

Rexed BA: Cytoarchitectonic atlas of the spinal cord in the cat. J Comp Neurol 100:297–379, 1954

Scheibel ME, Scheibel AB: Spinal motoneurons, interneurons and Renshaw cells: a Golgi study. Arch Ital Biol 104:328–353, 1966

Sindou M, Quoex C, Baleydier C: Fiber organization at the posterior spinal cord-rootlet junction in man. J Comp Neurol 153:15–26, 1974

Smith MC: Observations on the topography of the lateral column of the human cervical spinal cord. Brain 80:263–272, 1957

Szentágothai J: Neuronal and synaptic arrangement in the substantia gelatinosa Rolandi. J Comp Neurol 122:219–239, 1964

Szentágothai J: Pathways and subcortical relay mechanisms of visceral afferents. Acta Neuroveg (Wien) 28:103–120, 1966

Teng P: Ligamentum denticulatum: an anatomical review and its role in various neurosurgical problems of the spinal cord. Mt Sinai J Med NY 32:567–577, 1965

Thomas RC, Wilson VJ: Precise localization of Renshaw cells with a new marking technique. Nature 206:211–213, 1965

Wall PD: The sensory and motor role of impulses travelling in the dorsal columns towards cerebral cortex. Brain 93:505–524, 1970

White JC: Conduction of pain in man: observations on its afferent pathways within the spinal cord and visceral nerves. Arch Neurol Psychiatry 71:1–23, 1954

Brain Stem:
External Anatomy

The brain stem, as the term is used here, consists of the medulla oblongata, pons, and midbrain. Although each of the three regions has special features, they have certain fiber tracts in common and each region includes nuclei of cranial nerves. The fourth ventricle is partly in the medulla and partly in the pons. It is advantageous, therefore, to describe the medulla, pons, and midbrain together.

MEDULLA OBLONGATA

The medulla oblongata (or medulla) is about 3 cm long and widens gradually in a rostral direction. It rests on the basilar portion of the occipital bone and is concealed from above by the cerebellum. The junction of the spinal cord and medulla is at the upper rootlet of the first cervical nerve, which corresponds to the level of the foramen magnum. The spinal cord seems to pass imperceptibly into the medulla, in so far as surface markings are concerned, but there is in fact an abrupt and extensive rearrangement of the gray matter and white matter. The rostral limit of the medulla is clearly marked on the ventral surface by the border of the pons (Fig. 6–1). In dorsal view (Fig. 6–3), the medulla is seen to consist of a **closed portion** containing a continuation of the central canal of the spinal cord, and an **open portion** in which part of the fourth ventricle is located. The ventricle results from a flexure of the embryonal brain with a dorsal concavity (the pontine flexure) and subsequent development of the large cerebellum with its thick peduncles. These events caused a divergence of the dorsal

halves of the maturing brain stem, so that its lumen widened out to form the fourth ventricle bounded by the medulla, pons, and cerebellum. The junction of the medulla and pons dorsally may be taken as a line passing along the inferior edges of the middle cerebellar peduncles.

The longitudinal grooves previously described for the spinal cord continue on the medulla. The **ventral median fissure** is interrupted at the spinomedullary junction by small bundles of decussating fibers. These are corticospinal fibers crossing from the pyramid of the medulla to the opposite side of the cord where they constitute the lateral corticospinal tract. The **dorsal median sulcus** continues on the closed portion of the medulla, and the **ventrolateral** and **dorsolateral sulci** are in approximately the same position as they are in the spinal cord.

Three areas, all of which have important landmarks, are thereby outlined on each side. The ventral area is occupied by the **pyramid,** which consists of corticospinal fibers (Fig. 6–1). This is the origin of the term pyramidal tract as a synonym for corticospinal tract. The lateral area (Fig. 6–2) includes a prominent oval swelling, the **olive,** which marks the position of the inferior olivary nucleus. Rootlets of the glossopharyngeal, vagus, and accessory nerves are attached to the lateral area just dorsal to the olive. The **tuberculum cinereum** is that part of the lateral area intervening between the attachment of the above-mentioned nerves and the dorsolateral sulcus. The tuberculum cinereum marks the position of the spinal tract of the trigeminal nerve and the nucleus of the spinal tract, these being comparable to the zone

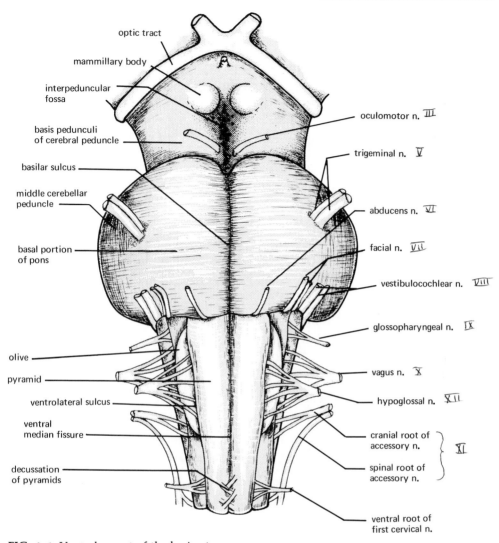

optic tract

mammillary body

interpeduncular
fossa

basis pedunculi
of cerebral peduncle

basilar sulcus

middle cerebellar
peduncle

basal portion
of pons

olive

pyramid

ventrolateral sulcus

ventral
median fissure

decussation
of pyramids

oculomotor n. III

trigeminal n. V

abducens n. VI

facial n. VII

vestibulocochlear n. VIII

glossopharyngeal n. IX

vagus n. X

hypoglossal n. XII

cranial root of
accessory n. } XI
spinal root of
accessory n.

ventral root of
first cervical n.

FIG. 6-1. Ventral aspect of the brain stem.

of Lissauer and the substantia gelatinosa in the spinal cord. The dorsal spinocerebellar tract is superficial to the trigeminal spinal tract in the rostral part of the tuberculum cinereum because the spinocerebellar fibers turn dorsally at this point to enter the inferior cerebellar peduncle. The **fasciculi gracilis** and **cuneatus** continue from the spinal cord into the dorsal area of the medulla (Fig. 6-3). The **clava,** a slight elevation at the rostral end of the fasciculus gracilis, is produced by the nucleus gracilis, in which fibers of the fasciculus end. At a slightly more rostral level, the **cuneate tubercle** marks the position of the nucleus cuneatus or terminal nucleus of the

fasciculus cuneatus. The apex of the V-shaped boundary of the inferior portion of the fourth ventricle is known as the **obex.**

Seven of the twelve cranial nerves are attached to the medulla or the junction of the medulla and pons (Figs. 6-1, 6-2, and 6-3). The **abducens nerve** emerges from the ventral surface between the pons and the pyramid of the medulla. The nerve passes forward in the subarachnoid space beneath the pons, traverses the cavernous venous sinus just lateral to the sphenoid bone, and enters the orbit through the superior orbital fissure. The **facial** and **vestibulocochlear nerves** are attached to the brain stem at the caudal border of the pons well out laterally,

FIG. 6–2. Lateral aspect of the brain stem.

the facial nerve being the more medial. The facial nerve has two roots, motor and sensory. The sensory root lies between the larger motor root and the vestibulocochlear nerve; it is therefore known as the **nervus intermedius** (of Wrisberg). The cochlear division of the vestibulocochlear nerve ends in the dorsal and ventral cochlear nuclei, which are situated on the base of the inferior cerebellar peduncle, whereas the vestibular division penetrates the brain stem deep to the root of the inferior cerebellar peduncle. The facial and vestibulocochlear nerves enter the internal acoustic meatus in the petrous temporal bone.

Roots of the **glossopharyngeal** and **vagus** nerves, as well as those of the cranial division on the **accessory nerve,** are attached to the medulla along a line between the olive and the tuberculum cinereum (the dorsoolivary sulcus). The accessory nerve is motor, whereas the glossopharyngeal and vagus nerves are mixed, having sensory and motor components. The cranial root of the accessory nerve is joined by the spinal root, and the glossopharyngeal, vagus, and accessory nerves leave the posterior cranial fossa through the jugular foramen. Roots of the **hypoglossal nerve,** a motor nerve, emerge along the ventrolateral sulcus between the pyramid and the olive, and the nerve leaves the posterior fossa through the hypoglossal canal.

pineal gland

superior colliculus

superior brachium

pulvinar

medial geniculate body

r brachium

erior colliculus

r medullary velum

minence

mitans

edullares

tibuli

l cochlear nucleus

obex

e tubercle

clava

dorsolateral sulcus

fasciculus cuneatus

tuberculum cinereum

fasciculus gracilis

lateral geniculate body

trochlear n.

position of lateral lemniscus

superior cerebellar peduncle

inferior cerebellar peduncle

middle cerebellar peduncle

hypoglossal triangle

vestibulocochlear n.

glossopharyngeal n.

vagal triangle

area postrema

vagus n.

dorsal median sulcus

cranial root of accessory n.

spinal root of accessory n.

dorsal root of first cervical n.

FIG. 6-3. Dorsal aspect of the brain stem.

PONS

This part of the brain stem owes its name to the appearance presented on the ventral surface (Fig. 6-1), which is that of a bridge connecting the right and left cerebellar hemispheres. However, the appearance is deceptive as far as the constituent nerve fibers are concerned, as noted below.

The pons consists of two quite different parts, known as the basal (ventral) and dorsal portions of the pons, as is seen clearly in sections (Figs. 7-8 and 7-9). The **basal portion** is distinctive of this part of the brain stem. Fibers from the cerebral cortex terminate ipsilaterally on nerve cells composing the pontine nuclei, and axons of the latter cells constitute the contralateral middle cerebellar peduncle. In effect the basal pons is a large synaptic or relay station, providing a connection between the cortex of a cerebral hemisphere and that of the opposite cerebellar hemisphere as part of a circuit contributing to maximal efficiency of voluntary movements. The cerebral cortex, basal pons, and cerebellum all increased in size during mammalian evolution and are best developed in the human brain. The corticospinal tracts traverse the basal portion of the pons before entering the pyramids.

The **dorsal portion** or **tegmentum** of the pons is similar to much of the medulla and midbrain in that it contains ascending and descending tracts and nuclei of cranial nerves. The dorsal surface of the pons contributes to the floor of the fourth ventricle.

The pons is about 2.5 cm in length. A shallow groove, the **basilar sulcus,** runs along its ventral surface in the midline. The pons merges laterally into the middle cerebellar peduncles, the attachment of the **trigeminal nerve** marking the transition between the pons and the peduncle (Figs. 6-1 and 6-2). The motor root of the trigeminal nerve is rostromedial to the larger sensory root. The trigeminal nerve enters the middle cranial fossa at the medial end of the petrous temporal bone, where the trigeminal ganglion is located. The three divisions of the nerve diverge from the ganglion, embedded in the dura mater. The ophthalmic division passes through the superior orbital fissure to reach the orbit. The maxillary division traverses the foramen rotundum, and the mandibular division the foramen ovale, both foramina being in the floor of the middle cranial fossa.

The rostral part of the pons is known as the **isthmus of the brain stem.** A slight bandlike elevation runs obliquely across the dorsolateral surface of the isthmus toward the inferior colliculus of the midbrain (Fig. 6-2). This elevation is produced by the underlying lateral lemniscus, which is the main auditory tract of the brain stem.

FOURTH VENTRICLE

The **floor of the fourth ventricle (rhomboid fossa)** is broad in its midportion, narrowing toward the obex and the aqueduct of the midbrain (Fig. 6-3). The floor is divided into symmetrical halves by a **median sulcus;** the **sulcus limitans** further divides each half into medial and lateral areas. The vestibular nuclear complex lies beneath most of the lateral area, which is therefore known as the **vestibular area** of the rhomboid fossa. Motor nuclei are located beneath the medial area, the caudal part of which is marked by two triangles or trigones. The rostral end of the dorsal nucleus of the vagus nerve lies beneath the

vagal triangle (ala cinerea), and the rostral end of the hypoglossal nucleus lies beneath the **hypoglossal triangle.** The appearance of this part of the rhomboid fossa suggested the tip of a pen to early anatomists, and the term calamus scriptorius (writing pen) was therefore applied to it.

The **area postrema** is a narrow strip between the vagal triangle and the margin of the ventricle. The tissue immediately beneath this area consists of neuroglial cells, a few nerve cells, and many blood vessels.

The **facial colliculus,** a slight swelling at the lower end of the **median eminence,** is formed by fibers from the motor nucleus of the facial nerve looping over the abducens nucleus. There is a small pigmented area, the **locus ceruleus** (blue place), at the rostral end of the sulcus limitans, indicating the site of a cluster of nerve cells containing melanin pigment. Delicate strands of nerve fibers emerge from the median sulcus, run laterally over the floor of the ventricle as the **striae medullares,** and enter the inferior cerebellar peduncle. The floor of the fourth ventricle is covered by ependymal epithelium, such as lines the whole of the ventricular system and the central canal of the spinal cord.

The tent-shaped roof of the fourth ventricle protrudes toward the cerebellum. The forepart of the roof is formed on each side by the superior cerebellar peduncles, which consist mainly of fibers proceeding from cerebellar nuclei into the midbrain. The V-shaped interval between the converging peduncles is bridged by the **superior medullary velum,** a thin sheet of tissue consisting of a layer of pia mater and one of ependyma, with some nerve fibers in between. The remainder of the roof consists of a thin pia-ependymal membrane, the **inferior medullary velum,** which often adheres to the undersurface of the cerebellum. A deficiency of variable size in the latter membrane constitutes the **median aperture of the fourth ventricle,** alternatively known as the **foramen of Magendie,** which provides the principal communication between the ventricular system and the subarachnoid space (Fig. 6-4).

The lateral walls of the fourth ventricle include the inferior cerebellar peduncles, which curve from the medulla into the cerebellum on the medial aspect of the middle peduncles (Fig. 6-3). Lateral recesses of the ventricle extend around the sides of the me-

FIG. 6-4. Median aperture of the fourth ventricle (foramen of Magendie), opening from the fourth ventricle into the cerebellomedullary cistern of the subarachnoid space. (× 2½)

FIG. 6-5. Lateral apertures of the fourth ventricle (foramina of Luschka). Tufts of choroid plexus **(arrows)** occupy the foramina, into which marker sticks have been inserted. (× 1 1/5)

facial nerve

vestibulocochlear nerve

glossopharyngeal, vagus, and accessory nerves

dulla and open ventrally as the **lateral apertures of the fourth ventricle** or the **foramina of Luschka,** through which cerebrospinal fluid enters the subarachnoid space (Fig. 6–5). These foramina are situated at the junction of the medulla, pons, and cerebellum (the cerebellopontine angles) near the attachment to the brain stem of the facial, vestibulocochlear, and glossopharyngeal nerves. The choroid plexus of the fourth ventricle is suspended from the inferior medullary velum; the plexus extends into the lateral recesses, and tufts even protrude into the foramina of Luschka.

MIDBRAIN

The ventral surface of the midbrain extends from the pons to the mammillary bodies of the diencephalon (Fig. 6–1). The prominent elevation on each side is formed by the **basis pedunculi** (crus cerebri), which consists of fibers of the pyramidal motor system and corticopontine fibers. Many small blood vessels penetrate the midbrain in the floor of the **interpeduncular fossa,** and this region is therefore known as the **posterior perforated substance.** The **oculomotor nerve** emerges from the side of the interpeduncular fossa and passes forward through the cavernous venous sinus into the orbit.

The dorsal surface of the midbrain bears four rounded elevations, the paired **inferior** and **superior colliculi** (corpora quadrigemina) (Figs. 6–2 and 6–3). The colliculi make up the **roof** or **tectum** and indicate the extent of the midbrain on the dorsal surface (about 1.5 cm long). The major role of the inferior colliculus is that of a relay nucleus on the auditory pathway to the thalamus and thence to the cerebral cortex. Fibers connecting the inferior colliculus with the specific thalamic nucleus for hearing (medial geniculate nucleus) form an elevation known as the **inferior brachium** (Figs. 6–2 and 6–3). The superior colliculus is primarily a reflex center for movements of the eyes and head in response to visual and other stimuli. The **superior brachium** contains fibers proceeding from cortex of the occipital lobe and from the retina to the superior colliculus. Other fibers in the superior brachium terminate in the pretectal nucleus just in front of the superior colliculus; the latter fibers are part of a pathway from the retina for the pupillary light reflex. The **trochlear nerve** emerges from the brain stem immediately caudal to the inferior colliculus, curves around the midbrain, and enters the orbit after traversing the cavernous venous sinus.

The lateral surface of the midbrain (Fig. 6–2) is formed mainly by the **cerebral peduncle,** which constitutes the major portion of this region of the brain stem on each side.

The posterior part of the thalamus grows beyond the plane of transition between the diencephalon and the midbrain during maturation of the brain (Fig. 6–3). Consequently transverse sections at the level of the superior colliculi include thalamic nuclei, in particular the medial and lateral geniculate nuclei and a prominent nucleus of the thalamus known as the pulvinar (Figs. 7–14 and 7–15).

7
Brain Stem:
Nuclei and Tracts of the
Medulla, Pons, and Midbrain

The principal nuclei and fiber tracts of the brain stem are identified and discussed in the present chapter. Long fiber tracts that traverse all, or most, of the brain stem are noted successively in the medulla, pons, and midbrain. A regional presentation of such tracts is not wholly desirable, and some pathways are reviewed as functional systems in Chapters 19 and 23. The larger nuclei of cranial nerves are included among the cell groups identified, although a description of the functional components of the cranial nerves is reserved for Chapter 8.

Sections stained by the Weigert method are used as illustrations, the levels of the sections being shown in Figure 7–1. The smaller tracts are difficult to identify in such sections, although their location has been established by experimental work using laboratory animals and clinicopathologic correlations in man. In the illustrations, therefore, the sites of some tracts are indicated even though they cannot be distinguished clearly from adjacent fasciculi.

The reticular formation is mentioned briefly at this point because it is necessary to use the term in the present chapter. The reticular formation of the brain stem consists of neurons in areas not occupied by prominent nuclei or tracts. Most of the constituent cells defy organization into easily identifiable groups, and histologic analysis therefore presents a formidable problem. The reticular formation has several functions of the first importance. These include the following, among others: 1) an influence on levels of consciousness and degrees of alertness (ascending reticular activating system); 2) a role

in the extrapyramidal motor system through afferents from the cerebral cortex and efferents to motor neurons of cerebrospinal nerves; and 3) a contribution to the autonomic nervous system through groups of neurons that function as cardiovascular and respiratory centers. In view of its special histologic characteristics and functional importance, the reticular formation is discussed separately in Chapter 9.

MEDULLA

There is an extensive rearrangement of gray matter and white matter in the transitional zone between the spinal cord and the medulla, this zone being coextensive with the pyramidal decussation. The ventral gray horns continue into the region of the decussation, where they include motor cells for the first cervical nerve and the spinal root of the accessory nerve, and where the gray matter is traversed obliquely by bundles of fibers passing from the pyramids to the lateral corticospinal tracts (Figs. 7–2 and 7–3). Dorsal expansions of the gray matter at the level of the pyramidal decussation form the nuclei gracilis and cuneatus. The medulla has a complex internal structure above the decussation, a structure that is entirely different from that of the spinal cord (Figs. 7–4 through 7–7). The inferior olivary nucleus is the most prominent feature of the rostral half of the medulla. Near the pons, the base of the inferior cerebellar peduncle appears as a distinctive area of white matter in the dorsolateral part of the medulla (Fig. 7–7).

FIG. 7-1. Key to levels of Weigert-stained sections of the brain stem shown in Figs. 7–2 through 7–10 and in Figs. 7–12 through 7–15 (see Fig. 6–2).

ASCENDING PATHWAYS

Dorsal Column System

It will be recalled that long dorsal column fibers reaching the medulla oblongata from the spinal cord transmit impulses for discriminative touch, proprioception, and vibration as an ipsilateral pathway. The **fasciculus gracilis** is concerned with these sensations for the leg and lower trunk, whereas impulses from the upper trunk, arm, and neck are transmitted in the **fasciculus cuneatus.**

The **nucleus gracilis,** in which fibers of the corresponding fasciculus terminate, is present throughout the closed portion of the medulla. The fibers of the fasciculus cuneatus end in the **nucleus cuneatus,** which first appears slightly rostral to the beginning of the nucleus gracilis and continues beyond the latter nucleus. There is a somatotopic representation in these dorsal column nuclei, *i.e.,* fibers entering the spinal cord in a specific segment synapse with a specific group of cells in the nuclei. Such a point-to-point projection of fibers on sensory nuclei is characteristic of pathways to the thalamus and cerebral cortex, forming an anatomic basis for recognition of the source of stimuli. The

less the convergence from primary to secondary to tertiary neurons in the pathway, the greater is the precision of localization and the quality of discrimination, maximal discrimination obviously being achieved by a 1:1:1 ratio. The system for fine touch, position and movement, and vibration is the most discriminative of the general sensory systems. There is therefore little convergence between successive neurons that constitute the pathway to the cerebral cortex.

The myelinated axons of cells in the dorsal column nuclei pursue a curved course to the median raphe as **internal arcuate fibers,** which are shown especially well in Figure 7–4. After crossing the midline in the **decussation of the medial lemniscus,** the fibers turn rostrally in the **medial lemniscus.** This is one of the more substantial tracts of the brain stem, occupying the interval between the median raphe and the inferior olivary nucleus in the medulla (Figs. 7–4 through 7–7). Fibers conducting data from the contralateral foot are most ventral, *i.e.,* adjacent to the pyramid. The opposite side of the body is then represented sequentially, so that fibers for the neck are in the most dorsal part of the medial lemniscus. After traversing the pons and midbrain, the tract ends in the thalamic nucleus for general sensation, which is the ventral posterior nucleus of the thalamus.

Spinothalamic and Spinotectal Tracts

The **lateral spinothalamic tract** for pain and temperature, and the **ventral spinothalamic tract** for light (simple) touch and pressure, on the opposite side of the body, continue into the medulla without appreciable change in position. This is also true of the **spinotectal tract,** which conveys somesthetic data to the superior colliculus of the midbrain. However, the three tracts soon merge to form the **spinal lemniscus,** which traverses the lateral area of the medulla dorsal to the inferior olivary nucleus (Figs. 7–4 through 7–7). The spinotectal fibers leave the spinal lemniscus in the rostral midbrain, and the spinothalamic fibers continue to the ventral posterior nucleus of the thalamus.

Spinoreticular Fibers

Spinoreticular fibers in the ventrolateral white matter of the cord continue into the brain stem, where they synapse with cells of

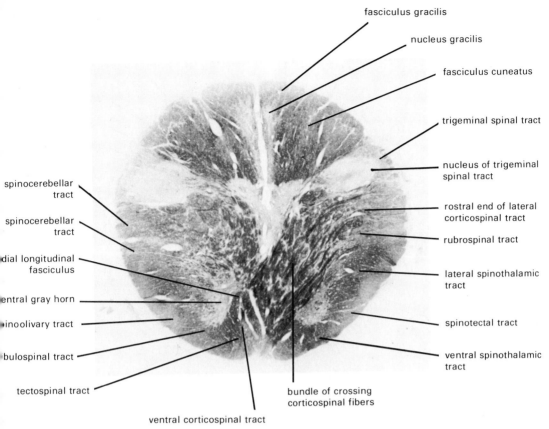

fasciculus gracilis

nucleus gracilis

fasciculus cuneatus

trigeminal spinal tract

nucleus of trigeminal spinal tract

rostral end of lateral corticospinal tract

rubrospinal tract

lateral spinothalamic tract

spinotectal tract

ventral spinothalamic tract

spinocerebellar tract

spinocerebellar tract

dial longitudinal fasciculus

entral gray horn

inoolivary tract

bulospinal tract

tectospinal tract

ventral corticospinal tract

bundle of crossing corticospinal fibers

7-2. Junction of the medulla and spinal cord. (Weigert stain, × 6½)

7-3. Medulla at the rostral end of the pyramidal decussation. (Weigert stain, × 5½)

fasciculus gracilis

nucleus gracilis

fasciculus cuneatus

nucleus cuneatus

trigeminal spinal tract

nucleus of trigeminal spinal tract

rubrospinal tract

ventral gray horn

lateral spinothalamic tract

spinotectal tract

vestibulospinal tract

ventral spinothalamic tract

al spinocerebellar tract

al spinocerebellar tract

medial longitudinal fasciculus

tectospinal tract

spinoolivary tract

pyramid

rostral end of pyramidal decussation

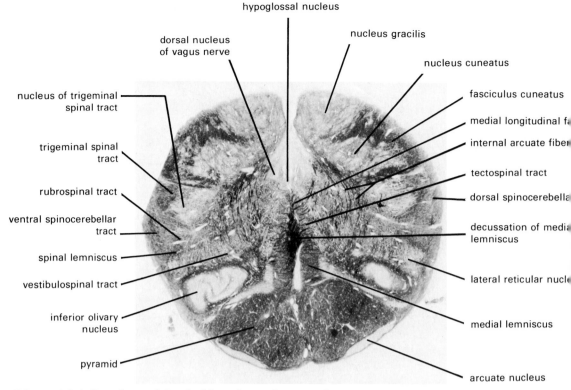

hypoglossal nucleus

dorsal nucleus
of vagus nerve

nucleus gracilis

nucleus cuneatus

nucleus of trigeminal
spinal tract

fasciculus cuneatus

medial longitudinal f

internal arcuate fiber

trigeminal spinal
tract

tectospinal tract

rubrospinal tract

dorsal spinocerebella

ventral spinocerebellar
tract

decussation of medi
lemniscus

spinal lemniscus

vestibulospinal tract

lateral reticular nucle

inferior olivary
nucleus

medial lemniscus

pyramid

arcuate nucleus

FIG. 7–4. Medulla at the caudal end of the inferior olivary nucleus. (Weigert stain, × 4 4/5)

FIG. 7–5. Medulla at the level of transition between its closed and open portions. (Weigert stain, × 4)

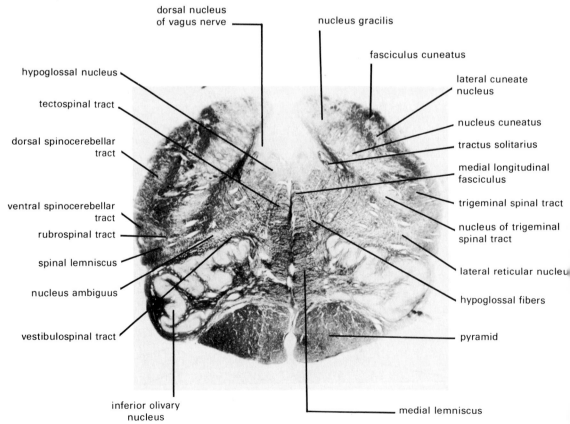

dorsal nucleus
of vagus nerve

nucleus gracilis

fasciculus cuneatus

hypoglossal nucleus

lateral cuneate
nucleus

tectospinal tract

nucleus cuneatus

tractus solitarius

dorsal spinocerebellar
tract

medial longitudinal
fasciculus

ventral spinocerebellar
tract

trigeminal spinal tract

rubrospinal tract

nucleus of trigeminal
spinal tract

spinal lemniscus

lateral reticular nucleu

nucleus ambiguus

hypoglossal fibers

vestibulospinal tract

pyramid

inferior olivary
nucleus

medial lemniscus

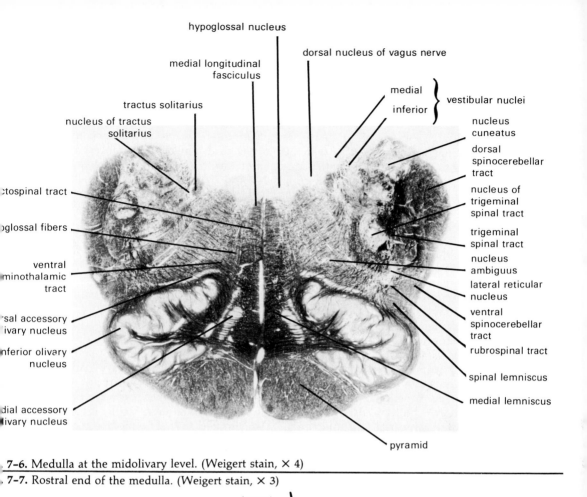

7-6. Medulla at the midolivary level. (Weigert stain, × 4)

7-7. Rostral end of the medulla. (Weigert stain, × 3)

Figure 7-6 labels:

hypoglossal nucleus

medial longitudinal fasciculus

dorsal nucleus of vagus nerve

medial / inferior } vestibular nuclei

tractus solitarius

nucleus of tractus solitarius

nucleus cuneatus

dorsal spinocerebellar tract

ctospinal tract

oglossal fibers

nucleus of trigeminal spinal tract

trigeminal spinal tract

ventral minothalamic tract

nucleus ambiguus

lateral reticular nucleus

ventral spinocerebellar tract

sal accessory ivary nucleus

nferior olivary nucleus

rubrospinal tract

spinal lemniscus

medial lemniscus

dial accessory livary nucleus

pyramid

Figure 7-7 labels:

dorsal cochlear nucleus

lateral / inferior / medial } vestibular nuclei

hypoglossal nucleus

dorsal nucleus of vagus nerve

base of inferior cerebellar peduncle

rigeminal spinal tract

medial longitudinal fasciculus

nucleus of trigeminal spinal tract

ventral lear nucleus

tractus solitarius

tectospinal tract

nucleus ambiguus

ventral spinocerebellar tract

sopharyngeal nerve

ivocerebellar fibers

central mental tract

rubrospinal tract

spinal lemniscus

inferior olivary nucleus

ventral trigeminothalamic tract

pyramid

medial lemniscus

the reticular formation. They transmit somesthetic data, especially of cutaneous origin, and data from the viscera. Spinoreticular fibers are rather diffusely disposed in the spinal cord and medulla; some intermingle with fibers of the spinal lemniscus, from which collateral branches ending in the reticular formation also arise. Axons of cells in the reticular formation project caudally to the spinal cord and rostrally to the diencephalon, and impulses transmitted by the ascending fibers influence neuronal activity throughout much of the cerebral cortex through thalamic relays.

There are, therefore, alternative routes for exteroceptive somesthetic conduction from the spinal cord to the thalamus and cerebral cortex. The direct lemniscal route proceeds without interruption to the ventral posterior thalamic nucleus. This is the more recent pathway, which became increasingly important as the thalamus and cerebral cortex increased in size and functional significance during mammalian evolution. Alternatively exteroceptive data reach certain thalamic nuclei through a polysynaptic, extralemniscal route involving the reticular formation. Although the latter pathway is related to early stages of phylogeny, through thalamocortical projections it has attained importance in man as part of the ascending reticular activating system which has an important influence on levels of consciousness and degrees of alertness.

As intimated earlier, detailed studies of a research nature were required to divide the reticular formation into aggregations of cells or nuclei because of the scattered disposition of its neurons. The **lateral reticular nucleus,** related functionally to the cerebellum, is an exception. This nucleus is situated dorsal to the inferior olivary nucleus and near the surface of the medulla; the constituent neurons form a compact aggregation, and the lateral reticular nucleus appears as a pale area in Weigert-stained sections (Figs. 7–4, 7–5, 7–6).

Spinocerebellar Tracts

The **dorsal** and **ventral spinocerebellar tracts** traverse the medulla in the periphery of the lateral area (Figs. 7–2 through 7–6). It will be recalled that the dorsal tract, which is uncrossed, originates in the nucleus dorsalis (nucleus thoracicus or Clarke's column) of the thoracic and upper lumbar segments of the spinal cord. The ventral tract, on the other hand, is crossed, and many of the cells of origin are in the lumbosacral enlargement of the cord. The dorsal spinocerebellar fibers enter the inferior cerebellar peduncle (Figs. 7–7 and 7–8), whereas the ventral spinocerebellar tract continues through the pons and enters the cerebellum by way of the superior cerebellar peduncle.

MEDULLARY NUCLEI CONNECTED WITH THE CEREBELLUM

Inferior Olivary Complex

Several nuclei in the medulla receive afferents from various sources and project to the cerebellum. These nuclei include the components of the inferior olivary complex. The largest component is the **inferior olivary nucleus,** which is shaped like a crumpled bag or purse with the hilus facing medially (Figs. 7–5 through 7–7). The **medial accessory olivary nucleus** lies between the medial lemniscus and the inferior olivary nucleus, and the **dorsal accessory olivary nucleus** is immediately dorsal to the inferior olivary nucleus (Fig. 7–6). The relatively small accessory nuclei are phylogenetically older than the inferior olivary or principal nucleus.

The **central tegmental tract,** which will be identified in the pons and midbrain, is in part a pathway from the midbrain to the inferior olivary complex. The constituent fibers originate in the red nucleus and the periaqueductal gray matter, and from neurons elsewhere in the tegmentum of the midbrain; these sources relay data from the cerebral cortex, the cerebellum, and other sites that have yet to be clearly identified. The terminal portion of the central tegmental tract forms a dense layer on the dorsal surface of the inferior olivary nucleus, best seen in Figure 7–7. The tract also contains numerous ascending fibers originating in the reticular formation of the brain stem and proceeding to the diencephalon.

Other afferents to the inferior olivary complex come from the cerebral cortex, spinal cord, and cerebellum. **Corticoolivary fibers** originate in the sensorimotor strip of cerebral cortex, lying on each side of the boundary between the frontal and parietal lobes. These fibers, which terminate mainly in the principal nucleus, accompany the corticospinal tract through the midbrain and pons. The inferior olivary nucleus receives impulses originating in proprioceptors by way of afferent fibers from the nuclei gracilis and cuneatus. The **spinoolivary tract** continues from the cord into the ventrolateral area of the medulla (Figs. 7–2 and 7–3), and most of its fibers end in the accessory olivary nuclei. A modest number of **cerebelloolivary fibers,** which are collateral branches of fibers entering the midbrain from the cerebellum through the superior cerebellar peduncle, convey impulses from the central nuclei of the cerebellum.

Olivocerebellar fibers constitute the projection from the inferior olivary complex. Fibers from the principal nucleus occupy its interior and leave through the hilus. After decussating in the median raphe, the strands of myelinated olivocerebellar fibers curve in a dorsolateral direction and enter the inferior cerebellar peduncle, of which they are the largest single component (Fig. 7–7). The phylogenetically older accessory olivary nuclei project to correspondingly older regions of the cerebellum. These regions constitute the archicerebellum, which is concerned with the maintenance of equilibrium, and the paleocerebellum, which functions in relation to the generally stereotyped movements of postural changes and locomotion. The inferior olivary nucleus projects to the neocerebellum—the major part of the cerebellum of man. Its role is to ensure efficiency of voluntary movements, especially those requiring precision. The inferior olivary complex is therefore important in the context of cerebellar control of movements, although its precise contribution to cerebellar physiology has yet to be determined.

Information is also scanty with respect to the effects of lesions involving the inferior olivary complex. A curious clinical observation is that of rhythmic movement of the soft palate (palatal myoclonus) when a degenerative lesion of the brain stem includes the inferior olivary nucleus. Instances of degeneration of the olivary nuclei, nuclei of the basal pons, and the cerebellum are well documented, although the etiology is unknown. The patients show a combination of motor deficits, including ataxia, that are characteristic of cerebellar dysfunction.

Arcuate Nucleus

The arcuate nucleus lies on the surface of the pyramid (Fig. 7–4) and receives collateral branches of corticospinal fibers. Fibers from the nucleus enter the cerebellum by way of the inferior cerebellar peduncle, which they reach by two routes. Some of them travel over the lateral surface of the medulla; the remainder run dorsally in the median raphe and then laterally in the striae medullares in the floor of the fourth ventricle. The connections of the arcuate nucleus are like those of the cell groups in the basal portion of the pons—both receive afferents from the cerebral cortex and project to the cerebellum.

Lateral Cuneate Nucleus

The lateral (accessory) cuneate nucleus is embedded in the fasciculus cuneatus external to the cuneate nucleus (Fig. 7–5). The afferents to the lateral cuneate nucleus are fibers of the fasciculus cuneatus that entered the spinal cord in cervical dorsal roots; many such afferents are in fact collateral branches of fibers ending in the cuneate nucleus. Efferents from the lateral cuneate nucleus, accompanied by a few fibers from the cuneate nucleus, enter the cerebellum by way of the inferior peduncle. These cuneocerebellar fibers reinforce the dorsal spinocerebellar tract as a pathway from proprioceptive and other sensory endings in the neck and upper limb. They provide the main route to the cerebellum for impulses entering the spinal cord in the upper four cervical nerves, from which no fibers reach Clarke's column.

DESCENDING TRACTS

Corticospinal Tract

The corticospinal (pyramidal) tract is among the larger and more important tracts of the human brain and spinal cord. About 40% of the parent cell bodies are situated in the dorsal two-thirds of the motor area (a strip of cortex along the posterior boundary of the frontal lobe), and the remainder are in the premotor area of the frontal lobe and cortex of the parietal lobe. The corticospinal fibers traverse the medullary center of the cerebral hemisphere and the internal capsule to reach the brain stem. The fibers continue as a compact fasciculus in the basis pedunculi of the midbrain, but the tract is broken up into many small bundles on entering the basal portion of the pons. The bundles coalesce in the caudal pons and the corticospinal tract is again a compact fasciculus in the pyramid of the medulla (Figs. 7–7 through 7–4).

Each pyramid contains approximately one million fibers of varying size. About 50% of the fibers are fine and very thinly myelinated, measuring 1μ in diameter, and 90% are less than 4μ in diameter. However, approximately 35,000, or roughly 3% of the pyramidal fibers are thickly myelinated and about 10μ in diameter. These rapidly conducting fibers are considered to come from the giant pyramidal cells of Betz in the motor area.

The proportion of fibers that cross over in the **decussation of the pyramids** varies among individuals, but on the average about 85% enter the decussation. The rostral limit of the pyramidal decussation appears in Figure 7–3, and a bundle of fibers passing through the gray matter from a pyramid to the opposite lateral corticospinal tract is shown in Figure 7–2. A few pyramidal fibers enter the lateral corticospinal tract of the same side. With this exception, the 15% of nondecussating fibers continues into the ventral white column of the cord as the ventral corticospinal tract. The bundles of corticobulbar fibers destined for motor nuclei of cranial nerves in the medulla are small and inconstant in position; no attempt has been made to identify them in the illustrations.

Tracts Originating in the Midbrain

The **rubrospinal tract** arises from the red nucleus and crosses to the opposite side of the brain stem at the level of origin. The tract runs caudally in the lateral area, dorsal to the inferior olivary nucleus, throughout most of the medulla (Figs. 7–7 through 7–4). The fibers of the pyramidal decussation turn caudally immediately dorsal to the rubrospinal tract (Fig. 7–2), and the lateral corticospinal and rubrospinal tracts continue into the lateral white column of the cord in this relationship.

The **tectospinal tract** originates in the superior colliculus of the midbrain, and the fibers cross at that level to the opposite side of the brain stem. The tract lies next to the median raphe and dorsal to the medial lemniscus throughout most of the medulla (Figs. 7–7 through 7–4). The decussating corticospinal bundles pass dorsal to the tectospinal tract, which is therefore deflected ventrally (Figs. 7–3 and 7–2) to take up a position in the ventral white column of the cord.

NUCLEI OF CRANIAL NERVES AND ASSOCIATED TRACTS

Hypoglossal, Accessory, Vagus, and Glossopharyngeal Nerves

The **hypoglossal nucleus** for innervation of the muscles of the tongue consists of a column of motor cells near the midline and coextensive with the inferior olivary nucleus. The hypoglossal nucleus is situated in the central gray matter in the closed part of the medulla (Fig. 7–4) and beneath the hypoglossal triangle of the rhomboid fossa (Figs. 7–5 through 7–7). The medullated axons leaving the nucleus are directed ventrally between the medial lemniscus and the inferior olivary nucleus (Figs. 7–5 and 7–6); they continue lateral to the pyramid and emerge as the hypoglossal nerve roots along the ventrolateral sulcus. The **nucleus ambiguus** is situated dorsal to the inferior olivary nucleus in the position shown in Figures 7–5 through 7–7. This important cell column supplies muscles of the soft palate, pharynx, larynx, and upper esophagus through the cranial root of the accessory nerve and the vagus and glossopharyngeal nerves. The **dorsal nucleus of the vagus nerve** is the largest of the parasympathetic nuclei in the brain stem; it contains the cell bodies of preganglionic neurons for smooth muscle and glandular elements of thoracic and abdominal viscera, as well as the heart. The nucleus lies lateral to the hypoglossal nucleus in the gray matter surrounding the central canal (Fig. 7–4), and extends rostrally beneath the vagal triangle of the rhomboid fossa (Figs. 7–5 through 7–7).

There is a bundle of visceral afferent fibers known as the **tractus solitarius,** which lies along the lateral side of the dorsal nucleus of the vagus nerve (Figs. 7–5 through 7–7). This tract consists of caudally directed fibers, whose cell bodies are in the inferior ganglia of the vagus and glossopharyngeal nerves and the geniculate ganglion of the facial nerve. The fibers terminate in the **nucleus of the tractus solitarius,** a column of cells that lies adjacent to, and partly surrounds, the tract. The vagal and glossopharyngeal afferents have an important role in visceral reflexes and transmit impulses for taste from the epiglottis and posterior one-third of the tongue. The fibers contributed by the facial nerve are for taste in the anterior two-thirds of the tongue and in the palate.

Vestibulocochlear Nerve

Nuclei in which the cochlear and vestibular divisions of the eighth cranial nerve terminate are situated in the most rostral part of the medulla. The **dorsal cochlear nucleus,** lying on the base of the inferior cerebellar peduncle, is shown in Figure 7–7, and a portion of the **ventral cochlear nucleus** appears lateral to the peduncle in the same figure. Fibers leaving the cochlear nuclei are noted later in the description of the pons. The **vestibular nuclear complex,** situated beneath the vestibular area of the rhomboid fossa, is divided into **superior, lateral, medial,** and **inferior vestibular nuclei** on the basis of cytoarchitecture and connections. The superior nucleus is in the pons, in the position shown in Figure 7–8, whereas the remaining nuclei are in the medulla (Figs. 7–6 and 7–7). The vestibular nerve penetrates the brain stem deep to the fibers of the inferior cerebellar peduncle. This occurs slightly rostral to the attachment of the cochlear nerve and the vestibular nerve is therefore not included in Figure 7–7. Most of the vestibular nerve fibers terminate in the vestibular nuclear complex, and the remainder enter the cerebellum through the inferior peduncle. Descending branches of vestibular nerve fibers that terminate in the inferior vestibular nucleus give this nucleus a stippled appearance in sections (Fig. 7–7).

In addition to the primary vestibulocerebellar fibers just mentioned, numerous secondary fibers proceed from the vestibular nuclei into the cerebellum through the inferior peduncle. Vestibular nuclei project to spinal motor neurons by means of two tracts. The larger of these is the **vestibulospinal tract,** for which the cells of origin are in the lateral vestibular (Deiters') nucleus. Vestibulospinal fibers run caudally, dorsal to the inferior olivary nucleus, in the position indicated in Figures 7–5 and 7–4. The tract is deflected ventrally at the level of the pyramidal decussation (Figs. 7–3 and 7–2) and continues into the ipsilateral ventral white column of the spinal cord.

Fibers from all the vestibular nuclei form the **medial longitudinal fasciculus,** which extends rostrally and caudally adjacent to the midline. The ascending fibers are identified later in the pons and midbrain. The parent cell bodies of the descending fibers are in the medial and inferior vestibular nuclei; they are both crossed and uncrossed, but predominantly the latter. The fasciculus is dorsal to the tectospinal tract until the level of the pyramidal decussation is reached (Figs. 7–7 through 7–4). The decussating pyramidal fibers intervene between the gray matter around the central canal and the medial longitudinal fasciculus, so that the latter assumes a more ventral position (Figs. 7–3 and 7–2) and continues into the spinal cord as a major component of the sulcomarginal fasciculus in the ventral white column. The tectospinal tract is similarly deflected ventrally by the pyramidal decussation. The fibers of the medial longitudinal fasciculus and the tectospinal tract are joined by the ventral corticospinal tract below the pyramidal decussation, and there is considerable intermingling of the three categories of fibers in the ventral white column of the cervical cord.

Trigeminal Nerve

The trigeminal nerve contributes an important tract and nucleus to the internal structure of the medulla. Many of the fibers of the trigeminal sensory root turn caudally on entering the pons. These fibers constitute the **trigeminal spinal tract,** so named because some of the fibers extend caudally as far as the third cervical segment of the spinal cord. The spinal tract transmits data for pain, temperature, light touch, and pressure from the extensive area of distribution of the trigeminal nerve. The fibers terminate in the subjacent **nucleus of the trigeminal spinal tract.** The tract and nucleus lie deep to the root of the inferior cerebellar peduncle and the dorsal spinocerebellar tract in the rostral part of the medulla (Figs. 7–7 through 7–4). More caudally, they lie under the surface area of the medulla known as the tuberculum cinereum (Figs. 7–3 and 7–2). Many of the descending fibers are unmyelinated or thinly myelinated, and the nucleus consists principally of small neurons. The trigeminal spinal tract and its nucleus are, therefore, similar in some respects both structurally and functionally to the dorsolateral fasciculus and substantia gelatinosa of the spinal cord. The **ventral trigeminothalamic tract** (Fig. 7–6) is a crossed fasciculus, which projects from the nucleus of the spinal tract (and the chief sensory nucleus in the pons) to the ventral posterior nucleus of the thalamus. Conducting sensory data from the head, the ventral trigeminothalamic tract is comparable functionally to the spinothalamic pathways for the body generally.

PONS

The main features in Weigert-stained sections through the pons are 1) the division of the pons into basal (ventral) and dorsal regions, and 2) the prominent cerebellar peduncles (Figs. 7–8 and 7–9). The basal portion consists of longitudinal fiber bundles, transverse fibers, and collections of nerve cells in the intervals between longitudinal and transverse fasciculi. The longitudinal bundles are numerous and small at rostral levels (Figs. 7–9 and 7–10), although many of them coalesce as they approach the medulla (Fig. 7–8). The inferior and middle cerebellar peduncles appear in Figure 7–8, and the superior peduncles in Figure 7–9.

DORSAL PORTION (Tegmentum)
OF THE PONS

The pontine tegmentum is similar structurally to the medulla and midbrain. There are therefore tracts that were described in the medulla to identify, together with components of several cranial nerves.

Ascending Tracts; Inferior and Superior Cerebellar Peduncles

The **medial lemniscus** "rotates" in passing from the medulla into the pons, where it takes up a position in the most ventral part of the tegmentum. The lemniscus has a roughly oval outline at the level shown in Figure 7–8; it moves laterally farther forward and becomes straplike in shape (Figs. 7–9 and 7–10). The medial lemniscus rotates in such a way that fibers from the nucleus cuneatus are medial to those from the nucleus gracilis. The somatotopic representation is therefore neck, arm, trunk, and leg, in a medial to lateral sequence. The **spinal lemniscus** is situated near the lateral edge of the medial lemniscus throughout the pons (Figs. 7–8 through 7–10). The **ventral spinocerebellar tract** traverses the most lateral part of the tegmentum (Fig. 7–8), then curves dorsally and enters the cerebellum through the superior peduncle (Figs. 7–9 and 7–11).

The **inferior cerebellar penduncles** enter the cerebellum from the caudal part of the pons. In this location, they are on the medial aspect of the middle cerebellar peduncles, forming the lateral walls of the fourth ventricle. The main part of the inferior cerebellar peduncle consists of the **restiform body** (Fig. 7–8), in which olivocerebellar fibers are the most numerous, followed by fibers of the dorsal spinocerebellar tract. Smaller components are contributed by cuneocerebellar fibers from the lateral cuneate nucleus, fibers from the arcuate nucleus and the reticular formation of the medulla, and others from the chief sensory nucleus and nucleus of the spinal tract of the trigeminal nerve. The region of the inferior cerebellar peduncle immediately adjoining the fourth ventricle is known as the **juxtarestiform body** (Fig. 7–8) and includes fibers entering the cerebellum from the vestibular nerve and vestibular nuclei. The juxtarestiform body also contains cerebellar efferents from portions of the cerebellum that are concerned with maintaining equilibrium; these fibers terminate in vestibular nuclei and in the reticular formation of the medulla and pontine tegmentum.

The **superior cerebellar peduncles** (Fig. 7–9) consist mainly of cerebellar efferent fibers, which constitute the **brachia conjunctiva.** The brachia originate in cerebellar nuclei and enter the brain stem immediately caudal to the inferior colliculi of the midbrain. The constituent fibers cross the midline at the level of the inferior colliculi in the **decussation of the brachia conjunctiva** (Figs. 7–10, 7–12, and 7–13); most of them continue forward to a thalamic nucleus (ventral lateral

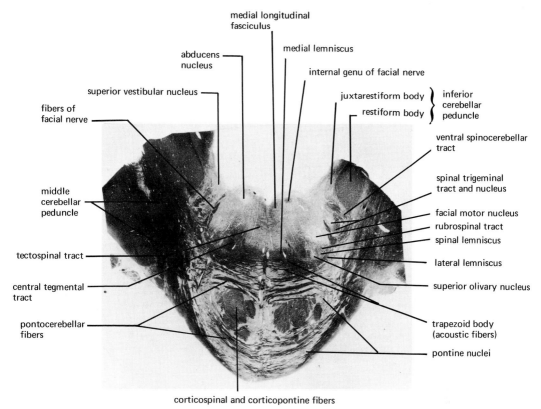

medial longitudinal
fasciculus

abducens
nucleus

medial lemniscus

internal genu of facial nerve

superior vestibular nucleus

juxtarestiform body ⎱ inferior
restiform body ⎰ cerebellar
peduncle

fibers of
facial nerve

ventral spinocerebellar
tract

middle
cerebellar
peduncle

spinal trigeminal
tract and nucleus

facial motor nucleus

rubrospinal tract

tectospinal tract

spinal lemniscus

lateral lemniscus

central tegmental
tract

superior olivary nucleus

pontocerebellar
fibers

trapezoid body
(acoustic fibers)

pontine nuclei

corticospinal and corticopontine fibers

FIG. 7–8. Caudal region of the pons. (Weigert stain, × 2 2/5)

FIG. 7–9. Pons at approximately midlevel. (Weigert stain, × 2⅓)

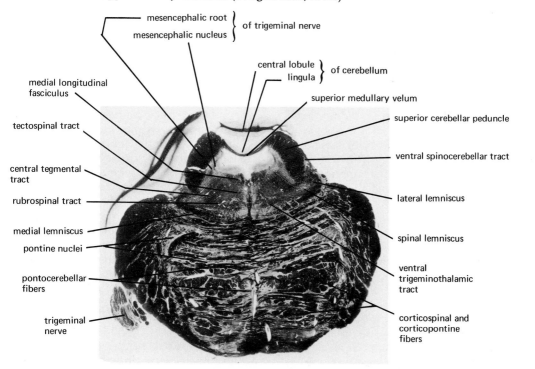

mesencephalic root ⎱
mesencephalic nucleus ⎰ of trigeminal nerve

central lobule ⎱ of cerebellum
lingula ⎰

medial longitudinal
fasciculus

superior medullary velum

superior cerebellar peduncle

tectospinal tract

ventral spinocerebellar tract

central tegmental
tract

lateral lemniscus

rubrospinal tract

medial lemniscus

spinal lemniscus

pontine nuclei

ventral
trigeminothalamic
tract

pontocerebellar
fibers

trigeminal
nerve

corticospinal and
corticopontine
fibers

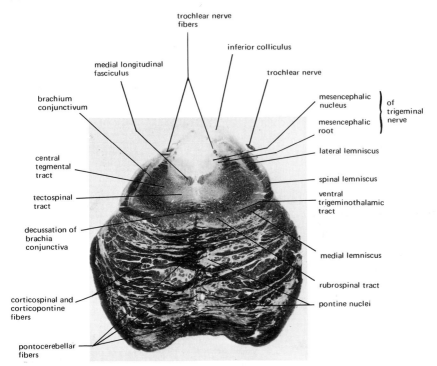

FIG. 7-10. Rostral portion of the pons including the isthmus region of the pontine tegmentum. (Weigert stain, × 2 1/5)

nucleus) from which fibers project to motor areas of cortex in the frontal lobe, and the remainder end in the red nucleus and the reticular formation. In addition to the brachium conjunctivum, the superior cerebellar peduncle contains fibers entering the cerebellum. These consist of the ventral spinocerebellar tract, and a few fibers from the red nucleus and a trigeminal nucleus known as the mesencephalic nucleus of the trigeminal nerve. Tectocerebellar fibers from the inferior colliculi run mainly in the superior medullary velum, which bridges the V-shaped interval between the superior peduncles.

Descending Tracts

Fibers from the red nucleus and other gray areas in the midbrain run in the **central tegmental tract** to the inferior olivary complex. This tract is situated medial to the fibers of the brachium conjunctivum at the level of the pontine isthmus (Fig. 7-10), in the central area of the tegmentum at midpons levels (Fig. 7-9), and just dorsal to the medial lemniscus in the caudal region of the pons (Fig. 7-8). As

noted previously the central tegmental tract includes fibers ascending from the reticular formation of the brain stem to the diencephalon.

The **rubrospinal tract** is situated deeply in the tegmentum; the tract shifts from a position near the midline to the lateral tegmentum while descending through the pons from its origin in the contralateral red nucleus (Figs. 7-10 through 7-8). The rubrospinal tract and the spinal lemniscus are close to one another at lower pontine levels. The **tectospinal tract** from the contralateral superior colliculus of the midbrain is situated near the midline in the pontine tegmentum (Figs. 7-10 through 7-8), a position that is maintained throughout the course of the tract in the medulla and spinal cord. Corticobulbar fibers proceeding to motor nuclei of cranial nerves in the pons and medulla are present in the tegmentum, but they are difficult to identify in Weigert-stained preparations.

Nuclei of Cranial Nerves and Associated Tracts

VESTIBULOCOCHLEAR NERVE. Fibers from the cochlear nuclei cross the pons to ascend in the lateral lemniscus of the opposite side.

FIG. 7-11. Portion of a section through the middle of the pons, at the level of the chief sensory and motor nuclei of the trigeminal nerve. (This particular level was missing from the series of Weigert-stained sections that illustrate this chapter. Fig. 7-11 is therefore substituted from another brain specimen.) (× 5½)

These slender bundles of auditory (acoustic) fibers are directed across the brain stem in the deepest part of the tegmentum, and it is difficult to distinguish them from nearby fascicles of pontocerebellar fibers. The transverse strands of acoustic fibers, some of which intersect the medial lemniscus, comprise the **trapezoid body** (Fig. 7-8). Some of the fibers from the cochlear nuclei end in the **superior olivary nucleus** (Fig. 7-8) of either side, from which efferent fibers are added to the auditory pathway. Fibers originating in the cochlear and superior olivary nuclei turn rostrally in the lateral part of the tegmentum to form the **lateral lemniscus** (Fig. 7-8). This tract is situated at the lateral edge of the medial lemniscus in the first part of its course (Fig. 7-9), then moves dorsally and ends in the inferior colliculus of the midbrain (Fig. 7-10). The auditory pathway continues through the inferior brachium to the medial geniculate nucleus of the thalamus, and then to the auditory area of cortex in the temporal lobe.

Of the four vestibular nuclei, only the **superior vestibular nucleus** is as far rostral as the level shown in Figure 7-8. Fibers from all the vestibular nuclei, some crossed and some uncrossed, ascend in the **medial longitudinal fasciculus,** which runs near the midline and close to the floor of the fourth ventricle throughout the pons (Figs. 7-8 through 7-10). The fibers terminate in the abducens, trochlear, and oculomotor nuclei; the connections thereby established have the important function of coordinating movements of the eyes with movements of the head.

FACIAL AND ABDUCENS NERVES. The **motor nucleus of the facial nerve** for the muscles of expression consists of a prominent group of typical motor neurons in the ventrolateral part of the tegmentum (Fig. 7-8). Fibers from the nucleus course in a dorsomedial direction, then form a compact bundle, the **internal genu,** which loops over the caudal end of the abducens nucleus beneath the facial colliculus of the rhomboid fossa. The bundle of fibers forming the genu then runs forward along the medial side of the abducens nucleus and curves again over its rostral end, where it appears on the right-hand side of Figure 7–8. After leaving the genu, the fibers pass between the nucleus of origin and the trigeminal spinal nucleus, emerging as the motor root of the facial nerve at the junction of the pons and medulla.

The **abducens nucleus,** for innervation of the lateral rectus muscle of the eye, is located beneath the facial colliculus, as noted above (Fig. 7–8). The efferent fibers of the nucleus proceed in a ventral direction, with a caudal inclination, and leave the brain stem as the abducens nerve between the pons and the pyramid of the medulla.

TRIGEMINAL NERVE. The **spinal trigeminal tract** and **nucleus** are situated in the lateral part of the tegmentum of the caudal portion of the pons (Fig. 7–8). The pontine tegmentum also contains two additional trigeminal nuclei, the chief sensory and motor nuclei (Fig. 7–11). The **chief sensory nucleus,** which receives trigeminal fibers for touch (especially discriminative touch), lies at the rostral end of the spinal trigeminal nucleus. Fibers from the chief sensory nucleus project to the thalamus, along with fibers from the nucleus of the spinal tract, in the **ventral trigeminothalamic tract** (Figs. 7–9 and 7–10). A **dorsal trigeminothalamic tract,** consisting of crossed and uncrossed fibers, originates in the chief sensory nuclei exclusively. Although not as well documented as its ventral counterpart, the dorsal tract appears to lie in a more dorsal position in the tegmentum, as its name suggests. (Alternatively all the trigeminothalamic fibers are said to comprise the trigeminal lemniscus.) The **motor nucleus,** which is situated medial to the chief sensory nucleus and is separated from it by trigeminal nerve fibers (Fig. 7–11), consists of typical motor neurons for the muscles of mastication.

The **mesencephalic nucleus of the trigeminal nerve** is a slender column of cells beneath the lateral edge of the rostral part of the fourth ventricle (Figs. 7–9 and 7–10) and extending into the midbrain. These cells are unusual because they are cell bodies of primary sensory neurons and the only such cells that are not in cerebrospinal ganglia. Fibers from the nucleus form the **mesencephalic root of the trigeminal nerve** (Figs. 7–9 and 7–10); most of them are distributed through the mandibular division of the nerve to proprioceptive endings in the muscles of masti-

cation and around the temporomandibular joint.

BASAL PORTION OF THE PONS

The basal or ventral portion of the pons (Figs. 7–8, 7–9, 7–10) is especially large in man because of its relationship to those parts of the cortex of the cerebral and cerebellar hemispheres that increased in size and functional importance during mammalian evolution.

The longitudinal fasciculi consist of fibers that entered the pons from the basis pedunculi of the midbrain. Many of them are **corticospinal fibers** passing through the pons to the pyramids of the medulla. The fasciculi also contain numerous **corticopontine fibers,** which originate in widespread areas of cerebral cortex and establish synaptic contact with cells of the **pontine nuclei** of the same side. Except in the caudal one-third of the pons, in which there are large regions of pontine gray matter (Fig. 7–8), the pontine nuclei are small groups of cells between the longitudinal and transverse fasciculi (Figs. 7–9 and 7–10). The pontine nuclei consist of small and medium-sized polygonal cells. Their axons cross the midline, forming the conspicuous transverse bundles of **pontocerebellar fibers,** and enter the cerebellum through the **middle cerebellar peduncle** (brachium pontis). These fibers are distributed to the cortex of the cerebellar hemispheres (neocerebellum). Corticopontine and pontocerebellar fibers acquire myelin sheaths during the first postnatal year. Data from the cerebral cortex, in which most of the neural events underlying volitional movements take place, are made available to the cerebellar cortex through the relay in the pontine nuclei. Activity in the neocerebellar cortex influences motor areas in the frontal lobe of the cerebral hemisphere through a pathway that includes the dentate nucleus of the cerebellum and the ventral lateral nucleus of the thalamus. The well-developed circuit linking the cerebral and cerebellar cortices provides for precision and efficiency of voluntary movements.

MIDBRAIN

The internal structure of the midbrain is illustrated in Figures 7–12 through 7–15. The sections shown in Figures 7–12 and 7–13 are

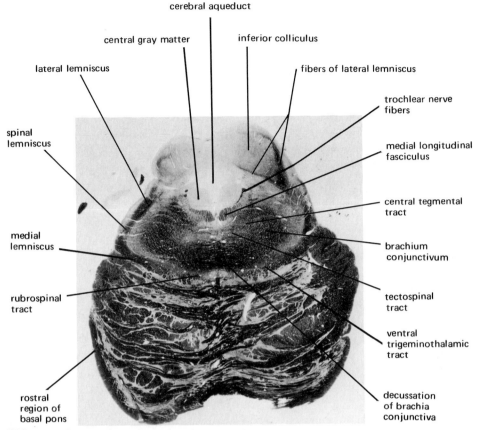

cerebral aqueduct

central gray matter   inferior colliculus

lateral lemniscus   fibers of lateral lemniscus

                                                     trochlear nerve
                                                     fibers
spinal
lemniscus   medial longitudinal
                                                     fasciculus

                                                     central tegmental
                                                     tract
medial
lemniscus   brachium
                                                     conjunctivum

rubrospinal   tectospinal
tract   tract

                                                     ventral
                                                     trigeminothalamic
                                                     tract

rostral   decussation
region of   of brachia
basal pons   conjunctiva

FIG. 7–12. Section through the basal pons and inferior colliculi of the midbrain. (Weigert stain, × 3)

through the inferior colliculi. The plane of the sections is such that Figure 7–12 includes the basal pons and Figure 7–13 shows the extreme rostral lip of the basal pons (see Fig. 7–1). Figures 7–14 and 7–15 illustrate more rostral levels that include the superior colliculi; the latter figure also includes certain thalamic nuclei that are in the transverse plane of the rostral midbrain.

For purposes of description the midbrain is divided into the following regions (Fig. 7–14 may be referred to for their identification): 1) the **tectum** or **roof,** which is special to this part of the brain stem, consists of the paired inferior and superior colliculi (corpora quadrigemina). 2) The **basis pedunculi** is a dense mass of descending fibers. 3) The **substantia nigra,** a motor nucleus, appears as a prominent zone of gray matter, immediately dorsal to the basis pedunculi. 4) The remainder of the midbrain comprises the **tegmentum,** which contains fiber tracts, the prominent

red nuclei, and a poorly-organized region of gray matter surrounding the cerebral aqueduct (aqueduct of Sylvius). The term **cerebral peduncle** refers to all of the midbrain, on each side, exclusive of the tectum.

TECTUM AND ASSOCIATED TRACTS

Inferior Colliculus

The inferior colliculus, which consists of a large nucleus made up of small and medium-sized cells, is incorporated in the auditory pathway to the cerebral cortex. Fibers of the lateral lemniscus envelop the nucleus and enter it from superficial and deep aspects (Fig. 7–12). Fibers from the nucleus of the inferior colliculus traverse the **inferior brachium** to reach the medial geniculate nucleus of the thalamus (Figs. 7–13 through 7–15), which in turn projects to the auditory area of cortex in the temporal lobe. There are commissural fibers between the inferior colliculi, accounting in part for the bilateral cortical projection from each ear.

cerebral aqueduct

fibers of lateral lemniscus

central gray matter

beginning of inferior brachium

inferior colliculus

trochlear nucleus

medial longitudinal fasciculus

spinal lemniscus

medial lemniscus

central tegmental tract

tectospinal tract

ventral trigeminothalamic tract

decussation of brachia conjunctiva

substantia nigra

basis pedunculi

rubrospinal tract

rostral lip of basal pons

interpeduncular fossa

FIG. 7-13. Midbrain at the level of rostral portions of the inferior colliculi. (Weigert stain, × 3)

Some fibers from the inferior colliculus pass forward into the superior colliculus. From the latter site, nerve impulses reach cranial nerve nuclei supplying the extraocular muscles and spinal motor neurons in the cervical region. A reflex pathway is thereby established for turning the eyes and head toward the source of a sound. Tectocerebellar fibers from the inferior colliculi enter the cerebellum by way of the superior medullary velum between the superior cerebellar peduncles and are distributed to the cerebellar cortex. The inferior colliculi evolved as increasingly significant structures in mammals concurrent with the development of the cortical area for hearing.

Superior Colliculus

The superior colliculi (Figs. 7-14 and 7-15) differ from the inferior colliculi in phylogenetic background and function. The optic lobes of the midbrain in lower vertebrates are homologues of the superior colliculi, and the optic lobes constitute an important integrating center for visual, acoustic, and somesthetic data. The visual pathway to the cerebral cortex bypassed the superior colliculi during mammalian evolution. Although the superior colliculi are relegated to the role of reflex centers, the importance of the optic lobes in lower vertebrates leaves an imprint in the form of a complex histologic structure, consisting of alternating layers of white matter and gray matter.

The cortex of the occipital lobe is the most important source of afferent fibers to the superior colliculus in man. Corticotectal fibers come mainly from visual association cortex in the occipital lobe; this cortex surrounds the visual area on which the retina projects after a synaptic relay in the lateral geniculate nucleus of the thalamus. Corticotectal fibers make up most of the **superior brachium,** which reaches the superior colliculus by passing between two thalamic nuclei, the

FIG. 7-14. Midbrain at the level of the superior colliculi. (Weigert stain, × 3)

FIG. 7-15. Midbrain at the level of the rostral portions of the superior colliculi. (Weigert stain, × 2)

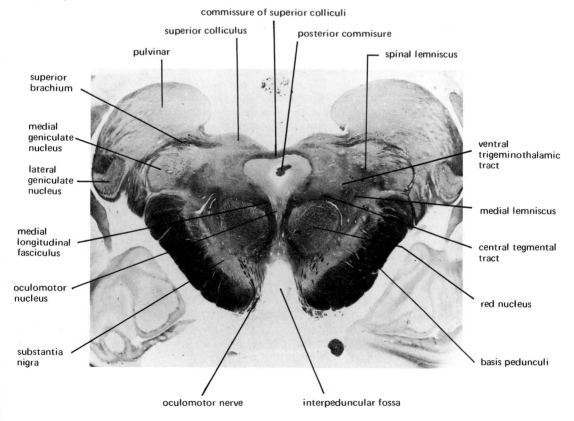

pulvinar and the medial geniculate nucleus (Figs. 7–14 and 7–15). Through collicular efferents to be described, the above connection between the cortex and the superior colliculus is responsible for reflex movements of the eyes and head, as in following objects passing across the visual field (automatic scanning movements). Corticotectal connections also appear to be of significance in the ocular responses for accommodation to near objects; these responses consist of convergence of the eyes, thickening of the lens, and pupillary constriction. A few fibers of the optic tract, originating in the retina, bypass the lateral geniculate nucleus and reach the superior colliculus by way of the superior brachium. These fibers constitute the afferent limb of a reflex arc which allows turning of the eyes and head toward the source of a sudden visual stimulus, together with closing the eyelids and perhaps raising the arms for protection against an approaching object.

Other afferents to the superior colliculus are indicative of its role as a sensory integrative center in lower forms. As previously mentioned, fibers from the inferior colliculus convey impulses of cochlear origin. In addition, spinotectal fibers terminate in the superior colliculus, transmitting data from general sensory endings, of which cutaneous endings are the most important. Reflex connections are thereby established for directing the eyes and head toward the source of acoustic and cutaneous stimuli.

Efferents from the superior colliculus are distributed to the spinal cord and nuclei of the brain stem. Fibers destined for the spinal cord curve around the periaqueductal gray matter, cross to the opposite side in the **dorsal tegmental decussation** (of Meynert), and continue caudally near the midline as the **tectospinal tract** (Figs. 7–12 and 7–13). Efferents to the brain stem (tectobulbar fibers) are directed for the most part bilaterally. Some of them terminate in the oculomotor, trochlear, and abducens nuclei for eye movement responses (mainly scanning) and in the motor nucleus of the facial nerve for protective closure of the eyelids when there is a sudden visual stimulus. Still other efferents terminate in the red nucleus and reticular formation of the brain stem. A projection to the cerebellum consists of tectopontine fibers to the dorsolateral region of the nuclei pontis (basal pons) and pontocerebellar fibers in the

middle cerebellar peduncle. The connections of the superior colliculus with neurons having motor functions are a further indication of its earlier role as an important sensory integrative center.

The superior colliculi are interconnected by the **commissure of the superior colliculi** (Figs. 7–14 and 7–15). The **posterior commissure** is a robust bundle running transversely, just dorsal to the transition between the cerebral aqueduct and the third ventricle. A small piece of the commissure in the midline is included in the section illustrated in Figure 7–15. In spite of the large size of the posterior commissure, the source and termination of its fibers are not well known. However, some have been identified as coming from the nucleus of the superior colliculus and the following small nuclei nearby: pretectal nucleus, habenular nucleus in the epithalamus of the diencephalon, and the interstitial nucleus of Cajal and the nucleus of Darkschewitsch, both of which are situated near the oculomotor nucleus.

Pretectal Nucleus

The pretectal nucleus is a small group of cells situated immediately in front of the lateral edge of the superior colliculus; the nucleus receives fibers from the retina by way of the optic tract and the superior brachium. Fibers leaving the pretectal nucleus pass around the periaqueductal gray matter to the Edinger-Westphal nucleus, a parasympathetic component of the oculomotor nucleus. The pretectal nucleus is included in a reflex pathway for the pupillary response to light, the pupil becoming smaller as the intensity of light increases.

TEGMENTUM

Fasciculi Proceeding to the Thalamus

The **medial lemniscus** continues to be a readily identifiable fasciculus as it traverses the midbrain in the lateral area of the tegmentum (Figs. 7–13 through 7–15). The **spinal lemniscus** is dorsolateral to the medial lemniscus, this spatial relationship being continued from the pontine tegmentum. Spinotectal fibers leave the spinal lemniscus to enter the superior colliculus; the lateral and ventral spinothalamic fibers continue into the diencephalon, where they end in the ventral posterior nucleus of the thalamus.

Red Nucleus and Associated Tracts

The red nucleus is a prominent motor component of the tegmentum. The nucleus is egg shaped (round in transverse section), extending from the caudal limit of the superior colliculus into the subthalamic region of the diencephalon. The nucleus has a pinkish hue in a fresh specimen because it is more vascular than the surrounding tissue. Myelinated nerve fibers traversing the nucleus give it a punctate appearance in Weigert-stained sections (Figs. 7–14 and 7–15).

The red nucleus is differentiated into two regions, which differ in cytoarchitecture and connections. The caudal region is the older part phylogenetically; it consists of large cells in the midst of small neurons and is known as the **pars magnocellularis.** The newer rostral portion is especially well developed in man; consisting of small cells only, it is called the **pars parvicellularis.**

Although some of the connections of the red nucleus are well known, the evidence for others is equivocal and they are still under investigation. Afferents from the cerebellum and the cerebral cortex are best documented. Fibers originating in cerebellar nuclei constitute the brachium conjunctivum and enter the midbrain. Some of these fibers terminate in the red nucleus, whereas the majority pass through and around it en route to a thalamic nucleus (the ventral lateral nucleus) which in turn projects to motor areas of the frontal lobe. These same areas give rise to numerous corticorubral fibers, and there are afferents to the red nucleus from the superior colliculus.

Of efferent connections of the red nucleus, fibers of the rubrospinal tract cross the midline at the level of the nucleus in the **ventral tegmental decussation** (of Forel). Impulses of motor significance from the various sources projecting to the red nucleus are also relayed to lower motor neurons through rubroreticular and reticulospinal connections. Numerous rubroolivary fibers proceed to the inferior olivary complex through the central tegmental tract. The red nucleus sends a few fibers to cerebellar nuclei through the superior peduncle, and there is evidence for reciprocal connections between the red nucleus and the substantia nigra.

Nuclei of Cranial Nerves and Associated Tracts

VESTIBULOCOCHLEAR NERVE. Certain tracts originating in sensory nuclei of cranial nerves continue into the midbrain, and two of them are associated with the vestibulocochlear nerve. The **lateral lemniscus** for auditory conduction was identified when discussing the inferior colliculus. The **medial longitudinal fasciculus** is situated adjacent to the midline (Figs. 7–12 through 7–15), in the same general position as at lower brain stem levels. Most of its fibers originate in vestibular nuclei, and those reaching the midbrain terminate in the trochlear and oculomotor nuclei. The fasciculus also contains association fibers connecting the abducens, trochlear, and oculomotor nuclei.

TRIGEMINAL NERVE. The **ventral trigeminothalamic tract,** which arises from the nucleus of the spinal tract and the chief sensory nucleus, continues through the midbrain near the medial lemniscus (Figs. 7–12 through 7–15). **Dorsal trigeminothalamic fibers** from the chief sensory nuclei of both sides traverse the midbrain tegmentum some distance dorsal to the ventral tract. The **mesencephalic nucleus** of the trigeminal nerve continues from the pons into the lateral region of the periaqueductal gray matter throughout most of the midbrain.

TROCHLEAR AND OCULOMOTOR NERVES. The **trochlear nucleus** is in the central gray matter at the level of the inferior colliculus, where it lies just dorsal to the medial longitudinal fasciculus (Fig. 7–13). Fibers from the nucleus curve dorsally around the central gray matter, with a caudal slope (Figs. 7–12 and 7–10). On reaching the dorsal surface of the brain stem, the fibers decussate and emerge as the trochlear nerves just behind the inferior colliculi. The trochlear nerve supplies the superior oblique muscle of the eye.

The **oculomotor nucleus** is in the ventral part of the central gray matter and coextensive with the superior colliculus; the paired nuclei have a V-shaped outline in sections (Figs. 7–14 and 7–15). Bundles of fibers from the nucleus pursue a curved course through the tegmentum, many of them traversing the red nucleus (Fig. 7–14), then emerge along the side of the interpeduncular fossa to form the oculomotor nerve (Fig. 7–15). The oculomotor nerve supplies the extraocular muscles, with the exception of the lateral rectus and superior oblique muscles, together with the striated fibers of the levator palpebrae superioris muscle. The oculomotor nucleus includes a parasympathetic component, the **Edinger–Westphal nucleus,** for the ciliary and sphincter pupillae muscles of the eye.

SUBSTANTIA NIGRA

The substantia nigra is a large motor nucleus, situated between the tegmentum and the basis pedunculi throughout the midbrain (Figs. 7–13 through 7–15) and extending into the subthalamic region of the diencephalon. The nucleus is rudimentary in lower vertebrates, makes its first definitive appearance in mammals, and is largest in the human brain. The neurons are multipolar and of medium size. The cells composing the **compact zone** adjacent to the tegmentum contain cytoplasmic inclusion granules of melanin pigment. These pigment-containing cells are most numerous in primates, especially in man. Melanin granules are scanty at birth, increase rapidly during childhood, and then more slowly throughout life. The pigment is said to be present in albinos. The region of the nucleus bordering the basis pedunculi is called the **reticular zone;** the cells here are lacking in pigment but contain significant amounts of iron compounds.

The connections of the substantia nigra are not fully known. There are corticonigral fibers from the frontal, parietal, and occipital lobes of the cerebral hemisphere, and reciprocal connections between the substantia nigra and the corpus striatum, red nucleus, and reticular formation. The substantia nigra sends fibers to thalamic nuclei of motor significance, *i.e.,* the ventral lateral and ventral anterior nuclei.

The importance of the substantia nigra as a motor center is manifest when one considers the disturbances of motor function in paralysis agitans or Parkinson's disease. In this crippling disorder there is muscular rigidity, a fine tremor, a slow and shuffling gait, masklike facies, and other abnormalities. The most consistent pathologic finding in Parkinson's disease is degeneration of the melanin-containing cells in the compact portion of the substantia nigra. Biochemical and histochemical studies offer a lead to therapy. Under normal circumstances dopamine is present in the pigmented cells of the substantia nigra and in the neostriatum of the corpus striatum, whereas it is virtually absent at these sites in Parkinson's disease. These observations led to the suggestion that the substantia nigra may have, as part of an undoubtedly complex role, a regulatory effect on nuclei to which it projects (especially the neostriatum) through the action of dopamine as a neurotransmitter substance. Administration of dopamine is an obvious form of biochemical therapy to explore. However, dopamine does not cross the blood-brain barrier, so a metabolic precursor that does gain access to brain tissue is used instead. This precursor is dihydroxyphenylalanine (dopa). The administration of L-dopa, which crosses the blood-brain barrier more readily than D-dopa and has fewer side effects, shows considerable promise as a therapeutic agent for ameliorating some of the abnormalities of motor function in Parkinson's disease.

The significance of melanin in the substantia nigra is not known, except that it is related chemically to the metabolic sequence that includes dopamine. Melanin pigment is produced by the action of the enzyme tyrosinase on dopa; this is the basis of the "dopa reaction" for the identification of melanocytes, or melanin-producing cells, in the skin or elsewhere. Melanocytes contain tyrosinase, and melanin is formed when dopa is made available as a substrate to tissue sections. Melanin pigment may be an inert byproduct of the essential biochemical reactions in the substantia nigra. The increase in amount of pigment with age is consistent with such a hypothesis.

BASIS PEDUNCULI

The basis pedunculi (crus cerebri) consists of fibers of the pyramidal and corticopontine systems (Figs. 7–13 through 7–15). **Corticospinal fibers** constitute the middle three-fifths of the basis pedunculi; the somatotopic arrangement is that of fibers for the neck, arm, trunk, and leg in a medial to lateral direction. **Corticobulbar fibers** for the oculomotor and trochlear nuclei proceed to these nuclei through the tegmentum of the midbrain; some of the corticobulbar fibers for other cranial nerves also leave the basis pedunculi and continue to their destination through the tegmentum of the midbrain and pons. Such corticobulbar fibers as remain continue caudally in the basis pedunculi, where they are situated between the corticospinal and frontopontine tracts. **Corticopontine fibers** are divided into two large fasciculi. The **frontopontine tract** occupies the medial one-fifth of the basis pedunculi. The lateral one-fifth consists of the **temporopontine tract,** which is inappropriately named because most of the constituent fibers originate in the cortex of the parietal lobe.

VISCERAL PATHWAYS IN THE BRAIN STEM

Central pathways related to visceral innervation are less well defined anatomically than many of the somatic sensory and motor pathways. For this reason, and because many of the constituent fibers are unmyelinated, identification of visceral pathways has presented technical problems.

Primary visceral afferent neurons at spinal cord levels accompany the parasympathetic division of the autonomic system in the sacral region and the sympathetic division in the thoracic and upper lumbar regions. In addition to their involvement in spinal visceral reflexes, the sacral afferents convey information related to the feeling of fullness in the bladder and rectum, and perhaps pain in pelvic viscera. The thoracic and upper lumbar afferents are concerned with pain of visceral origin, in addition to visceral reflex responses. The **ascending visceral pathway,** which consists in part of spinospinalis relays in the cord, continues through the brain stem as polysynaptic relays involving neurons of the reticular formation. By this means data of visceral origin reach several thalamic nuclei and the hypothalamus.

The more important visceral afferents physiologically reach the nucleus of the tractus solitarius in the medulla by way of the vagus and glossopharyngeal nerves. These nerves include general visceral afferents for visceral reflexes, in which the dorsal nucleus of the vagus nerve is the principal efferent component. The nucleus of the tractus solitarius also receives afferents for taste

through the vagus, glossopharyngeal, and facial nerves. Data for taste (a special visceral sense) are relayed to parasympathetic nuclei in the brain stem, notably the salivatory nuclei and the dorsal nucleus of the vagus nerve. In addition to the above reflex connections, fibers from the nucleus of the tractus solitarius join the internal arcuate fibers and ascend in the contralateral brain stem. These fibers travel rostrally near the medial lemniscus, probably in the region of the ventral trigeminothalamic tract, and conduction along this route is supplemented by relays in the reticular formation. The principal destinations are the hypothalamus and the ventral posterior thalamic nucleus. From the latter site information with respect to taste is relayed to a cortical taste area in the parietal lobe.

There are two descending fasciculi, whose cells of origin are located in the hypothalamus. **Mammillotegmental fibers** originate in the mammillary nucleus of the hypothalamus; they terminate in small nuclei associated with the reticular formation of the midbrain (dorsal and ventral tegmental nuclei), from where impulses reach autonomic nuclei through the dorsal longitudinal fasciculus or by means of relays in the reticular formation. Fibers from other hypothalamic nuclei run caudally in the **dorsal longitudinal fasciculus** (of Schütz), a bundle of unmyelinated fibers in the periaqueductal gray matter of the midbrain, and terminate in the autonomic nuclei and reticular formation of the brain stem. (Some of the ascending visceral fibers going to the hypothalamus are also in the dorsal longitudinal fasciculus.) Impulses of hypothalamic origin reach the intermediolateral cell column of the spinal cord and the sacral parasympathetic nucleus by way of reticulospinal connections.

ANATOMIC AND CLINICAL CORRELATIONS

Of the various pathologic conditions affecting the brain stem, vascular lesions are among the more important. Hemorrhage into the brain stem usually has serious consequences because of the presence of nuclei that control the vital functions of respiration and circulation. The neurologic signs resulting from vascular occlusion depend on the

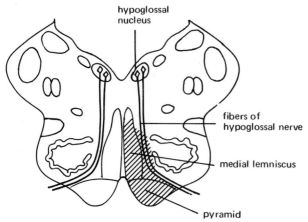

FIG. 7-16. Site of a lesion producing the medial medullary syndrome.

FIG. 7-17. Site of a lesion producing the lateral medullary syndrome.

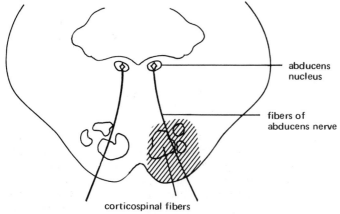

FIG. 7-18. Site of a basal pontine lesion involving the pyramidal tract and abducens nerve.

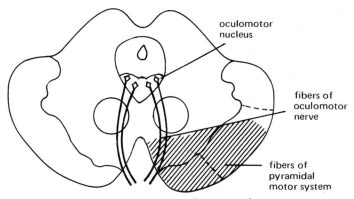

oculomotor
nucleus

fibers of
oculomotor
nerve

fibers of
pyramidal
motor system

FIG. 7-19. Site of a lesion in the midbrain involving the pyramidal tract and oculomotor nerve.

location and size of the affected region. The following examples are presented to show the correlation between neurologic signs and the location of the lesion.

The **medial medullary syndrome** results from occlusion of a medullary branch of the vertebral artery; the size of the infarction depends on the distribution of the particular artery involved. In the example shown in Figure 7-16 the affected area includes the pyramid and most of the medial lemniscus on one side. The lesion extends far enough laterally to include fibers of the hypoglossal nerve as they pass between the medial lemniscus and the inferior olivary nucleus. A patient with this particular lesion has contralateral hemiparesis; there is loss of sensations of position and movement, discriminative touch, and vibration on the opposite side of the body. Paralysis of the tongue muscles is ipsilateral, however, and the tongue deviates to the affected side on protrusion because the action of the healthy genioglossus muscle is unopposed. This is an example of crossed or alternating paralysis, in which the body is affected on the side opposite the lesion, whereas muscles supplied by a cranial nerve are affected on the same side as the lesion. The condition is therefore known as **alternating hypoglossal hemiplegia.**

Occlusion of a vessel supplying the lateral area of the medulla results in the **lateral medullary** or **Wallenberg's syndrome.** The occluded vessel may be the posterior inferior cerebellar artery, or a medullary branch of this artery or of the vertebral artery. The extent of the infarcted area is typically as shown in Figure 7-17. Inclusion of the spinal trigeminal tract and its nucleus is responsible for ipsilateral loss of pain and temperature sensibility in the area of distribution of the trigeminal nerve. Pain and temperature sensibility is absent on the opposite side of the body because of interruption of fibers of the lateral spinothalamic tract in the spinal lemniscus. The medial lemniscus being intact, touch sensation is diminished rather than abolished. Destruction of the nucleus ambiguus causes paralysis of muscles of the soft palate, pharynx, and larynx on the side of the lesion, with difficulty in swallowing and phonation. The pathway from the hypothalamus to the intermediolateral cell column of the spinal cord through the reticular formation may be included in the area of degeneration. The signs of a lateral medullary lesion may therefore include Horner's syndrome, which consists of a small pupil, slight drooping of the upper eyelid (ptosis), slight enophthalmos, and sometimes warm, dry, skin of the face, all on the side of the lesion. The infarcted region may extend dorsally to include the base of the inferior cerebellar peduncle and vestibular nuclei causing dizziness, cerebellar ataxia, and nystagmus. Cerebellar signs are more pronounced, of course, if infarction of part of the cerebellum is added to that of the medulla (posterior inferior cerebellar artery thrombosis).

Lesions in the basal region of the pons or the midbrain may produce alternating paralysis, similar to that described in the first example. Figure 7-18 illustrates an area of infarction in one side of the caudal region of the pons, resulting from occlusion of a pontine branch of the basilar artery. Interruption of corticospinal fibers causes contralateral hemiparesis, and inclusion of abducens nerve fibers in the lesion causes paralysis of the lateral rectus muscle on the ipsilateral side and a medial strabismus or squint.

The position of a vascular lesion in the basal region of a cerebral peduncle, such as might follow occlusion of a branch of the posterior cerebral artery, is shown in Figure 7–19. A lesion at this site causes **Weber's syndrome,** in which there is contralateral hemiparesis, due to interruption of pyramidal tract fibers, and ipsilateral paralysis of ocular muscles because of inclusion of oculomotor nerve fibers in the infarcted area. There is paralysis of all the extraocular muscles except the lateral rectus and superior oblique muscles. The most obvious signs are lateral strabismus and loss of ability to raise the upper eyelid, together with dilation of the pupil because of interruption of parasympathetic fibers supplying the sphincter pupillae muscle.

SUGGESTED READING

Armstrong DM: Functional significance of connections of the inferior olive. Physiol Rev 54:358–417, 1974

Barbeau A: L-dopa therapy in Parkinson's disease: a critical review of nine years' experience. Can Med Assoc J 101:791–800, 1969

Boesten AJP, Voogd J: Projections of the dorsal column nuclei and the spinal cord on the inferior olive in the cat. J Comp Neurol 161:215–237, 1975

Carptenter MB: Human Neuroanatomy, 7th ed. Baltimore, Williams & Wilkins, 1976

Carpenter MB, Nakano K, Kim R: Nigrothalamic projections in the monkey demonstrated by autoradiographic technics. J Comp Neurol 165:401–415, 1976

Cooke JD, Larson B, Oscarsson O, Sjölund B: Origin and termination of cuneocerebellar tract. Exp Brain Res 13:339–358, 1971

Courville J: Connections of the red nucleus with the cerebellum and certain caudal brain stem structures: a review with functional considerations. Rev Can Biol 27:127–144, 1968

Crosby EC, Humphrey T, Lauer EW: Correlative Anatomy of the Nervous System. New York, Macmillan, 1962

Currier RD, Giles CL, DeJong RN: Some comments on Wallenberg's lateral medullary syndrome. Neurology (Minneap) 11:778–791, 1961

Edwards SB: The ascending and descending projections of the red nucleus in the cat: an experimental study using an autoradiographic tracing method. Brain Res 48:45–63, 1972

Hopkins DA, Lawrence DG: On the absence of a rubrothalamic projection in the monkey with observations on some ascending mesencephalic projections. J Comp Neurol 161:269–293, 1975

Kuypers HGJM, Lawrence DG: Cortical projections to the red nucleus and the brain stem in the rhesus monkey. Brain Res 4:151–188, 1967

Lassek AM: The Pyramidal Tract. Springfield, IL, Thomas, 1954

Marsden CD: Pigmentation in the nuclei substantiae nigrae of mammals. J Anat 95:256–261, 1961

Massion J: The mammalian red nucleus. Physiol Rev 47:383–436, 1967

Miller RA, Burack E: Atlas of the Central Nervous System in Man. Baltimore, Williams & Wilkins, 1968

Miller RA, Strominger NL: Efferent connections of the red nucleus in the brain stem and spinal cord of the Rhesus monkey. J Comp Neurol 152:327–346, 1973

Olszewski J, Baxter D: Cytoarchitecture of the Human Brain Stem. Basel, Karger, 1954

Poirier LJ: Experimental and historical study of midbrain dyskinesias. J Neurophysiol 23:534–551, 1960

Poirier LJ, Bouvier G: The red nucleus and its efferent nervous pathways in the monkey. J Comp Neurol 128:223–243, 1966

Pollack M, Hornabrook RW: The prevalence, natural history and dementia of Parkinson's disease. Brain 89:429–448, 1966

Riley HA: An Atlas of the Basal Ganglia, Brain Stem and Spinal Cord. New York, Hafner, 1960

Rinvik E: The cortico-nigral projection in the cat: an experimental study with silver impregnation methods. J Comp Neurol 126:241–254, 1966

Stern G: The effects of lesions in the substantia nigra. Brain 89:449–478, 1966

Tolbert DL, Massopust LC, Murphy MG, Young PA: The anatomical organization of the cerebello-olivary projection in the cat. J Comp Neurol 170:525–544, 1976

Voorhoeve PE: Some neurophysiological aspects of Parkinson's disease. Psychiatr Neurol Neuro-chir 73:329–338, 1970

Cranial Nerves

The cranial nerves, listed in the order in which numbers are assigned to them, are as follows:

1. Olfactory	7. Facial
2. Optic	8. Vestibulocochlear
3. Oculomotor	9. Glossopharyngeal
4. Trochlear	10. Vagus
5. Trigeminal	11. Accessory
6. Abducens	12. Hypoglossal

In addition to motor and general sensory functions, five systems for the special senses are served by various cranial nerves. In these, the receptors are localized and highly specialized, in contrast to general sensory endings, which are scattered throughout the tissues of the body and are relatively simple in structure. Of the special senses, the olfactory system is an integral part of the forebrain and is discussed in Chapter 17. Discussion of the optic and vestibulocochlear nerves is set aside for the section on systemic neuroanatomy, in which the visual, auditory, and vestibular systems are described (Chapters 20, 21, and 22). There remains the special sense of taste (gustatory system), certain aspects of which are included in the present chapter because the primary sensory neurons for taste are included with sensory neurons having other functions in the facial, glossopharyngeal, and vagus nerves.

OCULOMOTOR, TROCHLEAR, AND ABDUCENS NERVES

The third, fourth, and sixth cranial nerves supply the extraocular muscles with motor fibers; their nuclei therefore consist of multipolar motor neurons and receive afferents from the same sources. The oculomotor nucleus includes a parasympathetic component, the Edinger–Westphal nucleus, for the sphincter pupillae and ciliary muscles of the eye.

OCULOMOTOR NERVE

The **oculomotor nucleus** is situated in the periaqueductal gray matter of the midbrain, ventral to the aqueduct and coextensive with the superior colliculus (Fig. 8–1). The paired nuclei have a triangular outline in transverse section and are bounded laterally by the medial longitudinal fasciculi. (The reader may wish to refer to illustrations in the preceding chapter for the topography of components of cranial nerves in Weigert-stained sections.) The cells for individual extraocular muscles (including the levator palpebrae superioris muscle) are localized in longitudinal groups; these subnuclei are represented bilaterally, except for one, which is situated dorsocaudally in the midline. According to Warwick's schema for the oculomotor nucleus of the monkey (Fig. 8–2), there are three laterally disposed cell groups, which supply the inferior rectus, inferior oblique, and medial rectus muscles. On the medial side of these there is a subnucleus for the superior rectus muscle. The unpaired cell group, which is called the caudal central nucleus, supplies the levator palpebrae superioris muscle on each side. Medullated axons from the oculomotor nucleus curve ventrally through the tegmentum, many of them traversing the red nucleus. The fibers emerge as a series of roots along the side of the interpeduncular fossa, and these roots converge immediately to form the oculomotor nerve.

Oculomotor fibers are partly crossed and partly uncrossed. Although full details are lacking for man, it appears that only uncrossed fibers supply the medial rectus, inferior rectus, and inferior oblique muscles. The superior rectus muscle receives crossed fibers only, and the levator palpebrae superioris muscle is supplied by the unpaired caudal central nucleus. (Smooth muscle fibers of the levator are innervated by sympathetic nerves.) The small size of the motor unit, in which about six muscle fibers are supplied by a nerve fiber, attests to the delicate neuromuscular mechanisms required for coordinated movement of the eyes in binocular vision.

The **Edinger–Westphal nucleus** is situated in the median plane, dorsal to the rostral two-thirds of the main oculomotor nucleus (Fig. 8–2). The cells are small and tend to be spindle-shaped, like other preganglionic parasympathetic neurons. Fibers from the Edinger–Westphal nucleus accompany other oculomotor fibers into the orbit, where they terminate in the ciliary ganglion. Postganglionic fibers then pass through short ciliary nerves to the sphincter pupillae and ciliary muscles of the eye.

A lesion interrupting fibers of the oculomotor nerve causes paralysis of all extraocular muscles except the superior oblique and lateral rectus muscles. The sphincter pupillae muscle in the iris and the ciliary muscle in the ciliary body are likewise paralysed. The consequences of such a lesion are lateral strabismus due to unopposed action of the lateral rectus muscle, inability to direct the eye medially or vertically, and drooping of the upper eyelid (ptosis). Interruption of the parasympathetic fibers causes dilation of the pupil because of unopposed action of the dilator pupillae muscle in the iris, which has a sympathetic innervation. There is no longer pupillary constriction in response to an increase of light intensity or in accommodation for near objects. Neither does the ciliary muscle contract to allow the lens to increase in thickness for focusing on a near object.

TROCHLEAR NERVE

The **trochlear nucleus** for the superior oblique muscle is immediately caudal to the oculomotor nucleus, at the level of the inferior colliculus (Fig. 8–3). Trochlear nerve fibers have an unusual course, and this is the only nerve to emerge from the dorsum of the brain stem. Small bundles of fibers curve around the periaqueductal gray matter with a caudal slope and decussate with fibers from the companion nucleus; the slender nerve emerges immediately caudal to the inferior colliculus. The superior oblique muscle, like the superior rectus, is therefore supplied by crossed fibers. Paralysis of the superior oblique muscle impairs ability to direct the eye downward and outward. The defect is difficult to detect on clinical examination, but a person so affected may experience difficulty in walking downstairs.

ABDUCENS NERVE

The **abducens nucleus** for the lateral rectus muscle is situated beneath the facial colliculus in the floor of the fourth ventricle (Fig. 8–4). A bundle of facial nerve fibers curves over the nucleus, contributing to the facial colliculus. Fibers from the abducens nucleus pass through the pons in a ventrocaudal direction, emerging from the brain stem at the junction of the pons and the pyramid. Interruption of the abducens nerve causes medial strabismus and inability to direct the affected eye laterally. Functional impairment of any of the extraocular muscles may cause diplopia (double vision).

AFFERENTS TO NUCLEI SUPPLYING EXTRAOCULAR MUSCLES

The main part of the oculomotor nucleus (*i.e.,* all but the parasympathetic component) and the trochlear and abducens nuclei receive fibers from the same sources, as is to be expected. **Tectobulbar fibers** from the superior colliculus function in connection with several ocular movements. These include scanning, reflex turning of the eyes toward the source of visual, acoustic, or cutaneous stimuli, and probably ocular changes during accommodation to near objects. The **medial longitudinal fasciculus,** which is adjacent to the three nuclei, transmits impulses from the vestibular nuclei and provides for coordinated movements of the eyes and head. Included in the fasciculus are axons of cells within the nuclei for extraocular muscles (or cells situated close to the nuclei). These fibers, which are crossed and uncrossed, pass from one nucleus to another. They have the important function of coordinating the action of extraocular muscles, precise coordination being essential to avoid diplopia in binocular vision. Cells in the reticular formation adjacent to the abducens nucleus are thought to con-

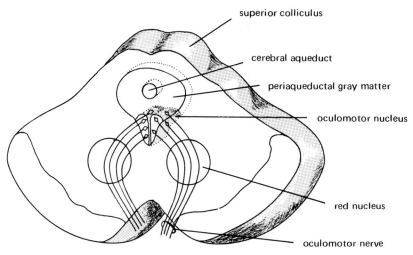

FIG. 8-1. Components of the oculomotor nerve in the midbrain.

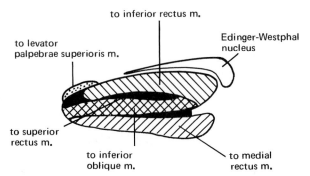

FIG. 8-2. Warwick's schema for the organization of the oculomotor nucleus (lateral view of the right oculomotor nucleus). (From Warwick R: J Comp Neurol 98: 449–504, 1953)

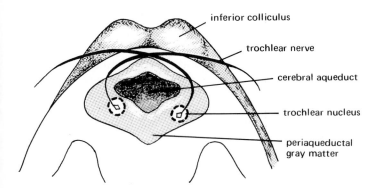

FIG. 8-3. The trochlear nerve in the midbrain.

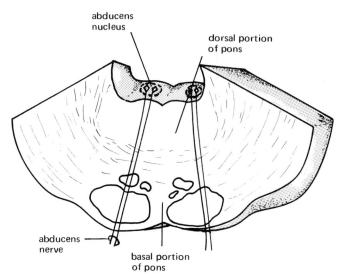

FIG. 8-4. The abducens nerve in the pons.

stitute a **parabducens nucleus,** which functions as a "center for lateral gaze." This nucleus sends fibers to the ipsilateral abducens nucleus and, through the medial longitudinal fasciculus, to those cells of the contralateral oculomotor nucleus that supply the medial rectus muscle. The actions of the medial and lateral recti muscles are thereby coordinated in horizontal movements of the eyes.

Corticobulbar fibers for voluntary eye movements originate mainly in the motor area of the frontal lobe. It is a general rule that small internuncial neurons in the brain stem intervene between corticobulbar fibers and motor nuclei of cranial nerves. Although corticobulbar fibers to the oculomotor, trochlear, and abducens nuclei are predominantly crossed, there is a substantial number of uncrossed fibers. Voluntary paralysis of the extraocular muscles is not, therefore, a feature of upper motor neuron lesions.*

* In the discussion of lesions of the spinal cord in Chapter 5 it was pointed out that voluntary movements involving the axial and limb musculature are mediated through both the corticospinal tract and extrapyramidal pathways. By extrapolation extrapyramidal pathways, in addition to the corticobulbar tract, may function in the voluntary control of muscles that are supplied by cranial nerves. Of several pathways that may be involved and which would be of interest in connection with an upper motor neuron lesion, there are corticorubral and corticoreticular connections, together with projections from the red nucleus and reticular formation to motor nuclei of cranial nerves. The neural mechanisms for voluntary

However, anterior to the motor area there is a cortical area known as the "frontal eye field," which has a special role in voluntary scanning movements. The pathway from the frontal eye field to the third, fourth, and sixth nerve nuclei has not been determined with certainty. The fibers are no doubt closely associated with the corticobulbar fibers already mentioned, but whether there is a relay in the superior colliculus has not been resolved. In any event, damage to the frontal eye field causes paralysis of contralateral gaze and transient deviation of the eyes to the side of an acute lesion.

CONNECTIONS OF THE EDINGER–WESTPHAL NUCLEUS

The Edinger–Westphal nucleus is a parasympathetic autonomic nucleus, and it therefore receives fibers from the hypothalamus through the **dorsal longitudinal fasciculus.** However, the more important afferents from the clinical point of view are those concerned with reflex responses to light and accommodation. An increase in the intensity of light falling on the retina causes constriction of the pupil. The afferent limb of the reflex arc consists of fibers in the optic nerve and optic tract reaching the **pretectal nucleus** by way of the superior brachium. The pretectal

control of some muscles of the head, in particular muscles lacking skeletal attachments, may differ from those for the muscles generally.

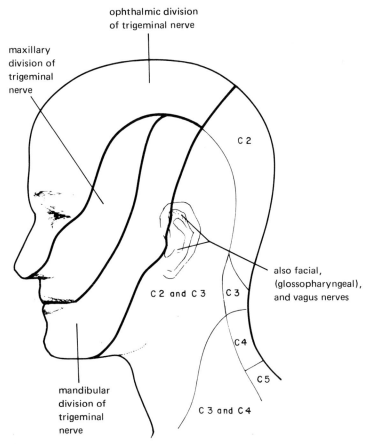

ophthalmic division
of trigeminal nerve

maxillary
division of
trigeminal
nerve

C 2

C 2 and C 3   C 3

also facial,
(glossopharyngeal),
and vagus nerves

C 4

C 5

mandibular
division of
trigeminal
nerve

C 3 and C 4

FIG. 8-5. Cutaneous innervation of the head and neck.

nucleus projects to the Edinger–Westphal nucleus, from which fibers traverse the oculomotor nerve to the ciliary ganglion in the orbital cavity. Postganglionic fibers travel through the short ciliary nerves to the sphincter pupillae muscle of the iris.

The reflex response to accommodation accompanies ocular convergence produced by voluntary fixation on a near object. The efferent limb of the reflex arc consists of pre- and postganglionic fibers from the Edinger–Westphal nucleus and the ciliary ganglion, respectively. The postganglionic fibers supply the ciliary muscle which, on contraction, allows the lens to increase in thickness, thereby increasing refractive power for focusing on a near object. The sphincter pupillae muscle contracts at the same time, sharpening the image by decreasing the diameter of the pupil and reducing spherical aberration in the refractive media.

The afferent side of the reflex pathway for accommodation is not entirely clear. The impulses appear to be cortical in origin, and the most probable source is cortex of the occipital lobe in which the visual area receiving data from the retina is located. The pathway may be from cortex of the occipital lobe to the superior colliculus and then to the oculomotor nucleus, or from occipital cortex to the motor cortex of the frontal lobe and then to the oculomotor nucleus through corticobulbar fibers. The pathways for pupillary responses to light and accommodation are obviously different because the reflexes may be disassociated by disease. For example in the Argyll Robertson pupil there is constriction of the pupil when attention is directed to a near object, although pupillary constriction in response to light is absent. The Argyll Robertson pupil is characteristically seen in patients with tabes dorsalis, a syphilitic disease of the central nervous system.

TRIGEMINAL NERVE

The trigeminal nerve is the principal sensory nerve for the head and the motor nerve for the muscles of mastication.

SENSORY COMPONENTS

The cell bodies of most of the primary sensory neurons are in the **trigeminal** (semilunar or gasserian) **ganglion,** the remainder being in the mesencephalic nucleus. The peripheral processes of trigeminal ganglion cells constitute the ophthalmic and maxillary nerves and the sensory component of the mandibular nerve. (The mandibular nerve in particular includes sensory fibers from the mesencephalic nucleus, as will be discussed presently.) The trigeminal nerve is responsible for general sensation from the skin of the face and forehead, the scalp as far back as the vertex of the head, the mucosa of the oral and nasal cavities and the paranasal sinuses, and the teeth (Fig. 8–5). The trigeminal nerve also contributes sensory fibers to most of the dura mater. The scalp of the back of the head and an area of skin at the angle of the jaw are supplied by the second and third cervical nerves. The external ear has a complicated and overlapping innervation. The anterior border of the ear, anterior wall of the acoustic canal, and anterior part of the tympanic membrane receive trigeminal fibers. The external ear in general, most of the acoustic canal and tympanic membrane, and a cutaneous area behind the ear are supplied by the facial and vagus nerves, in some instances by the glossopharyngeal nerve, and by the second and third cervical nerves.

Chief Sensory Nucleus

The central processes of trigeminal ganglion cells make up the large sensory root of the trigeminal nerve; these fibers enter the pons and terminate in the chief sensory nucleus and the nucleus of the trigeminal spinal tract. The chief sensory nucleus, also called the principal or superior nucleus, is in the dorsolateral area of the pontine tegmentum at the level of entry of the sensory fibers (Fig. 8–6). Fibers of large diameter for discriminative touch terminate in the chief sensory nucleus. Other fibers of medium caliber divide on nearing the chief sensory nucleus; one branch enters this nucleus and the other branch turns caudally in the spinal tract and ends in the nucleus of the spinal tract. These afferents are for light touch and pressure, and both nuclei must therefore participate in these modalities of sensation. The chief sensory nucleus is essentially a mammalian nucleus, developing along with encapsulated tactile endings.

Trigeminal Spinal Tract and Nucleus of the Spinal Tract

Large numbers of sensory root fibers of intermediate size and many fine, unmyelinated fibers turn caudally on entering the pons. These fibers for pain, temperature, light touch, and pressure combine with descending branches of afferents mentioned above to form the trigeminal spinal tract (Fig. 8–6). (As will be described later, the spinal tract includes a relatively small complement of fibers from the facial, glossopharyngeal, and vagus nerves. These fibers conduct general sensory data from the external ear and the mucosa of the posterior part of the tongue, the pharynx, and the larynx.) Some fibers of the spinal tract descend as far as the upper three segments of the cord, where they intermingle with fibers of the dorsolateral fasciculus or Lissauer's zone. There is a spatial arrangement of fibers in the sensory root and spinal tract, corresponding to the three divisions of the trigeminal nerve. In the sensory root, ophthalmic fibers are dorsal, mandibular fibers ventral, and maxillary fibers in between. There is a rotation of the fibers as they enter the brain stem, with the result that the mandibular fibers are dorsal and the ophthalmic fibers ventral in the trigeminal spinal tract.

Fibers of the spinal tract terminate in the subjacent nucleus of the spinal tract (Fig. 8–6). This nucleus extends from the chief sensory nucleus to the caudal limit of the medulla; the nucleus of the spinal tract and the dorsal portion of the dorsal gray horn are indistinguishable from one another in the upper three cervical segments of the spinal cord. Based on cytoarchitecture, the nucleus of the spinal tract is divided into three regions or subnuclei. In the **pars caudalis,** a layer of small cells identical with the substantia gelatinosa lies external to a zone containing larger neurons, the latter zone being similar cytologically to the chief nucleus of the dorsal horn. The pars caudalis receives

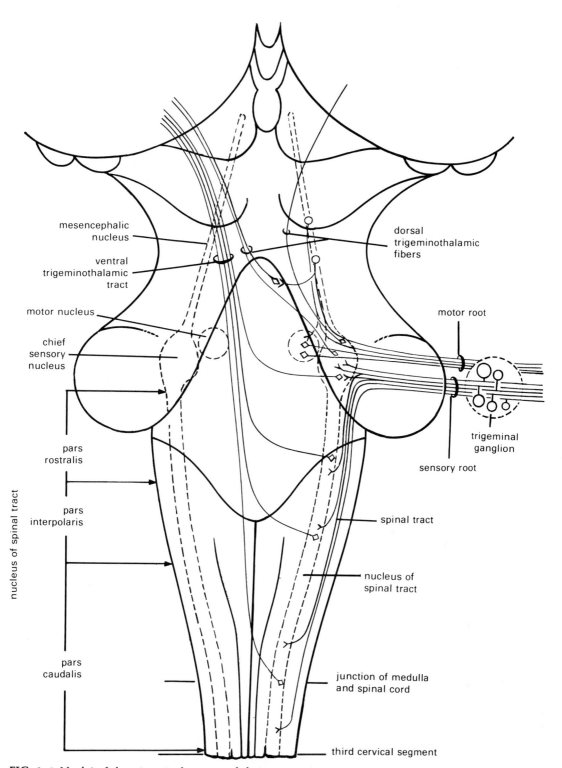

mesencephalic nucleus

ventral trigeminothalamic tract

motor nucleus

chief sensory nucleus

pars rostralis

nucleus of spinal tract

pars interpolaris

pars caudalis

dorsal trigeminothalamic fibers

motor root

trigeminal ganglion

sensory root

spinal tract

nucleus of spinal tract

junction of medulla and spinal cord

third cervical segment

FIG. 8–6. Nuclei of the trigeminal nerve and their connections.

107

fibers for pain, temperature, touch, and pressure, those for pain and temperature predominating. As in the substantia gelatinosa, there may be modification of sensory data during transmission through the nucleus of the trigeminal spinal tract. It will be apparent that the pars caudalis in the medulla is essentially a rostral extension of the dorsal region of the dorsal gray horn of the spinal cord. Similarly, the trigeminal spinal tract in the region of the pars caudalis is comparable to the dorsolateral fasciculus of the spinal cord. In the first three cervical segments these structures are concerned with pain and temperature in both the trigeminal area of distribution and that of the most rostral cervical nerves (neck and back of the head).

Of the remaining two regions of the nucleus of the spinal tract (Fig. 8-6), the **pars interpolaris** is characterized by the presence of rather large cells scattered among diffusely arranged small and medium-sized neurons. In the **pars rostralis** there is a more dense arrangement of cells of small and medium size. Fibers of the spinal tract terminating in these regions appear to be concerned in the main with light touch and pressure. Some of the fibers are descending branches of afferents that also send a branch to the chief sensory nucleus. There is still much to be learned about the functional properties of the pars interpolaris and pars rostralis and, indeed, the whole of the nucleus of the trigeminal spinal tract.

Efferent fibers from the sensory trigeminal nuclei proceed in various directions. Some of them terminate in motor nuclei of the trigeminal and facial nerves, the nucleus ambiguus, and the hypoglossal nucleus for reflex responses to stimuli arising in the area of distribution of the trigeminal nerve. For example, touching the cornea causes the eyelids to close reflexly; the afferent fibers are in the ophthalmic nerve and the efferent fibers of the reflex arc are in the facial nerve. As a further example, irritation of the nasal mucosa causes sneezing. For this reflex afferent impulses in the maxillary nerve are relayed to motor nuclei of the trigeminal and facial nerves, the nucleus ambiguus, the hypoglossal nucleus, and (through a reticulospinal relay) to the phrenic nucleus and motor cells in the spinal cord supplying the intercostal and other respiratory muscles.

Fibers from the sensory nuclei are also distributed to the reticular formation; they are an important source of cutaneous stimuli for the ascending reticular activating system. Other fibers enter the cerebellum through the inferior peduncle. The principal pathway from the chief sensory nucleus and nucleus of the spinal tract to the thalamus (ventral posterior nucleus) is the crossed **ventral trigeminothalamic tract** (Fig. 8-6), which ascends close to the medial lemniscus. Fewer crossed and uncrossed fibers proceed from the chief sensory nucleus to the thalamus in the **dorsal trigeminothalamic tract.**

Mesencephalic Nucleus

The mesencephalic nucleus consists of a slender strand of cells extending from the chief sensory nucleus through the midbrain (Fig. 8-6). The nucleus is located beneath the lateral edge of the floor of the fourth ventricle in the pons and in the lateral region of the periaqueductal gray matter in the midbrain. The unipolar cells are primary sensory neurons in an unusual location; they are the only such cells that are incorporated in the central nervous system, rather than being in cerebrospinal ganglia. Fibers from the nucleus constitute the slender **mesencephalic root** of the trigeminal nerve which runs alongside the mesencephalic nucleus. The single process of each cell divides into a peripheral and a central branch. Most of the peripheral branches enter the motor root of the trigeminal nerve and are distributed with the mandibular division (Fig. 8-6). These fibers end in deep receptors of proprioceptive type in the region of the temporomandibular joint and adjacent to the teeth of the lower jaw, and in neuromuscular spindles in the muscles of mastication. Some fibers from the mesencephalic nucleus traverse the sensory root and the trigeminal ganglion for distribution by way of the maxillary division to endings in the hard palate and adjacent to the teeth of the upper jaw. Central branches of the single processes of cells composing the mesencephalic nucleus terminate in the motor nuclei of the trigeminal nerve. This connection establishes the stretch reflex originating in neuromuscular spindles in the masticatory muscles, together with a reflex for control of the force of the bite. Other central branches synapse with cells of the reticular formation, from which fibers proceed to the ventral posterior thalamic nucleus along with dorsal trigeminothalamic fibers. In addition, a few fibers from the mesencephalic nucleus enter the cerebellum through the superior peduncle.

MOTOR COMPONENT

The **motor nucleus** of the trigeminal nerve, consisting of typical multipolar neurons, is situated medial to the chief sensory nucleus (Fig. 8-6). Fibers from the motor nucleus constitute the bulk of the motor root, which joins sensory fibers just distal to the trigeminal ganglion to form the mandibular nerve. This nerve supplies the muscles of mastication (masseter, temporal, and lateral and medial pterygoid muscles) and several small muscles. The latter consist of the tensor tympani, tensor veli palatini, digastric (anterior belly), and mylohyoid muscles. The motor nucleus receives afferents from the corticobulbar tract; most of these are crossed, but there is a significant proportion of uncrossed fibers. Afferents for reflexes come mainly from the sensory trigeminal nuclei, including the mesencephalic nucleus. Cells supplying the tensor tympani muscle receive acoustic fibers from the superior olivary nucleus. By reflex contraction, the tensor tympani muscle checks excessive movement of the tympanic membrane in response to loud sounds.

SOME CLINICAL COMMENTS

Of pathologic conditions affecting the trigeminal complex, major trigeminal neuralgia or **tic douloureux** is of special importance because of the excruciating pain. Tic douloureux is characterized by paroxysms of pain in the area of distribution of one of the trigeminal divisions, usually with periods of remission and exacerbation. The maxillary nerve is most frequently involved, then the mandibular, and least frequently the ophthalmic nerve. The paroxysm, which is of sudden onset, may be set off by mild stimulation of the face, such as touching the skin; there is often an especially sensitive "trigger zone." The cause of tic douloureux is not known. A pathologic process affecting the cells of the trigeminal ganglion has been suggested, and some believe that the disorder has a central basis, perhaps in the nucleus of the spinal tract.

Because medical management of tic douloureux is not always successful, various means of surgical intervention have been devised. The aim in most procedures is to interrupt the pain pathway from the affected cutaneous area to the nucleus of the spinal tract of the trigeminal nerve. It is important to preserve corneal sensitivity, which affords protection from damage that might lead to corneal ulceration.

The sensory and motor nuclei of the trigeminal nerve may be included in areas of degeneration in the brain stem, or the intracranial portion of the nerve may be affected by trauma, tumor growth, or other lesion. Interruption of the motor fibers causes paralysis and eventual atrophy of the muscles of mastication. The mandible deviates to the affected side because of the unopposed action of the normal lateral pterygoid muscle, the function of this muscle being to protrude the jaw. Interruption of corticobulbar fibers causes voluntary paresis of the masticatory muscles on the side opposite the lesion. Complete paralysis is lacking because the motor nucleus receives some uncrossed fibers from the motor cortex.

FACIAL NERVE

The facial nerve has two sensory components; one supplies taste buds and the other contributes cutaneous fibers to the external ear. There are also two motor or efferent components, one for the facial muscles of expression and one for the submandibular and sublingual salivary glands and the lacrimal gland.

SENSORY COMPONENTS

The cell bodies of primary sensory neurons are in the **geniculate ganglion,** situated at the bend of the nerve as it traverses the facial canal in the petrous temporal bone. The peripheral processes of cells for *taste*, these cells composing most of the ganglion, enter the chorda tympani branch of the facial nerve which joins the lingual branch of the mandibular nerve. The fibers are distributed to taste buds in the anterior two-thirds of the tongue, most of which are along its lateral border. Fibers for palatal taste buds follow a complicated route and, as is true also of

FIG. 8-7. Components of the facial nerve in the pons.

parasympathetic fibers in the facial and glossopharyngeal nerves, an understanding of the gross anatomy of the head is necessary in order to visualize their course. In brief, the sensory fibers in question leave the facial nerve in the greater petrosal branch at the level of the geniculate ganglion; this branch proceeds into the pterygopalatine fossa above the palate, where the fibers join palatine branches of the maxillary division of the trigeminal nerve. The trigeminal fibers of the palatine nerves provide for general sensation in the palate and inner surface of the gums, whereas the fibers from the facial nerve terminate in taste buds in the hard and soft palates.

Turning to the central processes of geniculate ganglion cells subserving taste, the fibers enter the brain stem in the sensory root of the facial nerve (nervus intermedius) and turn caudally in the tractus solitarius (Fig. 8-7). The facial nerve fibers in the fasciculus are joined more caudally by gustatory fibers from the glossopharyngeal and vagus nerves. Fibers from these three sources terminate in the **nucleus of the tractus solitarius,** consisting of a column of cells adjacent to, and partly surrounding, the tract. From this nucleus connections are established with efferent nuclei of the brain stem, especially the salivatory nuclei and the dorsal nucleus of the vagus nerve. There is also a discharge to the intermediolateral cell column of the spinal cord through the small solitariospinal tract. Ascending fibers from the nucleus of the tractus solitarius reach the hypothalamus and the ventral posterior thalamic nucleus by running close to the medial lemniscus. There is a further projection from the thalamus to the cortical area for taste which is located at the lower end of the general sensory strip in the parietal lobe.

With respect to the *cutaneous* sensory component, the fibers leave the facial nerve just after it leaves the facial canal. These fibers are distributed to the skin of the external ear, a small area behind the ear, the wall of the acoustic canal, and the external surface of the tympanic membrane. The central processes of the geniculate ganglion cells for cutaneous sensation enter the brain stem in the nervus intermedius and continue into the spinal tract of the trigeminal nerve (Fig. 8–7). They are joined in the tract by fibers from the glossopharyngeal and vagus nerves supplying the same cutaneous area. The combined fibers form a small bundle in the dorsal part of the spinal tract and terminate in the subjacent nucleus.

MOTOR COMPONENTS

For Supply of Striated Muscles

The motor component of the facial nerve for muscles of expression and certain additional small muscles is the most important part of the nerve from the clinical point of view. The **motor nucleus** is situated in the ventrolateral part of the pontine tegmentum, in its caudal one-third (Fig. 8–7). Efferent fibers of the nucleus pursue an unexpected course. Directed initially toward the floor of the fourth ventricle, the fibers form a compact bundle which runs forward along the medial side, and then over the rostral end, of the abducens nucleus. The fibers then proceed to the point of emergence of the motor root of the facial nerve by passing between the nucleus of origin and the nucleus of the trigeminal spinal tract. The configuration of the fiber bundle around the abducens nucleus is called the **internal genu,** the external genu of the facial nerve being in the facial canal at the level of the geniculate ganglion. The explanation given for the course of facial motor fibers in the pons is based on a migration of cells in the embryo. It has been suggested that neurons destined to form the abducens and facial nuclei are intermingled at an early embryonic stage. The facial neurons move subsequently in a ventrolateral direction under the influence of the trigeminal spinal tract and its nucleus. Concurrently the abducens neurons move dorsomedially toward the medial longitudinal fasciculus. The fibers extending from the facial nucleus to the region of the abducens nucleus indicate the direction and extent of the change in position of the nuclei during embryonic development. Such shifts in position of groups of nerve cells during development are said to be the result of neurobiotaxis, *i.e.,* the tendency of neurons to migrate toward major sources of stimuli.

The motor root of the facial nerve consists entirely of fibers from the motor nucleus. They supply the muscles of expression (mimetic muscles), the platysma and stylohyoid muscles, and the posterior belly of the digastric muscle. The facial nerve also supplies the stapedius muscle of the middle ear; this small muscle is inserted on the stapes and, by reflex contraction in response to loud sounds, prevents excessive movement of the stapes.

The motor nucleus receives afferents from several sources, including important connections for reflexes. Tectobulbar fibers from the superior colliculus complete a reflex pathway which provides for closure of the eyelids in response to intense light or a rapidly approaching object. Fibers from trigeminal sensory nuclei function in the corneal reflex and in chewing or sucking responses on placing food in the mouth. Fibers from the superior olivary nucleus on the auditory pathway permit reflex contraction of the stapedius muscle. Corticobulbar afferents are crossed, except for those terminating on cells that supply the frontalis and orbicularis oculi muscles which receive both crossed and uncrossed fibers. Contralateral voluntary paralysis of the *lower facial muscles* is therefore a feature of upper motor neuron lesions. However, under such circumstances the facial muscles continue to respond involuntarily to changing moods and emotions, probably because of impulses received by the motor nucleus from the hypothalamus. Emotional changes of facial expression are typically lost in Parkinson's disease (masklike facies), although voluntary use of the facial muscles is retained.

Parasympathetic Nuclei

The **superior salivatory** and **lacrimal nuclei** consist of indefinite clusters of small cells, partly intermingled, medial to the motor nucleus (Fig. 8–7). They contain the cell bodies of preganglionic neurons for the submandibular and sublingual salivary glands and the lacrimal gland. Fibers from the nuclei leave the brain stem in the nervus intermedius and continue in the facial nerve until branches are given off in the facial canal in the petrous temporal bone. The fibers follow devious routes to their destinations, running part of the way in branches of the trigeminal nerve. Briefly stated, fibers from the superior salivatory nucleus leave the facial nerve in the chorda tympani branch and join the lingual branch of the mandibular nerve to reach the floor of the oral cavity. There they terminate in the submandibular ganglion and on scattered nerve cells in the submandibular gland. Short postganglionic fibers are distributed to the parenchyma of the submandibular and sublingual glands, where impulses thus conveyed stimulate secretion and cause vasodilation. Fibers from the lacrimal nucleus leave the facial nerve in the greater petrosal branch and terminate in the pterygopalatine ganglion located in the fossa of the same name. Postganglionic fibers for stimulation of secretion and vasodilation reach the lacrimal gland through the zygomatic branch of the maxillary nerve. Other postganglionic fibers are distributed to glands in the mucosa lining the nasal cavity and the paranasal sinuses.

The superior salivatory nucleus comes under the influence of the hypothalamus through the dorsal longitudinal fasciculus, and of the olfactory system through relays in the reticular formation. Data from taste buds and the mucosa of the oral cavity are received by way of the nucleus of the tractus solitarius and sensory trigeminal nuclei, respectively. The chief sources of impulses to the lacrimal nucleus are the hypothalamus for emotional responses and the trigeminal spinal nucleus for lacrimation caused by irritation of the cornea and conjunctiva.

SOME CLINICAL COMMENTS

The facial nuclei and associated fiber bundles may be included in degenerative or other lesions of the brain stem, with facial paralysis and other signs. More frequently, however, the facial nerve is affected as it traverses the facial canal in the petrous temporal bone.

The usual condition, known as **Bell's palsy,** consists of weakness (paresis) or paralysis of the facial muscles on the affected side. The symptoms develop rapidly and the etiology is thought to be a viral infection, with edema of connective tissue lining the facial canal and pressure on the facial nerve. The signs of Bell's palsy depend not only on the severity of the viral infection (assuming this to be the cause), but also on where the facial nerve is affected in its passage through the facial canal. All functions of the nerve are lost if the damage is proximal to the geniculate ganglion. In addition to the paralysis of facial muscles, there is loss of taste sensation in the anterior two-thirds of the tongue and the palate of the affected side, together with impairment of secretion by the submandibular, sublingual, and lacrimal glands. In addition sounds are abnormally loud because of paralysis of the stapedius muscle.

In mild cases most of the nerve fibers are not so severely damaged as to result in wallerian degeneration and the outlook for recovery is good. Recovery is slow and frequently incomplete when it must rely on nerve fiber regeneration. Sensory fibers proceeding to the brain stem do not regenerate if the lesion is proximal to the geniculate ganglion. Also, in the case of a lesion in the proximal part of the nerve, some regenerating salivary fibers may find their way into the greater petrosal nerve and reach the pterygopalatine ganglion. This results in lacrimation (crocodile tears) when aromas and taste sensations cause stimulation of cells in the superior salivatory nucleus. When the nerve is affected in the distal part of the facial canal after the greater petrosal and chorda tympani branches are given off, the condition is limited to paresis or paralysis involving both the upper and lower facial muscles on the side of the lesion. The prospect for recovery is generally good.

GLOSSOPHARYNGEAL, VAGUS, AND ACCESSORY NERVES

The ninth, tenth, and eleventh cranial nerves have much in common functionally and share certain nuclei in the medulla. Although it is customary to discuss these nerves individually, repetition can be avoided by considering them as a group.

AFFERENT COMPONENTS

The glossopharyngeal and vagus nerves include sensory fibers for the special visceral sense of taste from the posterior one-third of the tongue, the pharynx, and the epiglottis, together with general visceral afferents from the carotid sinus, carotid body, and viscera of the thorax and abdomen. There are also sensory fibers for pain, temperature, and touch from the mucosa of the back of the tongue, the pharynx and nearby regions, and from the skin of the ear. The cell bodies of primary sensory neurons are in the superior and inferior ganglia of each of the nerves.

Visceral Afferents

The cell bodies for the **gustatory fibers** are in the inferior ganglia of the glossopharyngeal and vagus nerves. The fibers are distributed through the glossopharyngeal nerve to taste buds in the back of the tongue and, in few numbers, the pharyngeal mucosa. Vagal fibers supply taste buds on the epiglottis; these are unimportant because few persist into adult life. Central processes of the ganglion cells join the tractus solitarius and terminate in the corresponding nucleus (Figs. 8–8 and 8–9). The rostral portion of the nucleus of the tractus solitarius is concerned with taste, impulses being received by way of the facial, glossopharyngeal, and vagus nerves; it is frequently referred to as the **gustatory nucleus.** Projections from the nucleus for reflex responses and for awareness of taste are as described for the facial nerve.

The cell bodies of afferent neurons for **general visceral reflexes** are also in the inferior ganglia of the glossopharyngeal and vagus nerves. These fibers in the glossopharyngeal nerve supply the carotid sinus at the bifurcation of the common carotid artery and the adjacent carotid body. Nerve endings in the wall of the carotid sinus function as baroreceptors, which monitor arterial blood pressure, whereas the carotid body contains chemoreceptors that monitor oxygen tension in the circulating blood. Vagal fibers similarly supply baroreceptors in the aortic arch and chemoreceptors in the small aortic bodies adjacent to the arch. The vagus nerve contains many afferent fibers that are distributed to the viscera of the thorax and abdomen; impulses conveyed centrally are of importance in reflex control of cardiovascular, respiratory, and alimentary functions. The central processes of the primary sensory neurons for these reflexes descend in the tractus solitarius and end in the more caudal part of its nucleus (Figs. 8–8 and 8–9). From the latter site connections are established with the dorsal nucleus of the vagus nerve, visceral centers in the reticular formation, and cells of the reticular formation that project to the intermediolateral cell column of the spinal cord. Data of visceral origin are also relayed to the hypothalamus.

Other Afferent Fibers

The glossopharyngeal nerve includes fibers for the general sensations of pain, temperature, and touch in the mucosa of the posterior one-third of the tongue, upper part of the pharynx (including the tonsillar area), auditory or eustachian tube, and middle ear. The vagus nerve carries fibers having the same functions to the lower part of the pharynx, the larynx, and the esophagus. The areas thus supplied are of entodermal origin and in this respect the sensory neurons are visceral in nature. However, the sensations aroused are similar to those of cutaneous or somatic origin. There is some uncertainty, therefore, with respect to the central connections of these particular sensory fibers. The question has been resolved for fibers for pain (and probably for temperature). The pathway for pain from the areas just noted is interrupted by section of the spinal tract of the trigeminal nerve, a procedure used occasionally in the treatment of tic douloureux, indicating that fibers for pain in the glossopharyngeal and vagus nerves descend in the trigeminal spinal tract and end in its nucleus (Figs. 8–8 and 8–9). This being the case, the cell bodies are probably in the small superior ganglia of the glossopharyngeal and vagus nerves. Fibers for touch from the posterior part of the tongue, the pharynx, and adjacent areas may accompany visceral afferents to the nucleus of the tractus solitarius or they may terminate with somatic afferents in the nucleus of the trigeminal spinal tract. In either event, such afferents are important in the "gag reflex" through a reflex pathway that includes the nucleus ambiguus and the hypoglossal nucleus.

Finally the vagus nerve, through its auricu-

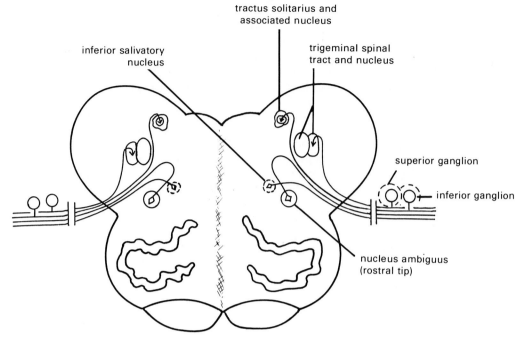

FIG. 8-8. Components of the glossopharyngeal nerve in the medulla.

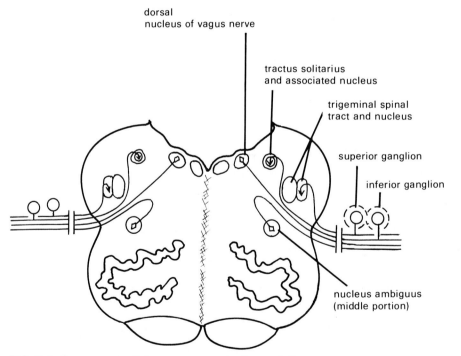

FIG. 8-9. Components of the vagus nerve in the medulla.

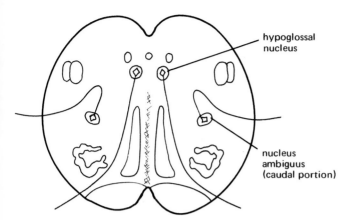

hypoglossal
nucleus

nucleus
ambiguus
(caudal portion)

FIG. 8–10. Hypoglossal nerve and origin of the cranial root of the accessory nerve in the medulla.

lar branch, contributes sensory fibers to the external ear, a small area behind the ear, the wall of the acoustic canal, and the tympanic membrane. The glossopharyngeal nerve contains a few such fibers, although inconstantly. The cell bodies are in the superior ganglia of the nerves and the central processes join other somatic afferent fibers in the spinal tract of the trigeminal nerve.

EFFERENT COMPONENTS

The ninth, tenth, and eleventh cranial nerves include motor fibers for striated muscles, and the ninth and tenth nerves contain parasympathetic efferents.

For Supply of Striated Muscles

The **nucleus ambiguus** is a column of typical motor neurons situated dorsal to the inferior olivary nucleus (Figs. 8–8 through 8–10). Fibers from the nucleus are directed dorsally at first. They then turn sharply to mingle with other fibers in the glossopharyngeal and vagus nerves, and constitute the entire cranial root of the accessory nerve. The nucleus ambiguus supplies muscles of the soft palate, pharynx, and larynx, together with striated muscle fibers in the upper part of the esophagus. The only muscle in the foregoing regions not supplied by this nucleus is the tensor veli palatini muscle, which is innervated by the trigeminal nerve.

A small group of cells in the rostral end of the nucleus ambiguus supplies the stylopharyngeus muscle through the glosso-

pharyngeal nerve (Fig. 8–8). A large region of the nucleus supplies the remaining pharyngeal muscles, the cricothyroid muscle (an external muscle of the larynx), and the striated muscle of the esophagus through the vagus nerve (Fig. 8–9). Fibers from the caudal part of the nucleus leave the brain stem in the cranial root of the accessory nerve (Fig. 8–10). They join the spinal root of the accessory nerve temporarily, then pass over to the vagus nerve in the region of the jugular foramen. These fibers supply muscles of the soft palate and the intrinsic muscles of the larynx. It would be simpler, although contrary to convention, to consider the cranial root of the accessory nerve as part of the vagus nerve, leaving the spinal root as the definitive accessory nerve.

The nucleus ambiguus receives afferents from sensory nuclei of the brain stem, most importantly the nucleus of the spinal tract of the trigeminal nerve and the nucleus of the tractus solitarius. These connections establish reflexes for coughing, gagging, and vomiting, the stimuli arising in the mucosa of the respiratory and alimentary passages. Corticobulbar afferents are both crossed and uncrossed; muscles supplied by the nucleus ambiguus are not paralyzed therefore in the event of a unilateral lesion of the upper motor neuron type.

Motor neurons for the sternocleidomastoid and trapezius muscles differentiate in the embryo near cells that are destined to form the nucleus ambiguus. The former cells migrate into the spinal cord (segments C1 through C6) and take up a position in the lateral part of the ventral gray horn. Arising as a series of rootlets along the side of the cord just dorsal to the denticulate ligament, the **spinal root of the accessory nerve** ascends alongside the spinal cord, thus retracing the migration of cells of origin. On reaching the side of the medulla by passing through the foramen magnum, the spinal and cranial roots unite and continue as the accessory nerve as far as the jugular foramen. Fibers from the nucleus ambiguus then join the vagus nerve as already noted, and those of spinal origin proceed to the sternocleidomastoid and trapezius muscles. Corticospinal fibers to the spinal accessory neurons are almost all crossed. There is therefore contralateral weakness (paresis) of the sternocleidomastoid and trapezius muscles as a result of an upper motor neuron lesion.

Parasympathetic Nuclei

There are parasympathetic fibers in the glossopharyngeal nerve, and these are especially numerous in the vagus nerve. The **inferior salivatory nucleus** for the parotid gland is a small collection of cells caudal to the superior salivatory nucleus and near the rostral tip of the nucleus ambiguus (Fig. 8–8). Fibers from the inferior salivatory nucleus are included in the glossopharyngeal nerve, enter its tympanic branch, and reach the otic ganglion by way of the tympanic plexus and the lesser petrosal nerve. Postganglionic fibers join the auriculotemporal branch of the mandibular nerve and thus reach the parotid gland. The parasympathetic supply to the parotid gland is secretomotor and vasodilator. The inferior salivatory nucleus is influenced by stimuli from the hypothalamus, olfactory system, nucleus of the tractus solitarius, and sensory trigeminal nuclei.

The main parasympathetic nucleus is the **dorsal nucleus of the vagus nerve.** This column of cells, which are mainly of medium size and spindle-shaped, extends through most of the medulla in the gray matter around the central canal and beneath the vagal triangle of the rhomboid fossa (Fig. 8–9). The portion of the nucleus for the heart and respiratory system lies beneath the floor of the fourth ventricle, whereas the caudal portion of the nucleus is for abdominal viscera. Preganglionic fibers in the vagus nerve are distributed to parasympathetic ganglia and plexuses in or near viscera, from where short postganglionic fibers continue to smooth and cardiac muscle and to secretory cells of glands. The dorsal nucleus of the vagus nerve receives afferents from several sources; the more important are the hypothalamus, the olfactory system, autonomic centers in the reticular formation, and the nucleus of the tractus solitarius.

Isolated lesions involving the ninth, tenth, or eleventh cranial nerves separately are uncommon. However, several pathologic events, most frequently of vascular origin, cause destruction of the central nuclei. A unilateral lesion of the nucleus ambiguus, for example, results in ipsilateral paralysis of the soft palate, pharynx, and larynx, with the expected signs of hoarseness and difficulty in breathing and swallowing. Extensive lesions, especially if bilateral, carry a poor prognosis. Complete laryngeal paralysis leads to asphyxia unless immediate precautions are taken to restore the airway. Interruption of the parasympathetic outflow causes visceral dysfunction, including cardiac acceleration.

HYPOGLOSSAL NERVE

The **hypoglossal nucleus,** consisting of motor cells like those of the ventral horn of the spinal cord, lies between the dorsal nucleus of the vagus nerve and the midline of the medulla (Fig. 8–10). The hypoglossal triangle of the rhomboid fossa marks the position of the rostral part of the nucleus. Fibers from the hypoglossal nucleus course ventrally on the lateral side of the medial lemniscus and emerge along the sulcus between the pyramid and the olive. The hypoglossal nerve supplies the intrinsic muscles of the tongue and the three extrinsic muscles (genioglossus, styloglossus, and hyoglossus). The nucleus receives afferents from the nucleus of the tractus solitarius and sensory trigeminal nuclei for reflex movements of the tongue in swallowing, chewing, and sucking in response to gustatory and other stimuli from the oral and pharyngeal mucosae. Corticobulbar afferents are predominantly crossed; a unilateral upper motor neuron lesion therefore causes paresis of the opposite side of the tongue, although demonstration of the muscle weakness may be difficult. Paralysis and eventual atrophy of the affected muscles follow destruction of the hypoglossal nucleus or interruption of the nerve. The tongue deviates to the weak side on protrusion because of the unopposed protrusor action of the healthy genioglossus muscle.

SENSORY NERVE SUPPLY OF MUSCLE SPINDLES

Sensory fibers originating in the mesencephalic nucleus of the trigeminal nerve supply neuromuscular spindles in muscles innervated by the mandibular division, together with other proprioceptors associated with the muscles of mastication and proprioceptive-like endings adjacent to the teeth and in the hard palate. The source of sensory fibers for spindles in muscles innervated by cranial nerves other than the trigeminal has not been established with certainty in all instances.

The extraocular muscles contain spindles of a special type. Their sensory fibers have been described as coming from the mesencephalic nucleus or, alternatively, from cells in the trigeminal ganglion whose central processes terminate in the nucleus of the spinal tract of the trigeminal nerve. In either case the fibers reach the orbit by way of the ophthalmic division, and their source may differ from one species of animal to another. Sensory fibers for spindles in laryngeal muscles have been identified in the vagus nerve; the cell bodies must be in the ganglia of the vagus nerve because the fibers persist after section of the nerve proximal to the ganglia. Spindles have been described in muscles of the tongue; the cell bodies of sensory neurons appear to be in the inferior ganglion of the vagus nerve, the fibers passing over to the hypoglossal nerve through an anastomotic connection. The situation with respect to facial muscles is especially obscure because the presence of spindles in these muscles has not been established conclusively. Proprioceptors in the sternocleidomastoid and trapezius muscles receive sensory fibers through the second, third, and fourth cervical nerves.

CLASSIFICATION OF COMPONENTS OF CRANIAL AND SPINAL NERVES

The spinal nerves and most of the cranial nerves have now been discussed and their components can be classified under seven headings. Of these, four are present in both spinal and cranial nerves; three more are added in the latter to include the special senses and to take cognizance of different embryologic origins of the muscles of the head. Cranial nerve nuclei in the brain stem are shown in Figure 8–11 according to the following classification.

AFFERENT COMPONENTS

General somatic afferent nuclei receive impulses from general sensory endings and are therefore concerned with pain, temperature, touch, pressure, proprioception, and vibration. The cells are in the dorsal gray horn of the spinal cord, the nuclei gracilis and cuneatus, and the sensory trigeminal nuclei. The **special somatic afferent** group consists of nuclei for those special senses that relate the body to the external environment. This group consists of the visual system (optic nerve) and the cochlear and vestibular divisions of the eighth cranial nerve. **General visceral afferent** components are for visceral reflexes and for sensations such as fullness of hollow organs and pain of visceral origin. The second order neurons are in the dorsal gray horn of the spinal cord and the caudal portion of the nucleus of the tractus solitarius. **Special visceral afferents** are for taste, with second order neurons located in the rostral part of the nucleus of the tractus solitarius (gustatory nucleus). The olfactory nerves are considered conventionally as visceral because of the influence of smell on visceral functions; they are therefore included under the heading of special visceral afferents.

EFFERENT COMPONENTS

Lower motor neurons included under the heading of **general somatic efferents** supply muscles that are derived from myotomes of the embryonic somites. They are the oculomotor, trochlear, abducens, and hypoglossal nuclei and ventral horn cells of the spinal cord. **General visceral efferents** are the preganglionic neurons of the autonomic nervous system. In the brain stem, they include the Edinger–Westphal nucleus, lacrimal nucleus, superior and inferior salivatory nuclei, and dorsal nucleus of the vagus nerve. In the spinal cord, this category consists of the intermediolateral cell column in the thoracic and

FIG. 8–11. Classification of the nuclei of cranial nerves.

upper lumbar segments and parasympathetic cells in the sacral cord. **Special visceral efferents** supply muscles derived from the branchial or gill arches of the embryo. They are classified as "visceral" because of the respiratory function of the gill arches in aquatic forms. There are three special visceral efferent nuclei: 1) the trigeminal motor nucleus for the muscles of mastication, which develop from the first branchial arch; 2) the facial motor nucleus for the muscles of expression, of second branchial arch derivation; and 3) the nucleus ambiguus for muscles of the palate, pharynx, larynx, and upper esophagus, these muscles being derived from the third, fourth, and fifth branchial arches.

SUGGESTED READING

Adata AK, Gehring EN: Proprioceptive innervation of the tongue. J Anat 110:215–220, 1971

Brodal A: The Cranial Nerves: Anatomy and Anatomicoclinical Correlations, 2nd ed. Oxford, Blackwell, 1965

Brodal A: Neurological Anatomy, 2nd ed. London, Oxford University Press, 1969

Carpenter MB, Strominger NL: The medial longitudinal fasciculus and disturbances of conjugate horizontal eye movements in the monkey. J Comp Neurol 125:41–65, 1965

Courville J: The nucleus of the facial nerve: the relation between cellular groups and peripheral branches of the nerve. Brain Res 1:338–354, 1966

Crosby EC, Humphrey T, Lauer EW: Correlative Anatomy of the Nervous System. New York, Macmillan, 1962

Denny-Brown D, Yanagisawa N: The function of the descending root of the fifth nerve. Brain 96:783–814, 1973

Eisenman J, Landgren S, Novin D: Functional organization in the main sensory trigeminal nucleus and in the rostral subdivision of the nucleus of the spinal trigeminal tract in the cat. Acta Physiol Scand [Suppl] 59 (214):1–44, 1963

Kerr FWL: The divisional organization of afferent fibers of the trigeminal nerve. Brain 86:721–733, 1963

Kerr FWL: The etiology of trigeminal neuralgia. Arch Neurol 8:15–25, 1963

Kugelberg E, Lindblom U: The mechanism of the pain in trigeminal neuralgia. J Neurol Neurosurg Psychiatry 22:36–43, 1959

Manni E, Palmieri G, Marini R: Peripheral pathway of the proprioceptive afferents from the lateral rectus muscle of the eye. Exp Neurol 30:46–53, 1971

Manni E, Palmieri G, Marini R: Pontine trigeminal termination of proprioceptive afferents from the eye muscles. Exp Neurol 36:310–318, 1972

Manni E, Palmieri G, Marini R: Central pathway of the extraocular muscle proprioception. Exp Neurol 42:181–190, 1974

Morest DH: Experimental study of the projections of the nucleus of the tractus solitarius and the area postrema in the cat. J Comp Neurol 130:277–299, 1967

Olszewski J: On the anatomical and functional organization of the spinal trigeminal nucleus. J Comp Neurol 92:401–413, 1950

Rhoton AL Jr, O'Leary JL, Ferguson JP: The trigeminal, facial, vagal, and glossopharyngeal nerves in the monkey. Arch Neurol 14:530–540, 1966

Schwartz HG, Roulhac GE, Lam RL, O'Leary JL: Organization of the fasciculus solitarius in man. J Comp Neurol 94:221–237, 1951

Sivanandasingham P: Somata of feline extra-ocular muscle proprioceptors. Acta Anat 99:152–159, 1977

Warwick R: Representation of the extra-ocular muscles in the oculomotor nuclei of the monkey. J Comp Neurol 98:449–503, 1953

Warwick R: The ocular parasympathetic nerve supply and its mesencephalic sources. J Anat 88:71–93, 1954

Reticular Formation

An attractive evolutionary concept of the reticular formation of the brain stem has been advanced, based on a long phylogenetic history. In the most primitive vertebrates, the brain consists in large part of neural tissue that is not well organized as nuclei and tracts; this diffuse arrangement of neurons is said to be "reticular" (forming a network). In the evolution of the brain the rostral part developed preferentially, with additions to the thalamus and the appearance of neocortex in mammals. Fiber tracts were acquired to connect the spinal cord and the forebrain, and the tracts of necessity traverse the brain stem. Large nuclei including the red nucleus, substantia nigra, and inferior olivary nucleus also appeared or increased in size in the mammalian brain stem. The primitive reticular formation did not disappear; on the contrary, it underwent further development to form an important component of the mammalian brain stem in those regions not occupied by tracts and nuclei.

The reticular formation is the recipient of data from almost all of the sensory systems and has efferent connections, direct or indirect, with all levels of the central nervous system. Constituting, in a sense, a central core of the brain, the reticular formation makes a significant contribution to several aspects of brain function, including a role in the sleep–arousal cycle. The reticular system of neurons is integrated into the motor system of the brain and spinal cord, and includes regions that regulate visceral functions. The primitive "reticular" characteristic is retained in the multineuronal or polysynaptic nature of intrinsic pathways.

CYTOARCHITECTURE

Histologic analysis of the reticular formation is difficult because the constituent neurons are not for the most part assembled in compact groups. Nevertheless a number of regions or nuclei are recognized on the basis of cellular characteristics and connections. Five such nuclei are present in the medulla (Figs. 9–1 and 9–2). The **lateral reticular nucleus** is exceptional in that it is sufficiently discrete to permit identification in Weigert-stained sections (Figs. 7–4 through 7–6). This nucleus is situated near the surface of the medulla and extends from a point caudal to the inferior olivary nucleus to the midolivary level. The **paramedian reticular nucleus** is adjacent to the midline of the medulla. The lateral and paramedian nuclei have connections with the cerebellum.

The remaining reticular nuclei in the medulla are in the region bounded ventrally by the inferior olivary nucleus, dorsally by the nuclei gracilis and cuneatus and the vestibular nuclear complex, and laterally by the nucleus of the spinal tract of the trigeminal nerve. Cells of the **ventral reticular nucleus** are scattered through the medial two-thirds of this area at the level of the caudal half of the inferior olivary nucleus (Fig. 9–1). Rostral to the ventral reticular nucleus, the reticular formation in the medial portion of the area just outlined consists of large neurons intermingled with smaller cells and is known as the **magnocellular reticular nucleus** (Fig. 9–2). The **parvicellular reticular nucleus,** in which the nerve cells are small, occupies an area bounded by the magnocellular nucleus, the nucleus of the spinal tract of the trigeminal nerve, and the vestibular nuclear complex, extending from the midolivary level to the rostral limit of the medulla (Fig. 9–2). As will be noted presently, the parvicellular nucleus receives sensory data from the spinal cord and trigeminal nuclei, and projects to more medial reticular nuclei. It is consequently regarded as part of the "sensory" or "association" region of the reticular formation.

Reticular nuclei in the tegmentum of the

pons are, by convention, described separately from those in the medulla, but two of them are in fact rostral extensions of medullary nuclei. The **caudal pontine reticular nucleus** (Fig. 9–3) is similar cytologically to the magnocellular nucleus in the medulla, of which it is essentially an extension. Farther forward in the pons, the **rostral pontine reticular nucleus** in the medial area of the tegmentum is lacking in the large neurons. The **parvicellular reticular nucleus,** situated in the lateral tegmentum of the pons (Fig. 9–3), is an extension of the same nucleus in the medulla and part of the sensory or association region of the reticular formation.

The reticular formation of the pons continues into the midbrain, where the **mesencephalic reticular nucleus** consists of scattered cells in an area bounded by the tectum, the red nucleus, and ascending lemnisci (Fig. 9–4). The reticular formation extends rostrally into the subthalamic region of the diencephalon, where it constitutes the zona incerta of the subthalamus (Chapter 11).

It is helpful from the functional point of view to consider the reticular formation as comprising three regions or nuclear groups. *Group 1* consists of the lateral and paramedian nuclei of the medulla, both of which have cerebellar connections. *Group 2* includes the parvicellular nuclei of the medulla and pons, constituting essentially a single nucleus in the lateral area of the brain stem. With afferents from several sensory systems, the parvicellular nuclei send fibers to the medial part of the reticular formation. *Group 3* consists of nuclei in the medial part of the medulla and pons, extending into the midbrain. This group therefore includes the ventral and magnocellular nuclei of the medulla, the caudal and rostral pontine nuclei, and the mesencephalic reticular nucleus, to which may be added the zona incerta of the subthalamus. These nuclei receive fibers from the lateral or sensory part of the reticular formation (parvicellular nuclei) and from other sources. Axons of cells of group 3 nuclei run longitudinally in the brain stem and give off numerous collateral branches as they ascend or descend. The branches synapse with other reticular neurons, forming the basis of the polysynaptic pathways which are characteristic of impulse conduction through the reticular formation.

FUNCTIONAL ORGANIZATION
CONNECTIONS WITH THE CEREBELLUM

The lateral reticular nucleus receives spinoreticular fibers and collaterals from the spinal lemniscus; efferent fibers enter the cerebellum through the inferior peduncle. There is thus established an auxiliary pathway for transmission of general sensory data to the cerebellum. The lateral reticular nucleus also receives fibers from the red nucleus and is therefore a cell station on a feedback circuit, the circuit being completed by fibers proceeding from cerebellar nuclei to the red nucleus. The paramedian reticular nucleus is on a simpler feedback circuit, receiving fibers from, and sending fibers to, the cerebellum.

ASCENDING RETICULAR ACTIVATING SYSTEM

The ascending activating system consists of the sensory input to the reticular formation and rostral transmission through polysynaptic pathways to certain thalamic nuclei, from which activity spreads to the cerebral cortex. The system has an important bearing on the sleep-arousal cycle and on alertness and attention.

All nuclei of the reticular formation, with the exception of the lateral and paramedian nuclei in the medulla, participate in the ascending activating system. Discussion of connections is simplified if the nuclei so involved are considered as forming two regions or areas. The **lateral area,** corresponding to group 2 nuclei, consists of the parvicellular nuclei in the medulla and pons. The **medial area** corresponds to group 3 nuclei, *i.e.,* the ventral and magnocellular nuclei in the medulla, the caudal and rostral pontine nuclei, and the mesencephalic reticular nucleus.

Sensory Input

The sensory input for the reticular activating system is as follows. The lateral reticular area receives collateral branches of fibers in the spinal lemniscus, and fibers from the nucleus of the spinal tract of the trigeminal nerve and the nucleus of the tractus solitarius. The reticular formation therefore receives impulses originating in receptors for pain, temperature, touch, and pressure throughout the entire body, and also impulses from sensory

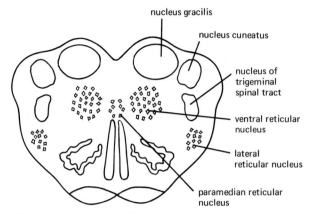

FIG. 9-1. Reticular nuclei at the level of the caudal portion of the inferior olivary nucleus.

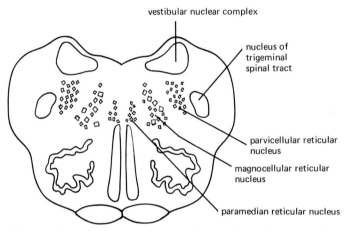

FIG. 9-2. Reticular nuclei at the level of the rostral portion of the inferior olivary nucleus.

FIG. 9-3. Reticular nuclei in the caudal region of the pontine tegmentum.

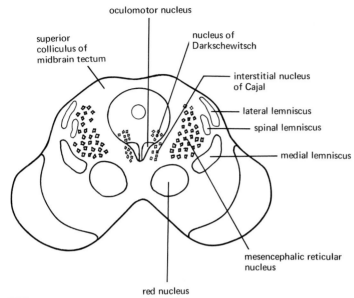

oculomotor nucleus

superior
colliculus of
midbrain tectum

nucleus of
Darkschewitsch

interstitial nucleus
of Cajal

lateral lemniscus

spinal lemniscus

medial lemniscus

mesencephalic reticular
nucleus

red nucleus

FIG. 9-4. Mesencephalic reticular nucleus and small nuclei in the rostral part of the midbrain.

endings in the viscera. The dorsal column system, which transmits data for the more discriminative aspects of general sensation, has no input to the reticular formation. The lateral area also receives afferents from vestibular nuclei and nuclei on the central auditory pathway. Axons from the lateral reticular area proceed to various parts of the medial area. The connections just described account for the expression "sensory or association part of the reticular formation," with respect to the parvicellular nuclei in the medulla and pons.

The remaining afferent fibers are not related specifically to the lateral area of the reticular formation. Spinoreticular fibers terminate mainly in the magnocellular part of the medial area, the remainder ending in the rostral pontine reticular nucleus and in the lateral area. The spinoreticular fibers represent a phylogenetically old ascending pathway, compared with the more recent spinothalamic tracts. Impulses of retinal origin reach various parts of the reticular formation through a relay in the superior colliculus. Olfactory impulses reach the reticular formation through several routes, including olfactotegmental fibers ending in the mesencephalic reticular nucleus. The reticular formation has an input therefore from all

sensory systems, somatic and visceral, with the exception of the dorsal column system for discriminative touch, proprioception, and vibration. Finally, corticoreticular fibers originate in widespread areas of the cerebral cortex, including the general sensory area. They end in various regions of the reticular formation and function in the well-known effect of psychic stimuli on attention.

Projections to Higher Centers

As mentioned previously, ascending axons of cells in the medial reticular area give off collateral branches which synapse with other reticular neurons. By repetition of relays, there is polysynaptic transmission of nerve impulses to the diencephalon. Many of the ascending fibers run in the central tegmental tract, and the last axons in the relay terminate in thalamic nuclei and the hypothalamus.

The thalamic nuclei receiving fibers from the reticular formation are the intralaminar nuclei and the nucleus of the midline (see also Chapter 11). A thin sheet of myelinated fibers (the internal medullary lamina) extends vertically through the thalamus in an anteroposterior plane. The lamina partially encloses several **intralaminar nuclei,** one of which, the **centromedian nucleus,** is especially well developed in man (Fig. 9–5). In addition to some fibers proceeding directly from the intralaminar nuclei to the cerebral

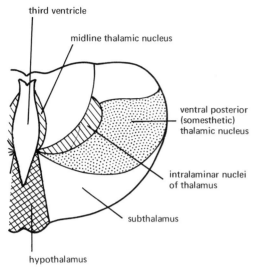

FIG. 9–5. Regions of the diencephalon receiving fibers of the lemniscal and extralemniscal systems.

cortex, there is an abundant projection to the cortex through relays in surrounding thalamic nuclei, thereby preserving the polysynaptic nature of the ascending reticular activating system. The general sensory nucleus of the thalamus (ventral posterior nucleus), which is the destination of the medial lemniscus, spinothalamic tracts, and trigeminothalamic tracts, projects to the somesthetic area of the parietal lobe. In contrast, the intralaminar nuclei project to widespread cortical areas, including nonspecific association areas and areas that are important with respect to emotions. The intralaminar nuclei have still other connections, notably with thalamic nuclei that participate in emotional aspects of brain function and with the corpus striatum, a large motor nucleus in the cerebral hemisphere.

The **nucleus of the midline,** which consists of groups of nerve cells in the medial part of the thalamus adjacent to the third ventricle (Fig. 9–5), represents the oldest part of the thalamus phylogenetically. The midline nucleus is immediately dorsal to the **hypothalamus.** Fibers from the reticular formation terminate in the hypothalamus, and impulses from the reticular formation also reach the hypothalamus through a relay in the nucleus of the midline. These connections contribute to the emotional and visceral responses that are associated with sensory stimuli reaching higher centers by way of the reticular formation.

Functions of the Reticular Activating System

The role of the reticular activating system is best understood when compared with that of the lemniscal system. Sensory information conveyed by the latter system, when projected from the ventral posterior nucleus of the thalamus to the somesthetic cortical area, is interpreted in a highly specific manner with respect to the nature of the sensory stimulus and its quantitative and discriminative aspects. The ascending reticular system is relatively nonspecific; the sensory modalities are merged in the polysynaptic pathway through the reticular formation and the thalamus, giving at best a vague awareness of any particular sensory modality. The cortex in general is stimulated, with a profound effect on levels of consciousness and on alerting reactions to sensory stimuli. When cortical stimulation by way of the reticular formation occurs during sleep, the electrical activity of the cortex (as seen on the electroencephalogram) changes from the large-wave random pattern of sleep to the small-wave pattern of the waking state. When one is awake, stimuli reaching the cortex through the activating system sharpen attentiveness and create optimal conditions for perception of sensory data conveyed through more direct pathways. Cutaneous stimuli appear to be especially important in maintaining consciousness, whereas visual, acoustic, and psychic stimuli have a special bearing on alertness and attention. Impulses from the trigeminal area of distribution have a significant influence on consciousness. This is the basis of methods found by experience to be useful in restoring a person from a "fainting spell." To cite a once popular example, smelling salts contain ammonia or other substances that stimulate trigeminal sensory endings in the nasal mucosa.

The reticular activating system is of considerable pharmacologic interest because general anesthetics are thought to suppress transmission through the polysynaptic pathway in the brain stem, although conduction continues along lemniscal routes. Similarly the site of action of tranquilizing drugs may be the reticular formation of the brain stem. As a corollary of the above, prolonged coma results from serious damage to the reticular formation.

The foregoing is a much simplified account of the ascending reticular activating system, and other systems of the brain are no doubt involved as well in the sleep–arousal cycle and related phenomena. Also, in addition to raising the level of consciousness and increasing alertness by the active process described, there may be a coexisting active process that induces sleep. Support for the existence of such a dual mechanism comes mainly from pharmacologic studies.

MOTOR FUNCTIONS

Numerous **reticulospinal fibers** originate in the medial area of the reticular formation, especially its magnocellular portion, and similar fibers functionally end in motor nuclei of cranial nerves. The medial area receives impulses of motor significance from motor areas of the cerebral cortex, the cerebellum, the red nucleus, and the substantia nigra. The reticular formation is thereby incorporated in important extrapyramidal motor pathways. Reticulospinal fibers synapse with both alpha and gamma motor neurons, and the gamma reflex loop has a significant role in producing the resulting motor responses.

VISCERAL CENTERS

Groups of neurons in the reticular formation regulate visceral functions through connections with nuclei of the autonomic outflow and, in the case of respiration, with motor neurons in the phrenic nucleus and thoracic region of the spinal cord. Respiratory and cardiovascular regions, commonly referred to as "centers," have been identified by electrical stimulation within the brain stem in experimental animals. Maximal inspiratory responses are obtained from the magnocellular nucleus in the medulla, whereas expiratory responses are evoked by stimulation of the parvicellular nucleus in the medulla. A pneumotaxic center in the pontine reticular formation controls normal respiratory rhythm. Stimulation of the ventral and mag-

nocellular reticular nuclei in the medulla has a depressor effect on the circulatory system, with slowing of the heart rate and lowering of blood pressure. The opposite or pressor effect is produced by stimulation of the lateral reticular area in the medulla. Damage to the brain stem is hazardous to life because of the presence of these centers controlling vital functions.

MISCELLANEOUS NUCLEI OF THE BRAIN STEM

Several small nuclei in the brain stem may conveniently be considered at this time, although not all of them are strictly components of the reticular formation.

The **area postrema** is a narrow strip of neural tissue in the caudal part of the rhomboid fossa between the vagal triangle and the margin of the fossa (Fig. 6–3). The most characteristic cell in the area postrema resembles astroblasts of the newborn; there are also astrocytes, a few oligodendrocytes, and a moderate number of nerve cells. The area is richly vascular and contains many large sinusoids; the "blood-brain barrier," which prevents certain substances from entering nervous tissue from capillary blood elsewhere, is lacking. The area postrema receives a few ascending visceral fibers from the spinal cord, and there are reciprocal connections with the nucleus of the tractus solitarius. It is thought to have a role in the physiology of vomiting and to send fibers to a "vomiting center" in the lateral area of the reticular formation. The area postrema has been shown in dogs to be an emetic trigger zone, serving as a chemoreceptor region for emetic drugs such as apomorphine and digitalis.

The **locus ceruleus,** at the rostral end of the floor of the fourth ventricle on each side, marks the position of a nucleus with a rich vascular supply, consisting of neurons containing melanin pigment. The nucleus is thought to have a role in the ascending reticular activating system and the control of respiration, together with other functions that have yet to be clarified.

There are several small nuclei worthy of brief mention in the midbrain. The **nucleus of Darkschewitsch** is situated in the central gray matter just dorsal to the oculomotor nucleus, and the **interstitial nucleus of Cajal** lies lateral to the oculomotor nucleus (Fig. 9–4). Among other possible connections, these nuclei receive fibers from the superior colliculus and from vestibular nuclei by way of the medial longitudinal fasciculus. Axons from the nuclei terminate in motor nuclei of cranial nerves and a small interstitiospinal tract is included in the sulcomarginal fasciculus in the ventral white column of the spinal cord.

Two additional midbrain nuclei are incorporated in a pathway originating in the olfactory and limbic systems. The **interpeduncular nucleus,** which is small in man, lies just above the interpeduncular fossa in the midline of the rostral end of the midbrain. The **dorsal tegmental nucleus** is located in the central gray matter, caudal to the nucleus of Darkschewitsch. The connections of the interpeduncular and dorsal tegmental nuclei are rather complicated. One pathway in which they participate begins in forebrain regions associated with the olfactory and limbic systems, from which fibers travel to the habenular nucleus in the epithalamus of the diencephalon. Habenulointerpeduncular fibers constitute the next link in this pathway. The interpeduncular nucleus then sends fibers to the dorsal tegmental nucleus, which influences autonomic nuclei either through fibers running in the dorsal longitudinal fasciculus or by means of relays in the reticular formation. Through these connections, data related to the sense of smell and the emotions reach autonomic nuclei in the brain stem and spinal cord—notably the salivatory nuclei, the dorsal nucleus of the vagus nerve, and the intermediolateral cell column of the spinal cord. (The habenular nucleus and its connections are described with the epithalamus in Chapter 11.)

The **ventral tegmental nucleus** occupies the same position as the interstitial nucleus of Cajal (Fig. 9–4) but is caudal to the latter and at the same level as the dorsal tegmental nucleus. The ventral tegmental nucleus is a minor component of the reticular formation of the midbrain, and its principal connections are with the hypothalamus. Finally, the **nucleus of the posterior commissure** lies dorsal to the periaqueductal gray matter at the rostral limit of the midbrain. This nucleus adjoins the posterior commissure and is a relay nucleus on connections utilizing this commissure.

SUGGESTED READING

Brodal A: The Reticular Formation of the Brain Stem: Anatomical Aspects and Functional Correlations. Edinburgh, Oliver & Boyd, 1957

Brodal A: Neurological Anatomy, 2nd ed. London, Oxford University Press, 1969

Jasper HH, Proctor LD, Knighton RS, Noshay WC, Costello RT (eds): Reticular Formation of the Brain. Boston, Little, Brown, 1958

Magoun HW: The Waking Brain, 2nd ed. Springfield, IL, Thomas, 1969

Merrill EG: The lateral respiratory neurones of the medulla: their associations with nucleus ambiguus, nucleus retroambigualis, the spinal accessory nucleus and the spinal cord. Brain Res 24:11–28, 1970

Morest DK: A study of the structure of the area postrema with Golgi methods. Am J Anat 107:291–303, 1960

Moruzzi G: Active processes in the brain stem during sleep. Harvey Lect 58:233–297, 1963

Moruzzi G, Magoun HW: Brain stem reticular formation and activation of the EEG. Electroencephalogr Clin Neurophysiol 1:455–473, 1949

Nygren L-G, Olson L: A new major projection from locus coeruleus: the main source of noradrenergic nerve terminals in the ventral and dorsal columns of the spinal cord. Brain Res 132:85–93, 1977

Olson L, Fuxe K: On the projections from the locus coeruleus noradrenaline neurons: the cerebellar innervation. Brain Res 28:165–171, 1971

Ramón-Moliner E, Nauta WJH: The isodendritic core of the brain stem. J Comp Neurol 126:311–335, 1966

Rossi GF, Zanchetti A: The brain stem reticular formation: anatomy and physiology. Arch Ital Biol 95:199–435, 1957

10

Cerebellum

Although the cerebellum has an abundant input from sensory receptors it is essentially a motor part of the brain, functioning in the maintenance of equilibrium and coordination of muscle action in both stereotyped and nonstereotyped movements. The cerebellum makes a special contribution to synergy of muscle action, *i.e.*, to the synchronization of muscles that make up a functional group, ensuring that there is contraction of the right muscles at the right time. It follows that cerebellar lesions become manifest as disturbances of motor function without voluntary paralysis. The cerebellum increased in size in the course of vertebrate evolution. Maximal development is found in the human brain, man having a particular need for synergy of muscles in learned activities that require precision.

The cerebellum consists of 1) a **cortex** or surface layer of gray matter contained in transverse folds or folia; 2) a **medullary center** of white matter; and 3) four pairs of **central nuclei** embedded in the medullary center. The paired **inferior, middle,** and **superior cerebellar peduncles,** composed of nerve fibers, connect the cerebellum with the medulla, pons, and midbrain, respectively.

GROSS ANATOMY

The superior cerebellar surface is elevated in the midline, conforming to the dural reflection or tentorium that forms a roof for the posterior cranial fossa. The inferior surface is grooved deeply in the midline; the remainder of this surface is convex on each side and rests on the floor of the posterior cranial fossa (Fig. 10-1).

Certain terms are useful for identifying regions of the cerebellar surface. The region in and near the midline is known as the **vermis** and the remainder as the **hemispheres.** The superior vermis is not demarcated from the hemispheres, but the inferior vermis lies in a deep depression (the vallecula) and is well delineated.

Three major regions, called the flocculonodular, anterior, and posterior lobes, are recognized in the horizontal plane (Fig. 10-1). The **flocculonodular lobe** (or lobule) is a small component, and the oldest phylogenetically, at the rostral edge of the inferior surface. The nodule is the rostral portion of the inferior vermis, and the flocculi are irregular-shaped masses on each side. The cerebellum is deeply indented by several transverse fissures. The **posterolateral fissure** along the caudal border of the flocculonodular lobe is the first of these to appear during embryologic development. The main mass of the cerebellum, *i.e.*, all but the flocculonodular lobe, is called the **corpus cerebelli** and consists of anterior and posterior lobes. The **anterior lobe** is that part of the superior surface rostral to the **primary fissure,** this being the second fissure to appear during embryologic development. The remainder of the cerebellum on both surfaces constitutes the **posterior lobe.**

The roof of the rostral part of the fourth ventricle is formed by the superior cerebellar peduncles and the superior medullary velum bridging the interval between them (Fig. 10-2). The remainder of the roof consists of the thin inferior medullary velum, formed by pia mater and ependyma. This membrane, in which a deficiency constitutes the median aperture of the fourth ventricle or foramen of Magendie (Fig. 6-4), frequently adheres to the inferior vermis. The three pairs of peduncles are attached to the cerebellum in the interval between the flocculonodular and anterior lobes.

Fissures that need not be identified by

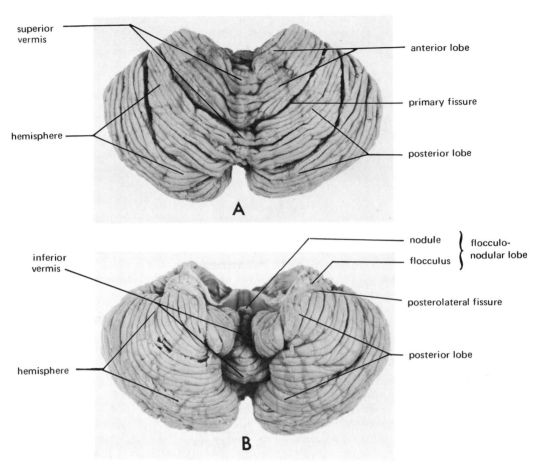

FIG. 10–1. **A.** Superior surface of the cerebellum. **B.** Inferior surface of the cerebellum. (× ⅔)

FIG. 10–2. Cerebellum viewed from in front and below, showing the cut surfaces of the cerebellar peduncles. (× ⅔)

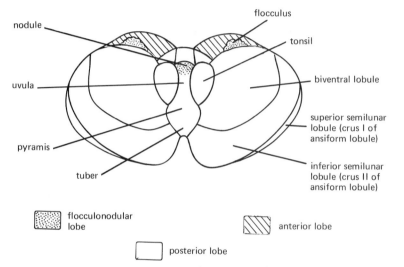

FIG. 10-3. Nomenclature for specific regions of the cerebellum.

name outline further subdivisions or lobules, especially in the posterior lobe. The names given to these lobules by early anatomists have no functional significance; neither is there uniform acceptance of a single system of nomenclature. Figure 10-3 is inserted for reference in the event that it is necessary to identify smaller subdivisions of the cerebellum. The lingula, not seen in Figure 10-3, is a small, flattened portion of the superior vermis beneath the central lobule and adherent to the superior medullary velum (Fig. 10-2).

The functional anatomy of the cerebellum is based primarily on the destination of different categories of afferent fibers. Viewed in this way there is a **vestibulocerebellum,** a **spinocerebellum,** and a **pontocerebellum.**

They are also called the **archicerebellum, paleocerebellum,** and **neocerebellum,** respectively, to signify the order of appearance in vertebrate evolution. The functional divisions are not reflected in corresponding differences in the cytoarchitecture of the cortex which, in fact, is the same in all parts of the cerebellum. The four central nuclei are likewise similar at the cellular level. The cortex and nuclei are therefore described at this point, after which the functional divisions will be considered.

CEREBELLAR CORTEX

Because of the extensive folding of the cerebellar surface in the form of thin transverse **folia,** 85% of the cortical surface is concealed. There is therefore a large cortical area, which is about three-quarters as extensive as that of the much larger cerebrum.

CORTICAL LAYERS

Three layers are evident in histologic sections. From the surface to the white matter of the folium, these are the molecular layer, the layer of Purkinje cells, and the granule cell layer (Figs. 10-4 and 10-5). The **Purkinje cell layer** consists of a single row (in sections) of bodies of Purkinje cells. The **molecular layer** contains relatively few nerve cells; it is largely a synaptic layer, made up of profusely branching dendrites of Purkinje cells and axons of the granule cells in the deepest layer. The term "molecular" is derived from the punctate appearance of this layer in sections stained for nerve fibers. The molecular layer includes scattered stellate cells near the surface and modified stellate cells, known as basket cells, at a deeper level. The **granule cell layer** consists of closely packed small neurons, from which axons extend into the molecular layer. There are scattered neurons known as Golgi cells in the outer zone of the granule cell layer.

There are two types of afferent fibers to the cortex. **Mossy fibers** terminate in synaptic contact with granule cells of the innermost layer, whereas **climbing fibers** enter the molecular layer and wind among the dendrites of Purkinje cells. The only fibers leaving the cortex are axons of Purkinje cells. These fibers terminate in central nuclei of the cerebellum, with the exception of some fibers from the cortex of the flocculonodular lobe that proceed to the brain stem.

CYTOARCHITECTURE

The five types of neuron in the cerebellar cortex establish a complex but remarkably regular pattern of intracortical circuits. The precise three-dimensional orientation of dendrites and axons, as shown by the Golgi staining method, has encouraged the study of cortical physiology at the cellular level by means of recording microelectrodes. The basic pattern of the neurons is indicated in Figure 10-6.

Granule Cells and Mossy Fibers

The granule cells are small and closely packed together in the deepest cortical layer.

Each cell has a spherical nucleus with a coarse chromatin pattern, and the scanty cytoplasm lacks clumps of Nissl substance. The short dendrites have claw-like endings which make synaptic contact with mossy fibers. The unmyelinated axon enters the molecular layer, where it bifurcates and runs parallel with the folium. Because of the density of the granule cell population, the whole of the molecular layer contains closely arranged parallel fibers. Each granule cell axon traverses the dendritic trees of some 450 Purkinje cells, with which it makes synaptic contacts. These axons also synapse with dendrites of stellate, basket, and Golgi cells in the molecular layer.

A large proportion of the afferent fibers to the cerebellum are mossy fibers terminating in synaptic relation with dendrites of granule cells. While still in the white matter, a mossy fiber divides into several branches which may enter the cortex of adjacent folia. On entering the granule cell layer, the fiber loses its myelin sheath and there is further terminal branching. Along the terminal portion of the fiber and at its end, there are swellings known as **rosettes,** with which the dendrites of several granule cells make synaptic contact (Fig. 10-7). The synaptic configuration that includes the rosette of a mossy fiber, dendrites of granule cells, and the axon of a Golgi cell (see Stellate and Golgi Cells) is known as a **glomerulus.**

Purkinje Cells and Climbing Fibers

Purkinje cells, the efferent cortical neurons, were described in Chapter 2 as an example of Golgi type I neurons. The number of Purkinje cells is of the order of 15 million. Their most remarkable characteristic is the profuse dendritic branching in the molecular layer, in a plane transverse to the folium. The primary and secondary branches are smooth, whereas the finer branches bear regularly spaced projections or spines, of which there are some 100,000 on each Purkinje cell dendrite. Electron micrographs show the spines indenting parallel fibers (axons of granule cells) to form synaptic junctions. The parallel arrangement of axons of granule cells and the transverse orientation of dendrites of Purkinje cells, with respect to a folium, provide maximal opportunity for a Purkinje cell to receive stimuli from a very large number of granule cells, and also allow a granule cell to contact

FIG. 10–4. Transverse section of cerebellar folia, showing the three layers of cortex and the white matter of the folia. (Cresyl violet stain, × 35)

FIG. 10–5. Transverse section of cerebellar folia, showing the three layers of cortex and the white matter of the folia. (Cajal silver nitrate method, × 35)

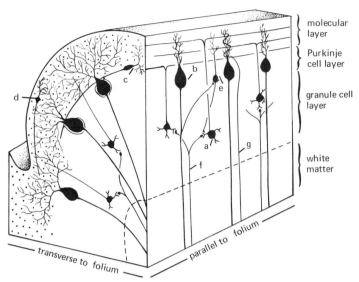

molecular
layer

Purkinje
cell layer

granule cell
layer

white
matter

transverse to folium

parallel to folium

FIG. 10-6. Cytoarchitecture of the cerebellar cortex. **a.** Granule cell; **b.** Purkinje cell; **c.** Basket cell; **d.** Stellate cell; **e.** Golgi cell; **f.** Mossy fiber; **g.** Climbing fiber.

about 450 Purkinje cells. The molecular layer is therefore a rich synaptic field, to which stellate, basket, and Golgi cells also contribute.

Axons of Purkinje cells traverse the granule cell layer, acquire myelin sheaths, and terminate in central cerebellar nuclei. Collateral branches given off by the axons synapse with adjacent Purkinje cells or, more frequently, with Golgi cells in the outer part of the granule cell layer.

As the mossy fibers have a special relationship with granule cells, so the climbing fibers have a special relationship with Purkinje cells. Climbing fibers enter the cortex from the medullary center, traverse the granule cell layer, and wind among the dendritic branches of Purkinje cells like a vine growing on a tree. Each climbing fiber makes synaptic contact with the smooth surface of the larger branches of a Purkinje cell dendrite. The synapse is excitatory, but the function of climbing fibers in a broader sense is still unknown. In addition, branches of climbing fibers synapse with stellate, basket, and Golgi cells. Although the sources of climbing fibers are perhaps not fully known, they are described as originating in the inferior olivary complex, the nuclei pontis, and the reticular formation of the brain stem.

Basket Cells

The basket cells are scattered in the molecular layer near the bodies of Purkinje cells. The dendrite of a basket cell branches in the transverse plane of the folium, making synaptic contact with many granule cell axons and also receiving stimuli from branches of climbing fibers. The axon of a basket cell is directed across the folium, and collateral branches form characteristic synapses with about 250 Purkinje cells. Each collateral branch forms a basketlike arrangement around the perikaryon of a Purkinje cell, the fibers concentrating around the origin of the Purkinje cell axon (Fig. 10-8). Because of an overlapping arrangement, collateral branches of several basket cell axons contribute to the synapse with a single Purkinje cell.

Stellate and Golgi Cells

The granule, Purkinje, and basket cells have special features, whereas the stellate and Golgi cells are similar to small neurons elsewhere in the nervous system.

There are scattered stellate cells in the superficial part of the molecular layer. Their dendrites are in contact with axons of granule cells and, to a lesser extent, with branches of climbing fibers. Axons of stellate cells synapse mainly with Purkinje cell dendrites; a few enter the innermost cortical layer and establish a feedback circuit by synapsing with granule cells. The Golgi cells are situ-

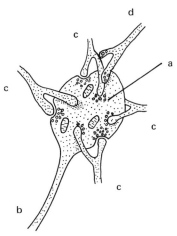

FIG. 10-7. A glomerulus in the granule cell layer. **a.** Rosette. **b.** Branch of a mossy fiber. **c.** Dendrites of granule cells. **d.** Axon of a Golgi cell.

ated in the outer portion of the granule cell layer; their dendrites extend into the molecular layer, where they make contact with parallel fibers. Other afferents to Golgi cells consist of collateral branches of Purkinje cell axons and branches of climbing fibers. Axons of Golgi cells enter glomeruli, where they synapse with the dendrites of granule cells (Fig. 10-7). In the main, therefore, Golgi cells form reverberating circuits with granule cells.

Intracortical Circuits

Recordings from microelectrodes inserted in the cerebellar cortex have yielded information about whether synapses between specific types of neurons produce an excitatory postsynaptic potential (EPSP) or an inhibitory postsynaptic potential (IPSP). These studies show that synapses between mossy fibers and granule cells, granule cells and Purkinje cells, and climbing fibers and Purkinje cells are all excitatory. The input to the cortex is therefore excitatory. However, this is modified by intracortical circuits that inhibit Purkinje cells and therefore suppress transmission from cortex to central nuclei. For example parallel fibers produce an EPSP in stellate and basket cells, but synapses between these and Purkinje cells produce an IPSP. Also parallel fibers excite Golgi cells, which inhibit granule cells. The inhibitory circuits include more synapses than the excitatory relays. Therefore afferent volleys to the cortex first produce an EPSP in Purkinje

cells, followed after 1-2 msec by an IPSP. The inhibitory circuits tend to limit the area of cortex excited and the degree of excitation resulting from an incoming volley.

CENTRAL NUCLEI

Four pairs of nuclei are embedded deep in the medullary center; in a medial to lateral direction they are the fastigial, globose, emboliform, and dentate nuclei (Fig. 10-9). The phylogenetic development of these nuclei was in the same order.

The **fastigial nucleus** is nearly spherical, close to the midline, and almost in contact with the roof of the fourth ventricle. The **globose nucleus** consists of two or three small cellular masses, and the larger **emboliform nucleus** is oval or plug-shaped. In mammals as high in the phylogenetic scale as the monkey, a single nucleus (the nucleus interpositus) is situated between the fastigial and dentate nuclei. In the highest primates,

FIG. 10-8. Cell body of a Purkinje cell situated between the molecular layer and the granule cell layer of the cerebellar cortex. The fibers surrounding the Purkinje cell body consist mainly of terminal branches of basket cell axons. (Cajal silver nitrate method, × 450)

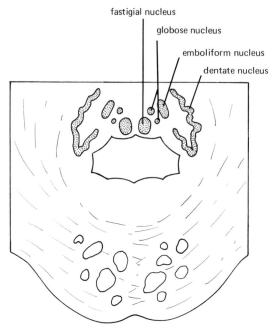

fastigial nucleus
globose nucleus
emboliform nucleus
dentate nucleus

FIG. 10–9. Central nuclei of the cerebellum.

including man, the nucleus interpositus is represented by the globose and emboliform nuclei. The **dentate nucleus** is the most prominent of the central nuclei; this mammalian nucleus is largest in primates, especially in man. The dentate nucleus has the irregular shape of a crumpled purse, like that of the inferior olivary nucleus, with the hilus facing medially. Its efferent fibers occupy the interior of the nucleus and leave through the hilus.

The input to the cerebellar nuclei is from two sources, the first being extracerebellar and the second from the Purkinje cells of the cerebellar cortex. The extrinsic input is still under investigation. Pontocerebellar and spinocerebellar fibers appear to be important, and some olivocerebellar fibers and fibers from the lateral reticular nucleus in the medulla end in the cerebellar nuclei. Some of these afferents are collateral branches of fibers proceeding to the cerebellar cortex. A few rubrocerebellar fibers end in the globose and emboliform nuclei, and the fastigial nucleus receives afferents from the vestibular nerve and nuclei. The fastigial nucleus discharges to the brain stem through the inferior cerebellar peduncle, whereas efferents from the remaining nuclei leave the cerebellum

through the superior peduncle, most of them terminating in the red nucleus and the thalamus.

Physiologic studies indicate that Purkinje cells inhibit neurons in the central nuclei and that the input from outside the cerebellum is excitatory. Crudely processed information in the central nuclei is infinitely refined by impulses received from the cortex. The combination of the two inputs maintains a tonic discharge from the central nuclei to the brain stem and thalamus. This discharge changes constantly according to the afferent input to the cerebellum at any given time.

MEDULLARY CENTER AND CEREBELLAR PEDUNCLES

The white matter is scanty in the region of the vermis, where it produces a branching, treelike pattern in a sagittal section (Fig. 10–10). Each hemisphere, however, contains a large medullary center in which the dentate nucleus is embedded (Fig. 10–11). This white matter consists of afferent fibers to the cortex, axons of Purkinje cells proceeding to the central nuclei, and efferent fibers of the nuclei. The afferent and efferent systems are discussed in connection with the functional divisions of the cerebellum. They are identified at this point only as components of the cerebellar peduncles.

The **inferior cerebellar peduncle** consists of two parts; the larger part is called the **restiform body,** on the medial side of which lies the **juxtarestiform body** (Fig. 7–8). The restiform body consists entirely of fibers entering the cerebellum, the largest component being those originating in the inferior olivary complex. The other components are the dorsal spinocerebellar tract and fibers from the lateral cuneate nucleus, the arcuate nucleus, the nucleus of the spinal tract of the trigeminal nerve, and the reticular formation in the medulla. The juxtarestiform body contains both afferent and efferent fibers with respect to the cerebellum. The afferent fibers come from the vestibular nuclei and vestibular nerve, and the efferent fibers proceed from the flocculonodular lobe and fastigial nucleus to the vestibular nuclei and the reticular formation in the medulla and pons.

The **middle cerebellar peduncle** or **brachium pontis** consists entirely of pontocere-

FIG. 10–10. Cerebellar surface in the median plane. The cut surface has been stained by a method which differentiates gray matter and white matter. (× 1½)

FIG. 10–11. Cerebellar surface in a sagittal plane through the hemisphere, stained to differentiate gray matter and white matter. The dentate nucleus is shown embedded in the medullary center of white matter. (× 1½)

bellar fibers. The **superior cerebellar peduncle** consists mainly of the **brachium conjunctivum,** which is made up of efferent fibers from the globose, emboliform, and dentate nuclei. The other components of the superior peduncle are afferent to the cerebellum. They include the ventral spinocerebellar tract on the dorsolateral surface of the brachium conjunctivum (Fig. 7–11), a small contingent of rubrocerebellar fibers, and fibers from the mesencephalic nucleus of the trigeminal nerve. There are also tectocerebellar fibers from the inferior colliculi, but most of these reach the cerebellum by running in the superior medullary velum.

FUNCTIONAL ANATOMY

Three functional divisions are recognized on the basis of the termination of afferent systems in the cortex and the sequence of phylogenetic development. The **vestibulocerebellum** or **archicerebellum** is the oldest part, constituting the entire cerebellum of fishes; it is concerned with maintenance of equilibrium. The **spinocerebellum** or **paleocerebellum** appeared next and is present in submammalian terrestrial vertebrates. In general the paleocerebellum influences muscle tonus and synergy of muscles during stereotyped movements such as those of postural changes and locomotion. A **pontocerebellum** or **neocerebellum** was added in mammals and is the largest part of the human cerebellum. Neocerebellar activity ensures the synergy and delicate adjustments of muscle tonus that are necessary for accuracy of nonstereotyped movements, especially those based on learning experience. The three divisions overlap to some extent in both the cortex and the central nuclei.

The following generalizations may be helpful as a background for the discussion of functional divisions. Firstly, olivocerebellar fibers are distributed to all parts of the cortex; the accessory olivary nuclei project to the flocculonodular lobe and vermis, and the inferior olivary nuclei to the hemispheres. The second generalization is concerned with the termination of Purkinje cells in the central nuclei. The cortex of the flocculus and vermis sends fibers to the fastigial nucleus; the cortex of the medial portion of the hemisphere (paravermal or intermediate zone) projects

on the globose and emboliform nuclei; and the large lateral region of hemispheral cortex sends fibers to the dentate nucleus.

ARCHICEREBELLUM

The archicerebellum (vestibulocerebellum) consists of the flocculonodular lobe, together with a region of the inferior vermis adjacent to the nodule known as the uvula (Figs. 10–3 and 10–12). A few vestibular fibers end in other parts of the vermis, so that archicerebellar and paleocerebellar areas partially overlap. Afferent impulses originate in the vestibular portion of the internal ear and are conveyed centrally by the vestibular nerve. Some fibers of the nerve enter the cerebellum, but these are outnumbered by indirect vestibular afferents from vestibular nuclei. The afferent fibers, which are included in the juxtarestiform body of the inferior cerebellar peduncle, terminate in the archicerebellar cortex and the fastigial nucleus.

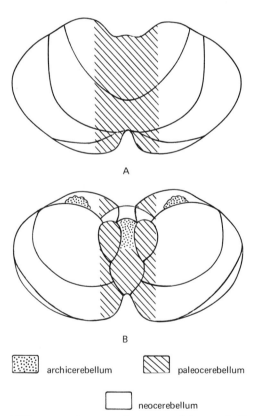

A

B

archicerebellum   paleocerebellum

neocerebellum

FIG. 10–12. Functional regions of the cerebellum. **A.** Superior surface. **B.** Inferior surface.

A proportion of Purkinje cell axons from archicerebellar cortex proceed to the brain stem (an exception to the general rule that such fibers end in central nuclei), and the remainder terminate in the fastigial nucleus. Fibers from the cortex and the fastigial nucleus traverse the juxtarestiform body to their termination in the vestibular nuclear complex and reticular formation of the medulla and pons. A bundle of fastigiobulbar fibers, known as the **uncinate fasciculus** (of Russell), has an aberrant course; the fasciculus curves over the root of the superior cerebellar peduncle and then joins the other efferent fibers of the archicerebellum in the juxtarestiform body of the inferior peduncle.

The archicerebellum influences lower motor neurons through the vestibulospinal tract, the medial longitudinal fasciculus, and reticulospinal fibers. It is concerned, as previously stated, with adjustment of muscle tonus in response to vestibular stimuli, and hence functions in maintaining equilibrium and in other motor responses to vestibular stimulation (see Chapter 22).

PALEOCEREBELLUM

The paleocerebellum (spinocerebellum) is defined as the portion receiving data from general sensory receptors, mainly through ascending fasciculi of the spinal cord. The area has been delineated in experimental animals, including the monkey, by establishing the course and termination of afferent fibers by neuroanatomic methods and by recording evoked potentials in the cortex during peripheral nerve stimulation. From these studies, with some supporting evidence for man, the paleocerebellum is considered to consist of the superior vermis, most of the inferior vermis, and the paravermal or intermediate zones on the superior and inferior surfaces of the hemispheres (Fig. 10–12).

The following afferent systems project specifically to paleocerebellar cortex. The dorsal and ventral spinocerebellar tracts convey data from proprioceptive endings and from touch and pressure receptors. The dorsal tract conveys information from the arm, trunk, and leg, whereas the ventral tract is involved mainly in conduction from the leg. Cuneocerebellar fibers from the lateral cuneate nucleus reinforce the dorsal spinocerebellar tract for conduction from the arm, and they constitute the main pathway for impulses originating in deep and cutaneous receptors in the neck. Data from cutaneous receptors are also carried by spinoreticular fibers to the lateral reticular nucleus, from which fibers project to the paleocerebellar cortex. Finally, the paleocerebellum receives fibers from sensory nuclei of the trigeminal nerve.

Each half of the body is represented in the ipsilateral cortex; if fibers cross the midline from cells of origin at lower levels, they cross again in the medullary center of the cerebellum. Studies in the monkey show a dual somatotopic representation, with one area on the superior surface and the other area on the inferior surface. The paleocerebellum also receives some pontocerebellar fibers, so that in this respect there is an overlap between paleocerebellum and neocerebellum. The principle underlying cerebellar cortical localization is not so much punctate topography, as in some areas of the cerebral cortex, but rather a localization that is in line with the computing function of the cerebellar cortex. Consistent with this there is an overlap of different inputs so that their influence is brought to bear on the same Purkinje cells.

The paleocerebellar cortex projects on the fastigial nucleus (from the vermis) and on the globose and emboliform nuclei (from the paravermal zone or medial portion of the hemisphere). Synergy of muscle action and control of muscle tonus are effected in part through fastigiobulbar connections, as described for the archicerebellum. Fibers from the globose and emboliform nuclei traverse the brachium conjunctivum and terminate in the red nucleus. Through this connection paleocerebellar activity is brought to bear on lower motor neurons by means of the rubrospinal tract, rubroreticular and reticulospinal fibers, and fibers from the red nucleus to motor nuclei of cranial nerves. The influence of the paleocerebellum on skeletal musculature is ipsilateral. For example the right half of the paleocerebellar cortical area, which receives sensory data from the right side of the body, influences lower motor neurons for right-sided muscles through compensating decussations, that of the brachium conjunctivum and the decussation of rubrospinal and rubroreticular fibers. Alpha and gamma motor neurons are both involved in the cerebellar control of muscle action.

Before reaching the red nucleus, some cerebellorubral fibers give off collateral branches which run caudally in the brain stem and end in the reticular formation, including the paramedian reticular nucleus of the medulla. These collaterals participate in feedback circuits between the brain stem and the cerebellum, and in a projection to lower motor neurons through reticulospinal connections.

In summary, the paleocerebellum receives information from proprioceptive endings and from exteroceptors for touch and pressure. Data thus received are processed by the computerlike circuitry of the cerebellar cortex and modify the discharge of nerve impulses from the central nuclei. Lower motor neurons are influenced through relays in the vestibular nuclei, the red nucleus, and the reticular formation. The end result is control of muscle tonus and synergy of collaborating muscles, as appropriate at any moment according to changes of posture and in many types of movement, including those of locomotion.

NEOCEREBELLUM

Pontocerebellar fibers constitute the whole of the middle cerebellar peduncle or brachium pontis. Originating in the nuclei pontis of the opposite side, these fibers are distributed throughout the cortex of the corpus cerebelli, i.e., to all of the cortex except that of the flocculonodular lobe. However, the greatest concentration of input from the nuclei pontis is to the large portions of the hemispheres that make up the neocerebellum (pontocerebellum) (Fig. 10–12). Through corticopontine tracts originating in widespread areas of the contralateral cerebral cortex (especially that of the frontal and parietal lobes) and the pontocerebellar projection, the cortex of a cerebellar hemisphere receives information concerning volitional movements which are about to take place or are in progress. As stated previously the inferior olivary complex projects to the cerebellar cortex generally, with fibers from the large principal nucleus being distributed to neocerebellar cortex.

Purkinje cell axons from the neocerebellar cortex terminate in the dentate nucleus, the efferent fibers of which make up most of the brachium conjunctivum. After traversing the decussation of the brachium conjunctivum, some of these fibers terminate in the red nucleus, from which impulses reach lower motor neurons. The majority, however, pass through or around the red nucleus, continuing forward to a thalamic relay nucleus (ventral lateral nucleus) which in turn projects to motor areas of cortex in the frontal lobe. These areas are an important source of pyramidal and extrapyramidal motor fibers. On entering the midbrain, some fibers originating in the dentate nucleus, and the globose and emboliform nuclei as well, give off collateral branches which end in the inferior olivary complex.

The neocerebellum may be thought of as a biologic computer which is especially well developed in man and designed for the refinement of voluntary movements. Data received from the cerebral cortex and other sources are subjected to a complex computerization in the neocerebellar cortex. The output from the dentate nuclei, which reaches motor areas of the cerebral cortex via the thalamus, constantly fluctuates according to the excitatory input to the dentate nuclei from extracerebellar sources and the all important refinement of discharge of the neurons comprising these nuclei by the inhibitory influence of Purkinje cells. The neocerebellum thereby ensures a smooth and orderly sequence of muscular contractions and the intended precision in the force, direction, and extent of volitional movements. A cerebellar hemisphere influences the musculature of the same side of the body because of the following compensating decussations: 1) the decussation of the brachia conjunctiva, and 2) the decussation of the corticospinal tracts and extrapyramidal motor pathways.

ADDITIONAL CEREBELLAR CONNECTIONS

Laboratory studies, including research using monkeys, show that impulses of acoustic and visual origin reach the cerebellar cortex. The area concerned is in the posterior part of the superior and inferior surfaces, including paleocerebellar cortex and the medial part of the neocerebellar cortex. There are two projections from the tectum of the midbrain to the cerebellum: tectocerebellar fibers in the superior medullary velum, and tectopontine and pontocerebellar fibers. The relay for the latter pathway is in the dorsolateral region of the nuclei pontis. There is evidence that the tectocerebellar fibers originate in the inferior colliculus and therefore convey acoustic data, and that the tectopontine fibers transmit visual data from the superior colliculus. Although a large proportion of corticopontine fibers originate in association areas of the cerebral cortex, there is an important contribution from primary cortical areas. It has been shown, again experimentally, that impulses from the visual and auditory areas reach the visuo-auditory area of cerebellar cortex, and that impulses from the somesthetic and motor areas reach paleocerebellar cortex.

Animal experiments also indicate that the cerebellum has a role in visceral functions. Under certain conditions electrical stimulation of paleocerebellar cortex produces respiratory, cardiovascular, pupillary, and urinary bladder responses. They are sympathetic in nature when the anterior lobe is stimulated and parasympathetic when the tonsils (Fig. 10–3) of the posterior lobe are stimulated. The pathways have not been identified with certainty, but it has been suggested that impulses are relayed to the hypothalamus through the reticular formation of the brain stem.

SIGNS OF CEREBELLAR DYSFUNCTION

Cerebellar disorders resulting from vascular occlusion, tumor growth, or other pathologic conditions are classified broadly into those affecting the vestibulocerebellum (flocculonodular lobe) and those affecting the main mass of the cerebellum (corpus cerebelli).

The vestibular portion of the cerebellum may be invaded by a tumor, typically a medulloblastoma occurring in childhood, and the resulting disorder of cerebellar function is known as the **archicerebellar syndrome.** The patient is unsteady, walks on a wide base, and sways from side to side. The signs are limited at first to a disturbance of equilibrium; reflexes and voluntary movements are not otherwise affected. However, additional cerebellar signs may appear if the tumor invades other parts of the cerebellum.

With respect to the corpus cerebelli, signs of cerebellar dysfunction accompany lesions that interrupt afferent pathways, cause destruction of the cortex and medullary center, or involve the central nuclei and efferent pathways in the brachium conjunctivum. There is considerable recovery with time because of compensation by intact regions and other motor systems. The motor disorder is more severe and more enduring when a lesion involves the central nuclei or the brachium conjunctivum. The signs of destructive lesions of the corpus cerebelli or its major afferent and efferent pathways are commonly referred to as the **neocerebellar syndrome,** although in many instances the paleocerebellum is also involved. When the lesion is unilateral, which is most frequently the case, the signs of motor dysfunction are on the same side of the body as the lesion. This follows from the compensating decussations that were just pointed out.

The following signs, in varying degrees of severity, are characteristic of the neocerebellar syndrome. Movements tend to be **ataxic** (intermittent or jerky). There is also **dysmetria;** for example, when reaching out with the finger to an object, the finger overshoots the mark or deviates from it **(past-pointing).** Rapidly alternating movements such as flexion and extension of the fingers or pronation and supination of the forearms are performed in a clumsy manner **(adiadochokinesia). Asynergy** is reflected in separation of voluntary movements that normally flow smoothly in sequence into a succession of mechanical or puppetlike movements **(decomposition of movements).** There may be **hypotonia of muscles,** and the muscles tend to tire easily. Cerebellar tremor is characteristically terminal, occurring at the end of a particular movement **(intention tremor).** Asynergy may involve muscles used in speech, which is then thick and monotonous. There may be **nystagmus,** especially if the lesion encroaches on the vermis, because of involvement of projections to the oculomotor, trochlear, and abducens nuclei via the vestibular nuclei and the red nucleus. The deficits noted are entirely motor and superimposed on volitional movements which are themselves basically intact.

SUGGESTED READING

Bloomfield S, Marr D: How the cerebellum may be used. Nature 227:1224–1228, 1970

Braitenberg V, Atwood RP: Morphological observations on the cerebellar cortex. J Comp Neurol 109:1–33, 1958

Carpenter MB: Human Neuroanatomy, 7th ed. Baltimore, Williams & Wilkins, 1976

Carpenter MB, Stevens GH: Structural and functional relationships between the deep cerebellar nuclei and the brachium conjunctivum in the rhesus monkey. J Comp Neurol 107:109–163, 1957

Courville J, Cooper CW: The cerebellar nuclei of Macaca mulatta: a morphological study. J Comp Neurol 140:241–254, 1970

Eccles JC: The dynamic loop hypothesis of movement control. In Leibovic KN (ed): Information Processing in the Nervous System. New York, Springer-Verlag, 1969, pp 245–269

Eccles JC, Ito M, Szentágothai J: The Cerebellum as a Neuronal Machine. New York, Springer, 1967

Evarts EV, Thach WT: Motor mechanisms of the CNS: cerebrocerebellar interrelations. Ann Rev Physiol 31:451–498, 1969

Flumerfelt BA, Otabe S, Courville J: Distinct projections to the red nucleus from the dentate and interposed nuclei in the monkey. Brain Res 50:408–414, 1973

Fox CA, Barnard JW: A quantitative study of the Purkinje cell dendritic branchlets and their relationship to afferent fibers. J Anat 91:299–313, 1957

Fox CA, Snider RS (eds): The cerebellum. Progr Brain Res 25:1–355, 1967

Gilbert PFC: A theory of memory that explains the function and structure of the cerebellum. Brain Res 70:1–18, 1974

Gray EG: The granule cells, mossy synapses and Purkinje spine synapses of the cerebellum: light and electron microscope observations. J Anat 95:345–356, 1961

Holmes G: The cerebellum of man. Brain 62:1–30, 1939

Koella WP: Some functional properties of optically evoked potentials in the cerebellar cortex of cats. J Neurophysiol 22:61–77, 1959

Meyer-Lohmann J, Hore J, Brooks VB: Cerebellar participation in generation of prompt arm movements. J Neurophysiol 40:1038–1050, 1977

Murphy MG, O'Leary JL, Cornblath D: Axoplasmic flow in cerebellar mossy and climbing fibers. Arch Neurol 28:118–123, 1973

Oscarsson O: Functional organization of spinocerebellar paths. In Iggo A (ed): Handbook of Sensory Physiology, II. Somatosensory System. New York, Springer-Verlag, 1973, pp 339–380

Rivera-Dominguez M, Mettler FA, Noback CR: Origin of cerebellar climbing fibers in the Rhesus monkey. J Comp Neurol 155:331–342, 1974

Snider RS: The cerebellum. Sci Am 199/2:84–90, 1958

Snider RS, Eldred E: Cerebro-cerebellar relationships in the monkey. J Neurophysiol 15:27–40, 1952

11

Diencephalon

The diencephalon and telencephalon together constitute the cerebrum, of which the diencephalon forms the central core and the telencephalon the cerebral hemispheres. Being almost entirely surrounded by the hemispheres, only the ventral surface of the diencephalon is exposed to view in a diamond-shaped area containing hypothalamic structures (Fig. 11–1). This area is bounded in front by the optic chiasma, and on each side by the optic tract and the region of continuity between the internal capsule and the basis pedunculi of the midbrain. The diencephalon is divided into symmetrical halves by the slitlike third ventricle. As seen in a median section (Fig. 11–2), the junction of the midbrain and diencephalon is represented by a line passing through the posterior commissure and immediately caudal to the mammillary body. The boundary between the diencephalon and the telencephalon is represented by a line traversing the interventricular foramen (foramen of Monro) and the optic chiasma.

GROSS FEATURES

SURFACES OF THE DIENCEPHALON

The surfaces of each half of the diencephalon have the following landmarks and relations. The **medial surface** forms the wall of the third ventricle (Fig. 11–2). A bundle of nerve fibers called the stria medullaris thalami forms an elevation along the junction of the medial and dorsal surfaces. The ependymal lining of the third ventricle is reflected from one side to the other along the striae medullares, forming the roof of the ventricle from which a small choroid plexus is suspended.

The **dorsal surface** is largely concealed by the fornix (Fig. 11–3); this robust bundle of

fibers originates in the hippocampus of the temporal lobe, curves over the thalamus, and ends mainly in the mammillary body. The fornices outline a triangular interval posteriorly which constitutes a rostral extension of the **transverse cerebral fissure** into the cerebrum, the remaining part of the fissure intervening between the cerebellum and the cerebral hemispheres. Between the fornices, the transverse fissure is roofed over by the corpus callosum, its floor being formed by a small area of the diencephalon and the roof of the third ventricle. The vascular connective tissue occupying the space just delineated is known as the **tela choroidea** and is continuous with the vascular core of the choroid plexuses of the lateral ventricles and the third ventricle. Lateral to the fornix, the dorsal surface of the thalamus forms the floor of the central portion of the lateral ventricle, much of which is concealed by the choroid plexus (Fig. 11–3).

The **lateral surface** is bounded by the thick internal capsule of white matter, consisting of fibers connecting the cerebral cortex with the thalamus and other parts of the central nervous system. The medial part of the **ventral surface** presents to the surface of the brain, as noted, and the lateral part is bounded by the internal capsule in the region of its continuity with the basis pedunculi of the midbrain.

MAJOR COMPONENTS OF THE DIENCEPHALON

The diencephalon consists of four components or regions on each side, named the thalamus, subthalamus, epithalamus, and hypothalamus. The **thalamus,** by far the largest component, is subdivided into several nuclei on the basis of fiber connections and the sequence of phylogenetic development. Cer-

141

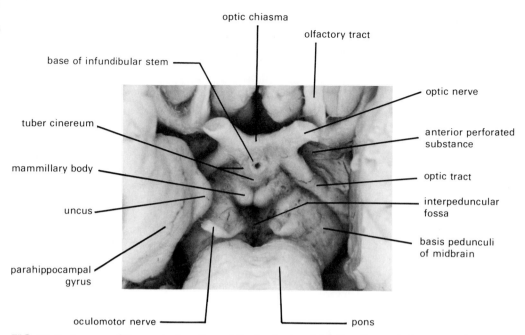

base of infundibular stem

optic chiasma

olfactory tract

optic nerve

tuber cinereum

anterior perforated substance

mammillary body

optic tract

uncus

interpeduncular fossa

parahippocampal gyrus

basis pedunculi of midbrain

oculomotor nerve

pons

FIG. 11-1. An area of the ventral surface of the brain, in which the diencephalon presents to the surface. (× 1½)

FIG. 11-2. Central region of the brain in median section. (× 1¼)

corpus callosum

fornix

septum pellucidum

cingulate gyrus

stria medullaris thalami

interventricu foramen

habenular commissure

anterior commissure

pineal gland

posterior commissure

medial olfac (septal) area

tectum of midbrain

lamina term

cerebral aqueduct

optic recess

optic chiasm

cerebral peduncle of midbrain

pons

median eminence

hypothalamic sulcus

tuber cinereum

mammillary body

FIG. 11-3. Dorsal aspect of the diencephalon, with the fornix and the choroid plexus removed on the right side. (× 1)

tain thalamic nuclei receive specific sensory input for the general senses, vision, and hearing; these nuclei project to corresponding sensory areas of the cerebral cortex. Other thalamic nuclei participate in emotional aspects of brain function, are functionally related to motor and association areas of cortex, or have a role in the ascending reticular activating system. The **subthalamus** is a complex region ventral to the thalamus; it includes a nucleus with motor functions (the subthalamic nucleus), sensory tracts terminating in the thalamus, and bundles of fibers proceeding from the cerebellum and corpus striatum to the thalamus. The reticular formation, red nucleus, and substantia nigra extend from the midbrain into the subthalamus. The **epithalamus,** situated dorsomedial to the thalamus and adjacent to the roof of the third ventricle, is a particularly old part of the diencephalon phylogenetically. It includes an endocrine organ (the pineal gland) and structures concerned with autonomic responses to olfactory stimuli and emotional changes. The **hypothalamus** occu-

pies the region between the third ventricle and the subthalamus; it is the main cerebral center for integrative control of the autonomic nervous system.

THALAMUS

The thalamus, measuring about 3 cm anteroposteriorly and 1.5 cm in the other two directions, makes up four-fifths of the diencephalon. Thin laminae of white matter outline the thalamus; the **stratum zonale** on the dorsal surface, best developed anteriorly (Fig. 11-11), is one such sheet of nerve fibers. The **external medullary lamina** is a thin layer of nerve fibers covering the lateral surface of the thalamus (Fig. 11-8). It consists of thalamocortical and corticothalamic fibers running along the surface of the thalamus briefly before entering or leaving the internal capsule. The external medullary lamina and internal capsule are separated by an attenuated layer of nerve cells constituting the reticular nucleus of the thalamus.

The **internal medullary lamina** (Figs. 11-4B and 11-8), consisting mainly of fibers passing from one thalamic nucleus to another, divides the thalamus into three gray masses. These are the lateral nuclear mass, the medial nucleus, and the anterior nucleus, the last named being enclosed by a bifurcation of the lamina. The lateral nuclear mass consists of ventral and dorsal tiers of nuclei which have been identified because of differing fiber connections (Fig. 11-4). Five nuclei are recognized in the ventral tier—the medial and lateral geniculate nuclei, and the ventral posterior, ventral lateral, and ventral anterior nuclei. (Alternatively the geniculate nuclei are described as composing the metathalamus.) The dorsal tier consists of the pulvinar, lateral posterior nucleus, and lateral dorsal nucleus. In the central part of the thalamus, the internal medullary lamina partially encloses the intralaminar nuclei, including the well-developed centromedian nucleus (Fig. 11-4C). The midline nucleus lies between the medial nucleus and the third ventricle.

On the basis of phylogeny, connections with other parts of the brain, and function, the thalamic nuclei may be classified according to the following scheme.

1. Reticular nucleus, which receives collateral branches of thalamocortical and corticothalamic fibers.

2. Midline and intralaminar nuclei, which receive afferents from the reticular formation of the brain stem and project mainly to other parts of the diencephalon.

3. Specific thalamic nuclei, comprising the ventral tier of the lateral nuclear mass and sending fibers to sensory and motor areas of cortex. The medial geniculate nucleus (hearing), lateral geniculate nucleus (vision), and ventral posterior nucleus (general sensations) are specific sensory nuclei. The ventral lateral nucleus and the ventral anterior nucleus are specific motor nuclei, in the sense that they receive data from the cerebellum, corpus striatum, and substantia nigra, and project to motor areas of cortex in the frontal lobe.

4. Nonspecific thalamic nuclei, which have reciprocal connections with association areas of cortex. This group includes the medial nucleus and the dorsal tier of the lateral nuclear mass, i.e., the pulvinar, lateral posterior nucleus, and lateral dorsal nucleus. The anterior nucleus is included conventionally under this heading, even though it is a thalamic component of the limbic system of the brain.

RETICULAR NUCLEUS

As noted already, the reticular nucleus consists of a thin sheet of nerve cells between the external medullary lamina and the internal capsule (Fig. 11-8). It has been considered as a final link on the pathway of the ascending reticular activating system to the cerebral cortex. However, more recent work indicates that the reticular nucleus does not project to the cortex. Instead axons of cells comprising the nucleus terminate in various parts of the thalamus, and the nucleus receives collateral branches of thalamocortical and corticothalamic fibers. The role of the reticular nucleus seems therefore to modify, in some as yet obscure way, neuronal activity in the thalamus.

MIDLINE AND INTRALAMINAR NUCLEI

Midline Nucleus

The **hypothalamic sulcus,** running from the interventricular foramen (foramen of Monro) to the opening of the cerebral aqueduct (Fig. 11-2), divides the wall of the third ventricle into thalamic and hypothalamic regions. The midline nucleus consists of clusters of nerve cells adjacent to the third ventricle, above the hypothalamic sulcus. The nucleus is prominent in lower vertebrates, but a minor part of the human thalamus. In 70% of brains the **massa intermedia** (interthalamic adhesion) forms a bridge of gray matter across the third ventricle and constitutes part of this primitive nuclear complex (Fig. 11-9).

The midline thalamic nucleus receives sensory data, notably from viscera and taste buds, through the polysynaptic pathway provided by the reticular formation of the brain stem. Unmyelinated and thinly myelinated fibers pass from the nucleus to the hypothalamus for autonomic responses. The midline nucleus also has connections with the medial and intralaminar nuclei of the thalamus, thereby participating in affective responses and the ascending activating system.

Intralaminar Nuclei

There are several nuclei, known collectively as intralaminar nuclei, in the region of the internal medullary lamina and partly surrounded by the lamina. Of these the **centro-**

Lateral View

Dorsal view

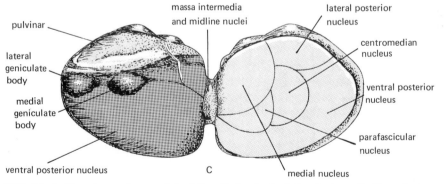

Posterior View
with right thalamus
seen in section.

FIG. 11–4. Drawings of a model of the thalami. **A.** Lateral view. **B.** Dorsal view. **C.** Posterior view with the posterior part of the right thalamus cut away. (Model prepared by Dr. D. G. Montemurro)

median nucleus is especially well represented in anthropoid apes and man (Figs. 11-4C and 11-6). A smaller **parafascicular nucleus** lies adjacent to the habenulointerpeduncular fasciculus; other intralaminar nuclei are too small in man to merit consideration.

The intralaminar nuclei receive afferents from the reticular formation of the brain stem, through which data from most of the sensory systems are relayed. Some spinothalamic and trigeminothalamic fibers also terminate in the intralaminar nuclei, although most of these fibers have the ventral posterior nucleus as their destination. Although some fibers from the intralaminar nuclei pass directly to the cerebral cortex, the main projection is to surrounding parts of the thalamus, i.e., to the lateral nuclear mass and the medial and anterior nuclei, which in turn project to widespread areas of cortex. This is the anatomic basis for the important effect of the reticular system on levels of consciousness and degrees of alertness. It also provides for vague awareness of sensory stimulation without specificity or discriminative qualities, but with emotional responses, especially to painful stimuli. The intralaminar nuclei, through thalamic nuclei having abundant cortical projections, constitute the key generator of much of the synchronized activity of the cerebral cortex, as shown in the electroencephalogram. The intralaminar nuclei are among the thalamic nuclei sending fibers to the corpus striatum.

Destruction of the intralaminar nuclei results in lethargy, somnolence, and diminished responses to sensory stimulation. An electrolytic lesion placed in the nuclei is reported to be effective in relief of intractable pain.

SPECIFIC THALAMIC NUCLEI

Medial Geniculate Nucleus

This nucleus on the auditory pathway forms a swelling (the medial geniculate body) on the posterior surface of the thalamus beneath the pulvinar (Figs. 7-14, 7-15, and 11-4). Afferent fibers to the medial geniculate nucleus constitute the inferior brachium coming from the inferior colliculus, which is the terminus of the lateral lemniscus. The nucleus receives data from the spiral organ (organ of Corti) of both sides, but predominantly from the opposite ear. This bilateral projection stems from the presence of a few ipsilateral fibers in the lateral lemniscus and decussating fibers in the commissure of the inferior colliculus. There is a topographic pattern in the medial geniculate nucleus with respect to pitch; the pattern simulates a spiral, corresponding to the configuration of the organ of Corti.

Fibers from the medial geniculate nucleus constitute the auditory radiation, which terminates in the auditory area of the temporal lobe (Fig. 11-12). Experimental evidence suggests that there is a general awareness of sounds at the thalamic level in subprimates and perhaps minimally in primates. With this possible exception, awareness of sounds is a function of the auditory cortex, and adjacent association cortex provides for discriminative aspects of hearing and recognition on the basis of past experience.

Lateral Geniculate Nucleus

The lateral geniculate body beneath the pulvinar marks the position of the lateral geniculate nucleus on the visual pathway to the cerebral cortex (Figs. 11-4 and 11-6). The nucleus consists of six layers of nerve cells, numbered consecutively from its ventral surface. Layers 1 and 2 consist of large neurons, whereas layers 3 through 6 are made up of small cells. The lateral geniculate nucleus is the terminus of all but a few of the fibers of the optic tract. The fibers originate in the ganglion cell layer of the retina; they are divided equally between those coming from the lateral half of the ipsilateral eye and from the medial half of the contralateral eye, the latter fibers having crossed the midline in the optic chiasma. Each nucleus therefore receives impulses related to the opposite field of vision. The crossed fibers terminate in layers 1, 4, and 6, and the uncrossed fibers end in layers 2, 3, and 5.

There is a detailed point-to-point projection of the retina on the lateral geniculate nucleus. In a more general way the superior retinal quadrants project to the medial portion of the nucleus, the inferior quadrants to the lateral portion, and the macular region for central vision to the posterior part of the nucleus. Axons of cells in the lateral geniculate nucleus constitute the geniculocalcarine tract, which terminates in the visual area of the occipital lobe adjacent to the calcarine sulcus (Fig. 11-12). At this site, and in the

6   7   8   9 10 11

Chap. 11

FIG. 11-5. Key to levels of Figures 11-6 through 11-11.

surrounding association cortex, there is awareness of visual stimuli, accompanied by discriminative and mnemonic aspects of vision.

Ventral Posterior Nucleus

The ventral posterior nucleus (Figs. 11-4, 11-6, and 11-7) functions as a thalamic relay nucleus for general sensations. The lateral and ventral spinothalamic tracts, the medial lemniscus, and the trigeminothalamic tracts all terminate in this nucleus. Fibers are also received from the gustatory nucleus in the brain stem, consisting of the rostral part of the nucleus of the tractus solitarius, and from the vestibular nuclear complex.

There is a detailed topographic projection of the opposite half of the body on the ventral posterior nucleus. The lower limb is represented in the dorsolateral part of the nucleus, the upper limb in an intermediate position, and the head most medially. The medial region receiving sensory data from the head is usually referred to as the **ventral posteromedial nucleus** (VPM), and the larger lateral portion for the remainder of the body

as the **ventral posterolateral nucleus** (VPL). The former is sometimes called the semilunar or arcuate nucleus because it conforms to the shape of the adjacent intralaminar nuclei (Fig. 11-4C). The image of the body is distorted in that the more important parts of the body with respect to sensory function, such as the hand and face, are disproportionately large. In addition, the more discriminative senses of fine touch and proprioception are represented further forward than the nociceptive senses of pain and temperature. Nevertheless, the topographic projection of the body on the ventral posterior nucleus (and on the somesthetic area of cortex) is the basis for precise recognition of the source of stimuli. Fibers originating in the gustatory nucleus terminate in the ventral posteromedial nucleus, and those from the vestibular nuclear complex terminate just lateral to this nucleus. The ventral posterior nucleus also receives general visceral information through the poorly-defined ascending visceral pathways of the spinal cord and brain stem.

Nerve fibers leave the lateral aspect of the ventral posterior nucleus in large numbers, traverse the internal capsule and medullary center of the cerebral hemisphere, and end in

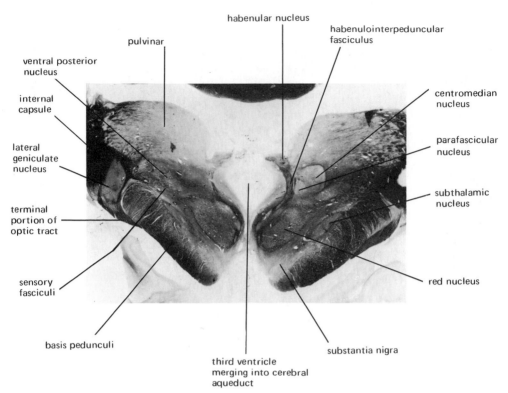

FIG. 11-6. Transverse section at the transition between the midbrain and the diencephalon, immediately caudal to the mammillary bodies. (Weigert stain, × 1 4/5)

FIG. 11-7. Diencephalon at the level of the mammillary bodies. (Weigert stain, × 1 4/5)

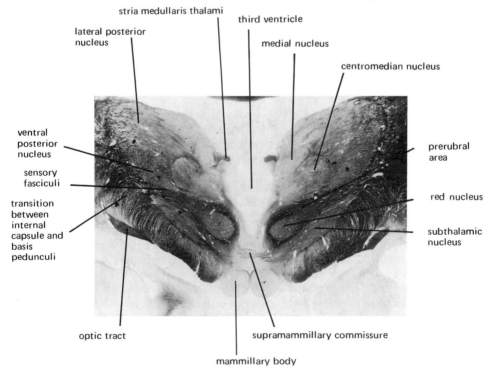

the general sensory area of cortex in the parietal lobe (Fig. 11–12). The opposite side of the body has an inverted representation in the somesthetic cortex, the portions assigned to the head and hand being disproportionately large, and the areas for taste and the vestibular system are adjacent to the head area (Chapter 15). Fibers from the ventral posterior nucleus also project to other thalamic nuclei, notably nuclei comprising the dorsal tier of the lateral mass of the thalamus and the medial nucleus. Experimental and clinical evidence shows that there is crude awareness of pain and temperature at the thalamic level. Localization is poor, discriminative aspects are lacking, and the sensations are not interpreted in the context of previous experience.

Ventral Lateral and Ventral Anterior Nuclei

The boundary between the ventral lateral and ventral anterior nuclei is arbitrary because they have overlapping connections (Figs. 11–4 and 11–8 through 11–11). Both nuclei receive fibers from the globus pallidus of the corpus striatum and the substantia nigra, and the ventral lateral nucleus receives fibers from the dentate nucleus of the cerebellum. Axons of neurons in both nuclei enter the internal capsule and proceed to motor and premotor cortical areas of the frontal lobe (Fig. 11–12). The symptoms of paralysis agitans (Parkinson's disease) may be ameliorated by a lesion placed in the nuclei surgically, although this form of therapy has been replaced to a considerable extent by administration of L-dopa. Several thalamic nuclei serve as relays between the intralaminar nuclei and the cerebral cortex. However, electrical stimulation of the ventral anterior nucleus is said to be especially effective in evoking changes in the electroencephalogram characteristic of cortical stimulation through the ascending reticular activating system. Some fibers from the ventral anterior nucleus terminate in the corpus striatum.

NONSPECIFIC THALAMIC NUCLEI

The dorsal tier of nuclei in the lateral mass of the thalamus, the medial nucleus, and the anterior nucleus constitute the nonspecific nuclei. Their cortical connections are mainly with areas other than the specific sensory and motor areas.

Dorsal Tier of Nuclei

The **pulvinar, lateral posterior nucleus,** and **lateral dorsal nucleus,** all situated in the dorsal part of the lateral nuclear mass (Figs. 11–4 and 11–6 through 11–8), have similar connections and functions. As noted previously, they receive fibers from other thalamic nuclei, including intralaminar nuclei and the ventral posterior nucleus. The three nuclei of the dorsal tier have reciprocal connections with association cortex of the parietal and occipital lobes and the posterior part of the temporal lobe (Fig. 11–12). The parieto-occipito-temporal association cortex is responsible for analysis of sensory input at the highest level and contributes to the neural substrate of the intellect. The activity of the cortex with respect to these extremely important functions is apparently reinforced by the nonspecific nuclei of the lateral thalamus.

Medial Nucleus

The medial thalamic nucleus (Figs. 11–4 and 11–9) includes several subnuclei; one of these, the **dorsomedial nucleus,** is well developed in man and occupies most of the medial nucleus.

The connections of the dorsomedial nucleus are varied and complex. Fibers enter the nucleus from other parts of the thalamus, including the lateral nuclear mass, intralaminar nuclei, and the midline nucleus. Sensory data, both somatic and visceral, are made available to the dorsomedial nucleus from those sources. There is a large reciprocal connection between the dorsomedial nucleus and association cortex of the frontal lobe (prefrontal cortex) (Fig. 11–12). In addition a bundle of fibers known as the **inferior thalamic peduncle** passes ventrally to the base of the hemisphere. This bundle provides reciprocal connections between the medial thalamic nucleus and various gray areas, including orbital cortex of the frontal lobe, gray matter underlying the anterior perforated substance, and the amygdaloid nucleus. Through these various connections the dorsomedial nucleus constitutes part of a system which contributes to those aspects of the emotions generally thought of as "moods" or

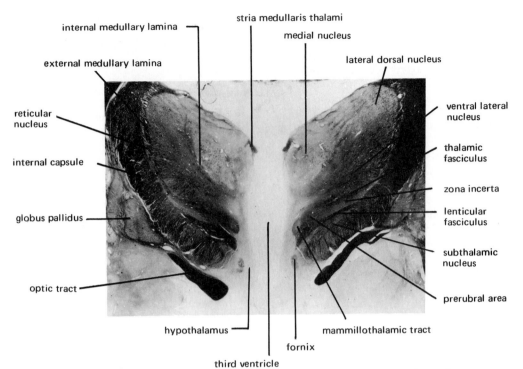

FIG. 11-8. Diencephalon at the level of the infundibular stem of the neurohypophysis. (Weigert stain, × 1 4/5)

FIG. 11-9. Diencephalon at the level of the optic chiasma. (Weigert stain, × 1 4/5)

stria medullaris thalami

medial nucleus

fornix

anterior nucleus

massa intermedia

midline nucleus

tail of caudate nucleus

lateral dorsal nucleus

external medullary lamina

internal capsule

ventral lateral nucleus

putamen

globus pallidus

third ventricle

hypothalamus

fornix

lamina terminalis

FIG. 11–10. Diencephalon rostral to the level of the optic chiasma. (Weigert stain, × 1 4/5)

"feeling tone." Depending on the nature of the present sensory input and past experience, the mood may be that of well being or malaise, or of euphoria or mild depression. Visceral changes may accompany changes in mood through reciprocal connections between the medial thalamic nucleus and the hypothalamus. The medial nucleus is another thalamic nucleus contributing afferents to the corpus striatum, along with the ventral anterior nucleus and intralaminar nuclei as already mentioned.

Severe anxiety states have been ameliorated by placing lesions in the dorsomedial nuclei, or more commonly, by severing the connections between these nuclei and the prefrontal cortices (leukotomy or prefrontal lobotomy). However, the procedure was sometimes followed by inappropriate social behavior and impairment of judgement and foresight, and this form of psychosurgery has been abandoned in favor of medical therapy.

The dorsomedial thalamic nucleus appears to play a role in memory. In Korsakoff's syndrome, in which amnesia is a characteristic symptom, the degenerative changes in the brain follow a variable pattern. However, the lesions are typically in regions surrounding the third ventricle, and the dorsomedial nucleus is reported as being affected most consistently. In addition memory deficits have been reported following surgical destruction of the dorsomedial thalamic nuclei.

Anterior Nucleus

The anterior thalamic nucleus (Figs. 11–4B and 11–11) is responsible for the anterior tubercle of the thalamus which, with the fornix, bounds the interventricular foramen or foramen of Monro (Figs. 11–2 and 11–3). This nucleus is included in the limbic system of the brain, which is concerned with basic emotions of importance in the preservation of the individual and the species and has a significant role in memory. The cortical components of the limbic system are the hippocampus, dentate gyrus, and parahippocampal

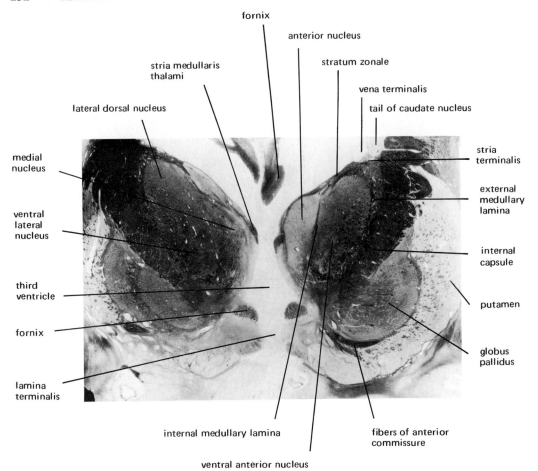

FIG. 11-11. Rostral region of the diencephalon. (Weigert stain, × 2)

gyrus (all in the temporal lobe), and the cingulate gyrus on the medial surface of the hemisphere above the corpus callosum. The diencephalic components are the hypothalamus (especially the mammillary bodies) and the anterior nucleus of the thalamus. The principal fiber bundles of the limbic system are the fornix, which projects from the hippocampus to the hypothalamus, and the mammillothalamic fasciculus (bundle of Vicq d'Azyr), through which reciprocal connections are established between the mammillary body and the anterior thalamic nucleus. This nucleus also has reciprocal connections with the cortex of the cingulate gyrus. (Additional components of the limbic system, e.g., the amygdaloid nucleus and its connections, are discussed in Chapter 18.)

THALAMIC SYNDROME

Aside from the motor aspects of the ventral lateral and ventral anterior nuclei, the thalamus is a sensory part of the brain and contributes to emotional responses to sensory experience. The thalamic syndrome is essentially a disturbance of these aspects of thalamic function, subsequent to a lesion (usually vascular in origin) involving the thalamus or its connections. The symptoms vary according to the location and extent of the lesion. The threshold for touch, pain, and temperature is usually raised on the opposite side of the body, but when the threshold is reached the sensations are exaggerated, perverted, and exceptionally disagreeable. For example, the prick of a pin may be felt as a severe burning sensation, and even music that is ordinarily pleasing may be disagreeable. There is spontaneous pain in some instances, which

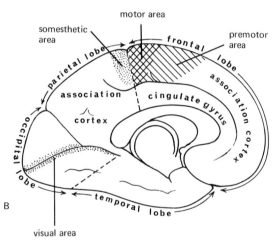

FIG. 11–12. Cortical areas receiving projections from specific thalamic nuclei. **A.** Lateral surface of a cerebral hemisphere. **B.** Medial surface of a cerebral hemisphere.

may become intractable to analgesics. There may also be emotional instability, with spontaneous or forced laughing and crying.

SUBTHALAMUS

The subthalamus contains sensory fasciculi, rostral extensions of midbrain nuclei, fiber bundles from the dentate nucleus of the cerebellum and the globus pallidus, and the subthalamic nucleus.

The **sensory fasciculi** are the medial lemniscus, the spinothalamic tracts, and the tri-

geminothalamic tracts. They are spread out immediately beneath the ventral posterior nucleus of the thalamus, in which the fibers terminate (Figs. 11–6 and 11–7).

The **substantia nigra** and the **red nucleus** extend from the midbrain part way into the subthalamus (Figs. 11–6 and 11–7). Dentatothalamic fibers of the brachium conjunctivum both surround and traverse the red nucleus, then continue forward in the **prerubral area** or **field H of Forel** (H, *Haube*, a cap) (Figs. 11–7 and 11–8). The dentatothalamic fibers contribute to the thalamic fasciculus (see next paragraph) and end in the ventral lateral nucleus of the thalamus.

Efferent fibers of the globus pallidus are contained in two bundles, the lenticular fasciculus and the ansa lenticularis. The **lenticular fasciculus** (Fig. 11–8) consists of fibers which cut across the internal capsule to reach the subthalamus, where they form a band of white matter known as **field H_2 of Forel.** The fibers reverse direction in the prerubral area, enter the **thalamic fasciculus (field H_1 of Forel),** and terminate in the ventral lateral and ventral anterior thalamic nuclei (Fig. 12–5). At a more rostral level the **ansa lenticularis** makes a sharp bend around the medial edge of the internal capsule, continues in the thalamic fasciculus, and ends in the ventral lateral and ventral anterior nuclei of the thalamus (Fig. 11–9). Only a very few fibers from the globus pallidus turn caudally; they terminate in a small nucleus in the tegmentum of the brain stem, at the junction of the midbrain and pons. The mesencephalic reticular formation extends into the subthalamus, where it appears as the **zona incerta** between the lenticular and thalamic fasciculi (Fig. 11–8). The **subthalamic nucleus** (nucleus of Luys), a motor nucleus best developed in primates, is biconvex in shape and lies against the internal capsule (Figs. 11–6, 11–7, 11–8). The connections of the subthalamic nucleus are varied, and not all of them have been established unequivocally. However, the major connection is with the globus pallidus; this consists of fibers running in both directions across the internal capsule and making up the **subthalamic fasciculus.** Fibers in the **supramammillary commissure** (Fig. 11–7) connect one subthalamic nucleus with the other.

A lesion in the subthalamic nucleus causes a motor disturbance on the opposite side of the body known as **hemiballismus.** The condition is characterized by involuntary movements, coming on suddenly and of great force and rapidity. The movements are purposeless and generally of a throwing or flailing type, although they may be choreiform or jerky. The spontaneous movements affect the proximal portions of the limbs most severely, especially the arms, and the muscles of the face and neck are sometimes involved.

EPITHALAMUS

The epithalamus consists of the habenular nuclei and their connections, and the pineal gland.

HABENULAR NUCLEUS

A slight swelling in the habenular trigone marks the position of the habenular nucleus (Figs. 11–3 and 11–6). Afferent fibers are received through the **stria medullaris thalami,** which runs along the dorsomedial border of the thalamus (Figs. 11–2, 11–3, and 11–8). Most of the cells of origin of the stria are situated in the medial olfactory (septal) area. This area is located on the medial surface of the frontal lobe beneath the rostral end of the corpus callosum (Fig. 11–2) and is part of both the olfactory and limbic systems of the brain. A few fibers of the stria terminalis (Fig. 11–11), originating in the amygdaloid nucleus in the temporal lobe, turn caudally in the region of the interventricular foramen and join the stria medullaris thalami.

The habenular nucleus gives rise to a well-defined bundle of fibers known as the **habenulointerpeduncular fasciculus** (fasciculus retroflexus of Meynert) (Fig. 11–6). The main destination of the fasciculus is the interpeduncular nucleus in the roof of the interpeduncular fossa of the midbrain. Fibers pass from the latter site to the dorsal tegmental nucleus, from which fibers proceed to the autonomic nuclei and reticular formation of the brain stem by way of the dorsal longitudinal fasciculus. The stria medullaris thalami, habenular nucleus, and habenulointerpeduncular fasciculus constitute part of a pathway through which primitive aspects of brain function, namely, basic emotional drives and the sense of smell, influence the viscera.

PINEAL GLAND

The pineal gland, also called the pineal body, has the shape of a pine cone and is about 5 × 7 mm in size; it is attached to the diencephalon by the pineal stalk, into which the third ventricle extends as the pineal recess (Figs. 11–2 and 11–3). The **habenular commissure** in the dorsal wall of the stalk includes fibers of the stria medullaris thalami that terminate in the opposite habenular nucleus. The ventral wall of the pineal stalk is attached to the **posterior commissure.** Although the pineal gland contains no nerve cells and is a proper subject for endocrinology, its close relationship with the nervous system justifies further discussion in a neurologic context.

Few structures have undergone such remarkable evolutionary changes as the pineal gland. In fish, amphibians, and reptiles it is situated immediately beneath the dorsum of the head, and it contains photoreceptors which respond to changes in light intensity because of the translucence of overlying tissues. The output of melatonin by the pineal depends on the level of illumination in the immediate environment. Melatonin has the property of clumping granules of melanin pigment in cutaneous melanocytes, thereby providing protective changes in the lightness or darkness of the animal.

The pineal gland of mammals contains no photoreceptors and its function has changed from that of submammalian vertebrates. Histologically the parenchymatous cells (pinealocytes) are arranged as cords separated by connective tissue. These cells have a granular cytoplasm and processes which end in bulbous expansions close to blood vessels at the surface of the cellular cords or in the intervening connective tissue septa. The cords contain a smaller population of neuroglial cells resembling astrocytes. After the age of about 16 years, granules of calcium and magnesium salts appear in the gland. These calcareous granules coalesce later to form larger particles (brain sand); the deposits may be a useful landmark in x-ray films for determining whether the pineal gland is displaced by a space-occupying lesion.

Clinical observations of long standing suggest an antigonadotropic function for the pineal gland in man because a pineal tumor developing around the time of puberty may alter the age of onset of pubertal changes. Puberty may be precocious if the tumor is of a type that destroys parenchymatous cells, or delayed if the tumor is derived from the functional cells of the gland. It is only in recent years that experimental work has placed these observations on a sounder basis, although many details remain for clarification.

Pinealectomy in experimental animals stimulates the genital system, with genital hypertrophy, precocious opening of the vagina in immature females, and changes in the estrous cycle. Administration of pineal extracts has the contrary effect through inhibition of the gonads. Chemical extraction of bovine pineal glands has produced several possible active principles, including melatonin and serotonin. Melatonin appears to be specific to the pineal because this is the only mammalian organ known to contain the enzyme required for its synthesis. However, administration of pure melatonin does not produce all the effects of pineal extracts, and related compounds may also serve as pineal hormones.

In mammals, as in lower vertebrates, the activity of the pineal gland is influenced by light; its antigonadotropic activity is highest when the animal is in the dark and lowest when in a light environment. The pathway for the influence of light on the gland is known to originate in the retina; it is also known that perivascular sympathetic fibers from the superior cervical ganglion have an inhibitory effect on the gland. A connection between the retina and the intermediolateral cell column in the upper thoracic segments of the spinal cord is therefore required. This connection has been shown in the rat to begin as fibers leaving the optic tract near the optic chiasma, these fibers terminating in the reticular formation of the midbrain. Reticulospinal fibers presumably complete the pathway.

The site of action of the pineal hormone(s) is under continued investigation. The target cells may be in the gonads or in the pars distalis of the pituitary gland. Alternatively they may be neurosecretory cells in the hypothalamus which produce releasing factors for the gonadotropin-producing cells of the pituitary, or neurons that project to the hypothalamus. Recent work tends to implicate cells of the central nervous system, either hypothalamic cells or neurons in the reticular formation of the midbrain projecting to the hypothalamus. In addition to the antigonadotropic function, there is some evidence that pineal hormones influence pituitary cells producing the growth (somatotropic) hormone (STH), the thyroid-stimulating hormone (TSH), and the adrenocorticotropic hormone (ACTH). The importance of the pineal gland in human physiology has yet to be assessed.

HYPOTHALAMUS

The hypothalamus, occupying only a small part of the brain and weighing about 4 g, has a functional importance that is quite out of proportion to its size. The hypothalamus is at a crossroads between the thalamus and cerebral cortex (especially that of the limbic system) and ascending fiber systems from the brain stem and spinal cord. Input from the thalamus and the limbic system has a special emotional significance, and the ascending fibers convey information that is largely of visceral origin. However, the hypothalamus is not influenced solely by neuronal systems; the constituent nerve cells respond to properties of the circulating blood, including temperature, osmotic pressure, and the levels of various hormones. Hypothalamic function becomes manifest through efferent pathways to autonomic nuclei in the brain stem and spinal cord, and through an intimate relationship with the hypophysis or pituitary gland by means of neurosecretory cells. These cells elaborate the hormones of the neurohypophysis and produce releasing factors which control the hormonal output of the adenohypophysis. By these means the hypothalamus has a major role in producing responses to emotional changes and to needs signaled by hunger and thirst, and it is instrumental in maintaining a constant internal environment (homeostasis).

The hypothalamus surrounds the third ventricle ventral to the hypothalamic sulci (Fig. 11-2). The **mammillary bodies** (also spelled mamillary bodies) are distinct swellings on the ventral surface (Fig. 11-1). The region bounded by the mammillary bodies, optic chiasma, and beginning of the optic tracts is known as the **tuber cinereum.** The **infundibular stem** arises from the **median eminence** just behind the optic chiasma and expands to form the **infundibular process** or pars nervosa of the pituitary gland. The median eminence, infundibular stem, and infundibular process have similar cytologic and functional characteristics; together they constitute the **neurohypophysis.**

The columns of the fornix traverse the hypothalamus to reach the mammillary bodies and serve as points of reference for sagittal planes dividing each half of the hypothalamus into **medial** and **lateral zones.** The medial zone is subdivided into three regions, **suprachiasmatic, tuberal,** and **mammillary,** with ventral structures as landmarks. The medial zone consists of gray matter in which several nuclei are recognized on the basis of cellular characteristics and connections. It also includes a thin layer of fine myelinated and unmyelinated fibers beneath the ependymal lining of the third ventricle. The lateral zone or area contains fewer nerve cells, but there are many nerve fibers, most of them running in a longitudinal direction.

HYPOTHALAMIC NUCLEI

The lamina terminalis represents the rostral end of the embryonal neural tube and limits the third ventricle anteriorly (Fig. 11–13). The lamina extends from the optic chiasma to the anterior commissure, which consists of a bundle of fibers connecting areas of the right and left temporal lobes, and includes some commissural fibers connecting the olfactory bulbs. The lamina terminalis and the anterior commissure are telencephalic structures. The gray matter immediately behind the lamina terminalis is also derived from the telencephalon of the embryo. However, it is included with the hypothalamus for convenience and is called the **preoptic area** of the hypothalamus.

Medial Zone

Within the medial zone (Fig. 11–13), the suprachiasmatic region contains the supraoptic, paraventricular, and anterior nuclei. The **supraoptic nucleus** consists of large cells and is best developed above the junction of the optic chiasma and optic tract. The **paraventricular nucleus** is characterized by large cells in a matrix of smaller neurons. These nuclei are conspicuous in Nissl-stained sections and have a plentiful supply of capillaries. The cells of the supraoptic and paraventricular nuclei elaborate neurohypo-

physial hormones, and secretory granules in the cytoplasm are evidence of neurosecretory activity. Axons from the nuclei constitute the hypothalamohypophysial tract, whose fibers terminate throughout the neurohypophysis where the hormones are released into capillary blood. The **anterior nucleus** is similar to the preoptic area cytologically, and they are not clearly demarcated from one another.

The tuberal region contains the **ventromedial, dorsomedial,** and **infundibular (arcuate) nuclei,** each nucleus consisting of small nerve cells. The mammillary region includes the **mammillary body** and the **posterior nucleus.** In man the mammillary body is occupied almost entirely by a medial mammillary nucleus, the remainder consisting of an intermediate nucleus and a lateral nucleus. The cells of the lateral nucleus are large, whereas the bulk of the mammillary body is made up of small neurons. The posterior nucleus consists of large neurons in a background of small nerve cells.

Lateral Zone

The large nerve cells throughout the lateral zone are relatively sparse and collectively constitute the **lateral nucleus** of the hypothalamus. The cells are interspersed with longitudinally running nerve fibers passing to or from hypothalamic nuclei or through the area. This zone includes the **lateral tuberal nucleus,** which consists of several groups of nerve cells near the surface of the tuber cinereum. The hypothalamus of man is characterized by the large size of the medial mammillary nucleus, the well defined lateral tuberal nucleus, and the presence of large neurons in the posterior and lateral nuclei.

AFFERENT CONNECTIONS OF THE HYPOTHALAMUS

As mentioned previously, the hypothalamus receives information from diverse sources in order to serve as the main integrator of the autonomic nervous system.

Ascending visceral afferents convey data of visceral origin, and include fibers for the special visceral sense of taste. The pathways are not well defined, compared with somatic sensory tracts leading to the thalamus, and consist in part of relays through the reticular formation of the brain stem and the midline

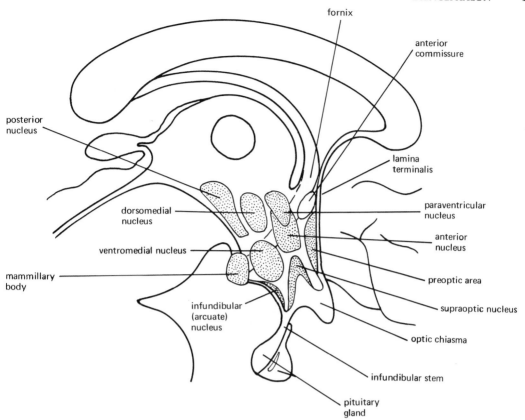

FIG. 11–13. Nuclei in the medial zone of the hypothalamus.

nucleus of the thalamus. Some of the ascending fibers are included in the dorsal longitudinal fasciculus, which also contains efferent fibers of the hypothalamus. Somatic sensory information, especially from erotogenic zones such as the nipples and genitalia, also reaches the hypothalamus.

The cells of origin of the **medial forebrain bundle** are chiefly in the septal or medial olfactory area, other fibers coming from the intermediate and lateral olfactory areas (Chapter 17). The medial forebrain bundle runs caudally in the lateral zone of the hypothalamus, giving off fibers to hypothalamic nuclei. Other fibers of the bundle continue through the hypothalamus to the reticular formation of the midbrain. The afferents just described are related to basic emotional drives and the sense of smell. The medial forebrain bundle is small in the human brain, in comparison with the brains of animals that rely heavily on the sense of smell. A second input related to smell and emotional drives comes from the amygdaloid nucleus. This

nucleus is situated in the temporal lobe in the region of the uncus, a small gyral configuration on the ventral surface (Fig. 11–1). A slender strand of fibers known as the **stria terminalis** arises from the amygdaloid nucleus, arches over the thalamus along the medial side of the caudate nucleus (Fig. 11–11), and terminates in part in the preoptic area and the anterior nucleus of the hypothalamus.

The **fornix,** originating in the hippocampus of the temporal lobe, is the largest of the fiber bundles ending in the hypothalamus. As mentioned earlier, the fornix arches over the thalamus and into the hypothalamus, where the fibers terminate mainly in the mammillary body (Fig. 11–14). The mammillary body also receives fibers from the anterior thalamic nucleus through the mammillothalamic fasciculus and is therefore in communication with the cortex of the cingulate gyrus. The hypothalamus is an integral part of the limbic system of the brain and essential to the intimate relationship between basic emotional drives and visceral function, which

mammillothalamic fasciculus   anterior tubercle
of thalamus

interventricular
foramen

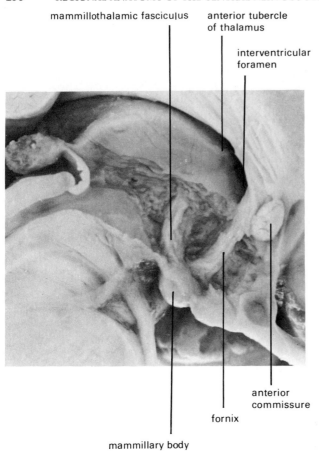

anterior
commissure

fornix

mammillary body

FIG. 11-14. Dissection demonstrating the fornix
and the mammillothalamic fasciculus. (× 2)

is an important aspect of the physiology of
the limbic system.

The hypothalamus receives fibers from the
medial thalamic nucleus and is thereby
brought under the influence of the prefrontal
cortex. These parts of the brain, it will be recalled, contribute to states of mind commonly referred to as moods, among other
functions. There are also direct **corticohypothalamic fibers,** especially from cortex on
the orbital surface of the frontal lobe.

EFFERENT CONNECTIONS OF THE HYPOTHALAMUS

There are two principal pathways from the
hypothalamus to the brain stem. The first of
these begins as thinly myelinated and unmyelinated **periventricular fibers** beneath
the ependyma of the third ventricle, continu-

ing into the **dorsal longitudinal fasciculus** in
the periaqueductal gray matter of the midbrain. Partly through relays in the reticular
formation, impulses of hypothalamic origin
reach parasympathetic nuclei in the brain
stem, *i.e.,* the salivatory and lacrimal nuclei
and the dorsal nucleus of the vagus nerve.
Reticulospinal fibers complete the pathway
to autonomic nuclei in the spinal cord. Lower
motor neurons supplying striated muscles
are also recipients of impulses of hypothalamic origin. These include cells in the motor
nuclei of the trigeminal and facial nerves, the
nucleus ambiguus, and the hypoglossal nucleus, in connection with the role of the hypothalamus in feeding and drinking. Motor
neurons of the spinal cord are influenced by
the hypothalamus in temperature regulation,
as in shivering to raise the body temperature.

The fibers of a second descending pathway, the **mammillotegmental fasciculus,** accompany the mammillothalamic fasciculus

briefly, then turn caudally and end in the reticular formation in the tegmentum of the midbrain. Impulses originating in the mammillary body reach autonomic nuclei in the brain stem and spinal cord through synaptic relays in the reticular formation. Finally, axons of some hypothalamic neurons enter the lateral zone and reach the midbrain along with fibers of the medial forebrain bundle.

Activity within the hypothalamus is transmitted to the thalamus and cerebral cortex, where it has an influence on affective states, both basic emotions of a primitive nature and those more closely related to moods. The large **mammillothalamic fasciculus** (bundle of Vicq d'Azyr) establishes reciprocal connections between the mammillary body and the anterior nucleus of the thalamus, which in turn has reciprocal connections with the cortex of the cingulate gyrus (Fig. 11–14). As noted previously, the anterior thalamic nucleus and the cingulate cortex share with other components of the limbic system responsibility for those emotions and aspects of behavior that are related to preservation of the individual and the species. The hypothalamus contributes to the subjective experience of these emotions through projections to the thalamus and cortex, and to visceral manifestations of emotions through the autonomic nervous system. A supplementary contribution to the affect, in particular to an individual's mood, derives from reciprocal connections between the hypothalamus and the medial thalamic nucleus, and between the latter and prefrontal cortex.

SOME FUNCTIONAL CONSIDERATIONS

Autonomic and Related Aspects

Electrical stimulation of the hypothalamus in experimental animals shows that some regions give parasympathetic, and others sympathetic, responses. Parasympathetic responses are most regularly elicited by stimulation of the anterior hypothalamus, notably the preoptic area and anterior nucleus. The responses include slowing of the heart rate, vasodilation, lowering of blood pressure, salivation, increased peristalsis in the gastrointestinal tract, contraction of the urinary bladder, and sweating. Sympathetic responses, most readily elicited by stimulation in the region of the posterior and lateral nuclei, include cardiac acceleration, elevation of blood pressure, cessation of peristalsis in the gastrointestinal tract, dilation of the pupils, and hyperglycemia.

With respect to the role of the hypothalamus in maintaining homeostasis, regulation of body temperature is an instructive example. Certain hypothalamic cells act as a thermostat, monitoring the temperature of blood flowing through the capillaries and initiating the responses necessary to maintain a normal body temperature. Thermosensitive neurons in the parasympathetic region of the anterior hypothalamus respond to an increase in temperature of the blood. Mechanisms that promote heat loss, such as cutaneous vasodilation and sweating, are activated. A lesion in the anterior hypothalamus may therefore result in hyperthermia in a hot environment or under states of high metabolic rate. Cells in the sympathetic region, especially the posterior hypothalamic nucleus, respond to a lowering of blood temperature. Responses such as cutaneous vasoconstriction and shivering are triggered for conservation and production of heat, and a lesion in the posterior hypothalamus interferes with temperature regulation in a cold environment. A lesion in the posterior part of the hypothalamus may not only destroy cells involved in conservation and production of heat, but also interrupt fibers running caudally from the heat-dissipating region. This results in a serious impairment of temperature regulation in either a cold or a hot environment.

Hypothalamic regulation of food and water intake has also been demonstrated by electrical stimulation and by placing small electrolytic lesions in the hypothalamus. A hunger or feeding center has been located in the lateral zone, and a satiety center (inhibiting food intake) has been demonstrated in the region of the ventromedial nucleus. These centers are influenced by the glucose level of the blood, visceral afferent fibers, the olfactory system, and by thalamic and cortical regions concerned with the emotions. Destruction of the satiety center in an experimental animal, such as the rat, results in excessive food intake and obesity. Naturally-occurring lesions affecting this center in man may also result in obesity, and hypothalamic cells which increase the output of gonadotropic hormones by the adenohypophysis may be destroyed at the same time. The combination of obesity and deficiency of secondary sex characteristics is known as the adiposogenital or Frölich's syndrome. Centers which inhibit or promote water intake have also been identified in the lateral and ventromedial nuclei, although not coinciding precisely with the centers for food intake.

Relations of the Hypothalamus with the Pituitary Gland (Hypophysis)

Neurohypophysial hormones are elaborated in the hypothalamus, and hormone production by the adenohypophysis is controlled by chemical substances synthesized in hypothalamic cells. The nervous system, through the neurosecretory function of hypothalamic cells, has therefore an intimate relation with the entire endocrine system. With the exception of the special conditions inherent in the nervous control of the pineal gland, only the adrenal medulla is regulated by direct nervous connections. These are preganglionic sympathetic fibers, the cells of the adrenal medulla having the same embryologic origin as cells of sympathetic ganglia. Only the major points concerning hypothalamic–hypophysial relationships are discussed here; the subject is a large one, comprising the specialty of neuroendocrinology.

NEUROHYPOPHYSIS. As noted previously, the neurohypophysis consists of the median eminence, infundibular stem, and infundibular process, all of which are of diencephalic origin in the embryo (Fig. 11–15). Although hormones enter the blood stream from the neurohypophysis, they are not elaborated there, but rather in the cells of the supraoptic and paraventricular nuclei. The hormones are vasopressin and oxytocin. Vasopressin has two properties, vasoconstrictor and antidiuretic, the former of which is of comparatively little physiologic and clinical importance. The antidiuretic effect results from the action of the hormone on the distal convoluted tubules of the kidney, with increased absorption of water from the glomerular filtrate. Oxytocin stimulates the smooth muscle of the uterus when it is sensitized by estrogen and not depressed by progesterone, and it causes contraction of myoepithelial cells surrounding the secretory alveoli of the mammary gland. In experimental animals

vasopressin is produced in the supraoptic nucleus and oxytocin in the paraventricular nucleus.

Processes of cells in the supraoptic and paraventricular nuclei constitute the **hypothalamohypophysial tract** and terminate as small expansions adjacent to capillaries in all parts of the neurohypophysis (Fig. 11–15). The secretory function of the cells is evident in the secretory granules present in the cytoplasm of the cell bodies. The neurosecretions are carried distally by axoplasmic flow, and vasopressin and oxytocin enter the blood stream by way of the capillary bed throughout the neurohypophysis.

The supraoptic nucleus serves as an osmoreceptor, the secretory activity of its cells being influenced by the osmolarity of the blood flowing through this highly vascular nucleus. A slight elevation of osmotic pressure causes the cells to synthesize antidiuretic hormone (vasopressin) more rapidly, and an increased amount of the hormone enters the capillary blood of the neurohypophysis. Resorption of water from the distal convoluted tubules of the kidney is then accelerated, and the osmolarity of the blood plasma returns to normal. A delicate mechanism is thereby provided to ensure homeostasis with respect to water balance. Destruction of the supraoptic nucleus or the neurohypophysis results in diabetes insipidus, which is characterized by excretion of large quantities of dilute urine (polyuria) and excessive thirst and water intake to compensate (polydipsia). A lesion restricted to the infundibular process of the pituitary gland is not as a rule followed by diabetes insipidus, because antidiuretic hormone enters the blood stream from the median eminence and infundibular stem.

PITUITARY PORTAL SYSTEM. The following hormones are produced in the pars distalis of the adenohypophysis: 1) follicle-stimulating hormone (FSH), 2) luteinizing hormone (LH), 3) luteotropic hormone (LTH), 4) thyrotropic or thyroid-stimulating hormone (TSH), 5) adrenocorticotropic hormone (ACTH), and 6) growth or somatotropic hormone (STH). The first three mentioned are gonadotropic hormones. FSH promotes growth of ovarian follicles and spermatogenesis. LH promotes ovulation, converts the ruptured ovarian follicle into a corpus luteum, and stimulates in-

FIG. 11–15. The hypothalamohypophysial tract.

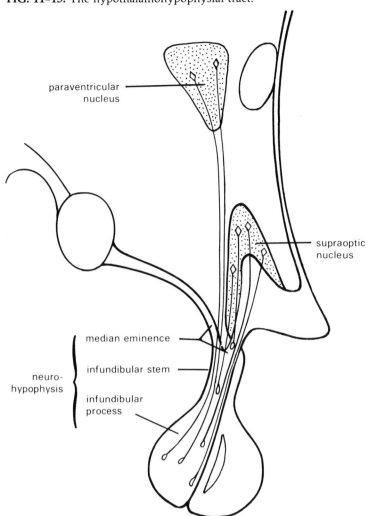

paraventricular
nucleus

supraoptic
nucleus

median eminence

infundibular stem

neuro-
hypophysis

infundibular
process

terstitial cells of the testis. LTH stimulates the corpus luteum to secrete progesterone and promotes secretion of milk in the lactating breast (hence also known as the lactogenic hormone or prolactin). Secretion of hormones by the pars distalis is under the control of the hypothalamus, but by a vascular route rather than nervous connections.

The pituitary portal system begins with the superior hypophysial artery, which arises from the internal carotid artery at the base of the brain and breaks up into capillary tufts and loops in the median eminence (Fig. 11–16). The capillaries are drained by veins which enter the adenohypophysis, where they empty into the large capillaries or sinusoids of the pars distalis. The hypothalamus contains cells that produce tripeptide or polypeptide releasing factors and at least one inhibiting factor, specifically for prolactin. There is a separate releasing factor for each hormone of the pars distalis, and there is probably a topographic pattern of cells producing different factors. The releasing factors pass by axoplasmic flow in the axons of the cells producing them and enter the capillaries of the portal system in the median eminence to reach the pars distalis, thereby bringing the synthesis and release of hormones by the pars distalis under hypothalamic control. Cells producing releasing factors are influenced by the various afferent fiber connections of the hypothalamus. Their activity is also regulated by hormones of the target

FIG. 11–16. The pituitary portal system.

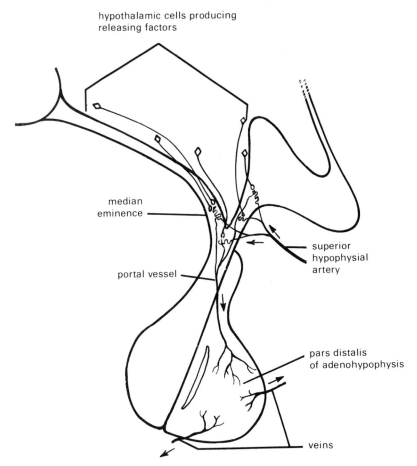

hypothalamic cells producing
releasing factors

median
eminence

portal vessel

superior
hypophysial
artery

pars distalis
of adenohypophysis

veins

organs for pituitary hormones. For example, when the blood titer of sex hormones is high, hypothalamic cells producing the releasing factor for FSH are suppressed. Conversely in hypogonadal conditions these hypothalamic cells produce an excess of the releasing factor, and FSH secretion is elevated.

THIRD VENTRICLE

The diencephalic part of the ventricular system consists of the narrow third ventricle (Fig. 11-2). The anterior wall of this ventricle is formed by the lamina terminalis; the anterior commissure crosses the midline in the dorsal part of the lamina terminalis. The rather extensive lateral wall is marked by the hypothalamic sulcus, separating the thalamus from the hypothalamus. A massa intermedia (interthalamic adhesion) bridges the ventricle in 70% of brains. The floor of

the third ventricle is indented by the optic chiasma. There is an optic recess in front of the chiasma, and behind the chiasma the infundibular recess extends into the median eminence and the proximal part of the infundibular stem. The floor then slopes upward to the cerebral aqueduct of the midbrain, the posterior commissure forming a slight prominence above the entrance to the aqueduct. A pineal recess extends into the stalk of the pineal gland, and the dorsal wall of the stalk accommodates the small habenular commissure. The membranous roof of the third ventricle is attached along the striae medullares thalami, and a small choroid plexus is suspended from the roof. Cerebrospinal fluid enters the third ventricle from each lateral ventricle through the interventricular foramen (foramen of Monro). The foramen is bounded by the fornix and the anterior tubercle of the thalamus and is closed posteriorly by a reflexion of ependyma between the fornix and the thalamus. The fluid leaves the third ventricle by way of the cerebral aqueduct of the midbrain, through which it reaches the fourth ventricle and then the subarachnoid space surrounding the brain and spinal cord.

SUGGESTED READING

Axelrod J: The pineal gland. Endeavour 29:144–148, 1970

Bowsher D: Termination of the central pain pathway in man: the conscious appreciation of pain. Brain 80:606–622, 1957

Carpenter MB: Ventral tier thalamic nuclei. In Williams D (ed): Modern Trends in Neurology. London, Butterworth, 1967, pp 1–20

Carpenter MB, Nakano K, Kim R: Nigrothalamic projections in the monkey demonstrated by autoradiographic technics. J Comp Neurol 165:410–415, 1976

Crosby EC, Humphrey T, Lauer EW: Correlative Anatomy of the Nervous System. New York, Macmillan, 1962

Harris GW: Neural Control of the Pituitary Gland. London, Arnold, 1955

Harris GW, Reed M, Fawcett CP: Hypothalamic releasing factors and the control of anterior pituitary function. Br Med Bull 22:266–272, 1966

Haymaker WE, Anderson E, Nauta WJH: The Hypothalamus. Springfield, IL, Thomas, 1969

Haywood JN: Functional and morphological aspects of hypothalamic neurons. Physiol Rev 57:574–658, 1977

Kelly DE: Pineal organs: photoreception, secretion, and development. Am Sci 50:597–625, 1962

Kuhlenbeck H: The Human Diencephalon. Basel, Karger, 1954

Miller RA, Burack E: Atlas of the Central Nervous System in Man. Baltimore, Williams & Wilkins, 1968

Montemurro DG: Neural relationships in pituitary function. Can Cancer Conf 6:82–108, 1966

Purpura DP, Yahr MD (eds): The Thalamus. New York, Columbia University Press, 1966

Reiter RJ, Fraschini F: Endocrine aspects of the mammalian pineal gland: a review. Neuroendocrinology 5:219–255, 1969

Scharrer E, Scharrer B: Neuroendocrinology. New York, Columbia University Press, 1963

Scheibel ME, Scheibel AB: The organization of the nucleus reticularis thalami: a Golgi study. Brain Res 1:43–62, 1966

Scheibel ME, Scheibel AB: Structural organization of nonspecific thalamic nuclei and their projection toward cortex. Brain Res 6:60–94, 1967

Spiegel EA, Wyeis HT, Orchinik CW, Freed H: The thalamus and temporal orientation. Science 121:771–772, 1955

Tasker RR: Thalamotomy for pain: lesion localization by detailed thalamic mapping. Can J Surg 12:62–74, 1969

Victor M: The amnesic syndrome and its anatomical basis. Can Med Assoc J 100:1115–1125, 1969

Von Euler C: Physiology and pharmacology of temperature regulation. Pharmacol Rev 13:361–398, 1961

Wurtman RJ, Axelrod J, Kelly DE: The Pineal. New York, Academic Press, 1968

12

Corpus Striatum

The corpus striatum is a substantial region of gray matter near the base of each cerebral hemisphere. It consists of the **caudate nucleus** and the **lenticular nucleus,** the latter being divided into the **putamen** and the **globus pallidus.** The corpus striatum, claustrum, and amygdaloid nucleus are sometimes referred to as the basal "ganglia" of the telencephalon. The claustrum is a thin sheet of gray matter lateral to the putamen; its connections are not fully known and its function is obscure. The amygdaloid nucleus in the temporal lobe is a component of the olfactory and limbic systems, which are discussed in Chapters 17 and 18, respectively. In clinical contexts the term basal ganglia is usually applied to the corpus striatum, subthalamic nucleus, and substantia nigra. The three nuclei are grouped under the common heading because they share an importance in motor disturbances called dyskinesias, characterized by involuntary, purposeless movements.

PHYLOGENETIC DEVELOPMENT

The corpus striatum of man is best understood against a phylogenetic background, even if stated in the most general terms. In fish and amphibians, the forerunner of the mammalian corpus striatum receives olfactory stimuli, a source which is of decreasing importance in higher animals and insignificant in man. This nucleus constitutes the **paleostriatum** in reptiles, birds, and mammals. A new component, the **neostriatum,** appeared on the lateral side of the paleostriatum in the reptilian stage of evolution and forms the largest part of the corpus striatum in mammals.

Another morphologic change occurred with the appearance of neocortex (nonolfac-

tory cortex), which is essentially a mammalian part of the cerebral hemisphere. Fibers connecting the neocortex with subcortical centers traverse the neostriatum and run along the medial side of the smaller paleostriatum (globus pallidus) as the internal capsule. The neostriatum is thereby divided into the caudate nucleus on the medial side of the itinerant fibers, and the putamen lateral to the globus pallidus (Fig. 12–1). The globus pallidus and the putamen constitute the lenticular nucleus. The two parts of the neostriatum remain connected at the base of the hemisphere, and by means of strands of gray matter running across the internal capsule. The gross division of the corpus striatum into caudate and lenticular nuclei is of secondary importance; the significant components remain the paleostriatum and the neostriatum.

The neostriatum is also called the **striatum,** and the globus pallidus is then referred to as the **pallidum.** The shorter forms are useful in naming afferent and efferent connections (*e.g.,* corticostriate and pallidothalamic fibers). The following correlations may be helpful in understanding the use of terms:

neostriatum = striatum = putamen + caudate nucleus

paleostriatum = pallidum = globus pallidus

lenticular nucleus = globus pallidus + putamen

LENTICULAR AND CAUDATE NUCLEI

It is desirable to understand the configuration and relations of the lenticular and caudate nuclei, even though the division of the corpus striatum into paleostriatum and neostriatum has a greater relevance to the affer-

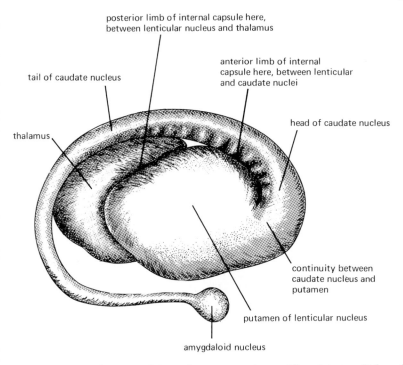

posterior limb of internal capsule here, between lenticular nucleus and thalamus

tail of caudate nucleus

anterior limb of internal capsule here, between lenticular and caudate nuclei

thalamus

head of caudate nucleus

continuity between caudate nucleus and putamen

putamen of lenticular nucleus

amygdaloid nucleus

FIG. 12–1. Lateral aspect of the right corpus striatum. The globus pallidus of the lenticular nucleus is concealed by the larger putamen.

FIG. 12–2. Horizontal section of the cerebrum, stained by a method which differentiates gray matter and white matter, showing the components and relations of the corpus striatum. (× 4/5)

corpus callosum

anterior horn of lateral ventricle

external capsule

head of caudate nucleus

insula

anterior limb

extreme capsule

internal capsule

genu

posterior limb

claustrum

putamen

tail of caudate nucleus

globus pallidus

thalamus   pineal gland

corpus callosum

lateral ventricle

septum pellucidum

caudate nucleus

internal capsule

external capsule

putamen

extreme capsule

insula

lateral medullary
lamina

claustrum

anterior commissure

amygdaloid nucleus

globus pallidus

medial medullary
lamina   fornix

optic tract

FIG. 12–3. Coronal section of the cerebrum anterior to the thalamus, stained by a method which differentiates gray matter and white matter, showing the components and relations of the corpus striatum. (× 4/5)

ent and efferent connections of this part of the brain.

LENTICULAR NUCLEUS

The lenticular nucleus (lentiform nucleus) is wedge shaped and has been described as having the approximate size and shape of a Brazil nut (Figs. 12–2 and 12–3). The narrow part of the wedge facing medially is occupied by the **globus pallidus,** which is divided into medial and lateral parts by a **medial medul-**

lary lamina consisting of nerve fibers. The globus pallidus of man may have three divisions. The **putamen** forms the lateral portion of the lenticular nucleus and extends beyond the globus pallidus in all directions except at the base of the nucleus. The two components of the lenticular nucleus are separated by a **lateral medullary lamina** of nerve fibers.

The lenticular nucleus is bounded laterally by a thin layer of white matter constituting the **external capsule** (Figs. 12–2 and 12–3). This is followed by the **claustrum,** which consists of a thin sheet of gray matter coextensive with the putamen. The **extreme capsule** separates the claustrum from the **insula** (island of Reil), an area of cortex buried in the depths of the lateral fissure of the cerebral hemisphere, also known as the fissure of Sylvius. The claustrum appears to be derived from the insula and has connections with the cortex of the frontal, parietal, and temporal lobes. The role of the claustrum is obscure; it has no demonstrable functional relationship with the corpus striatum. The medial surface of the lenticular nucleus lies against the internal capsule. The ventral surface is close to such structures at the base of the hemisphere as the anterior perforated substance, the optic tract, and the amygdaloid nucleus.

CAUDATE NUCLEUS

The caudate nucleus consists of an anterior portion or **head,** which tapers into a slender **tail** extending backward and then forward into the temporal lobe (Fig. 12–1). The extension of the caudate nucleus into the temporal lobe terminates at the amygdaloid nucleus, with which the caudate nucleus has no functional relationship, and consists of an attenuated, interrupted strand of gray matter in some human brains.

The head of the caudate nucleus bulges into the anterior horn of the lateral ventricle, and the first part of the tail lies along the lateral margin of the body or central part of the lateral ventricle (Figs. 11–9 through 11–11). The tail follows the contour of the lateral ventricle, as noted previously, continuing into the roof of the inferior or temporal horn of the ventricle. Two structures lie along the medial side of the tail of the caudate nucleus. These are the **stria terminalis,** a slender bundle of fibers originating in the amygdaloid nucleus, and the **vena terminalis,** which drains the caudate nucleus, thalamus, internal capsule, and nearby structures (Fig. 11–11).

The anterior limb of the internal capsule intervenes between the head of the caudate nucleus and the lenticular nucleus, and the tail of the caudate nucleus is adjacent to the internal capsule as the latter merges with the medullary center of the hemisphere. However, the cortical afferent and efferent fibers constituting the internal capsule do not separate the two components of the neostriatum entirely. The head of the caudate nucleus and the putamen are continuous with one another through a bridge of gray matter beneath the anterior limb of the internal capsule (Fig. 12–1). In addition numerous strands of gray matter joining the head and tail of the caudate nucleus with the putamen cut across the internal capsule.

CONNECTIONS

There are certain differences with respect to the connections of the putamen and the caudate nucleus because of the spatial separation of these two parts of the neostriatum. Similarly, the connections of the medial and lateral divisions of the globus pallidus are not precisely alike. In order to avoid excessive detail, the connections of the neostriatum and paleostriatum are described without reference to their anatomic subdivisions.

NEOSTRIATUM (Fig. 12–4)

The caudate nucleus and the putamen are similar histologically, as is to be expected. They consist mainly of small neurons forming intranuclear connections or projecting to the globus pallidus. Only about 1 cell in 20 is of relatively large size; these cells send fibers to the globus pallidus and the substantia nigra.

The neostriatum receives fibers from the cerebral cortex, thalamus, and substantia nigra. **Corticostriate** fibers originate in widespread areas of cortex, including that of all four lobes, but especially the frontal and parietal lobes. Most of the fibers enter the neostriatum from the internal capsule, some being collateral branches of corticobulbar and corticospinal fibers, although a substantial number enter the putamen from the external capsule. **Thalamostriate** fibers originate in the medial, ventral anterior, and intralaminar nuclei of the thalamus. **Nigrostriate** fibers from the substantia nigra constitute an important afferent connection of the corpus striatum. The functional and biochemical relationship between the substantia nigra and the striatum is prominent in current work on the pathogenesis and therapy of Parkinson's disease.

Most of the fibers leaving the neostriatum are **striopallidal,** bringing the globus pallidus under the influence and control of the neostriatum. The remaining efferents are **strionigral,** terminating in the substantia nigra.

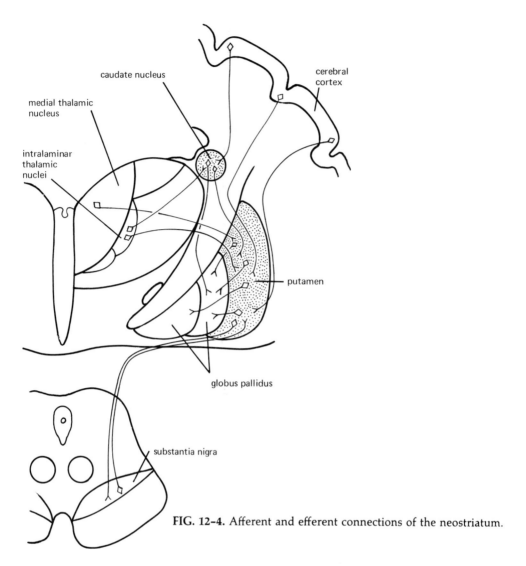

FIG. 12-4. Afferent and efferent connections of the neostriatum.

PALEOSTRIATUM (Fig. 12-5)

The globus pallidus, which is the principal efferent part of the corpus striatum, consists of moderately large, multipolar neurons. Their axons are well myelinated, accounting for the pallor of the nucleus in fresh sections and for the name "globus pallidus." Conversely, the globus pallidus is darker than the putamen and the caudate nucleus in Weigert-stained sections.

The **striopallidal** fibers noted previously are the principal afferents to the globus pallidus. **Corticopallidal** and **nigropallidal** fibers have been described, but these are unimportant compared with the projection from the cortex and substantia nigra to the striatum.

Efferent fibers of the globus pallidus take either of two routes initially. Some fibers cross the internal capsule and appear as the **lenticular fasciculus** (field H_2 of Forel) in the subthalamus, dorsal to the subthalamic nucleus. Other fibers curve around the medial edge of the internal capsule, forming the **ansa lenticularis.** These fasciculi consist almost entirely of **pallidothalamic fibers.** They enter the prerubral area of the subthalamus (field H of Forel), turn laterally into the thalamic fasciculus (field H_1 of Forel), and terminate in the ventral lateral and ventral anterior nuclei of the thalamus. These nuclei project to

FIG. 12–5. Afferent and efferent connections of the paleostriatum.

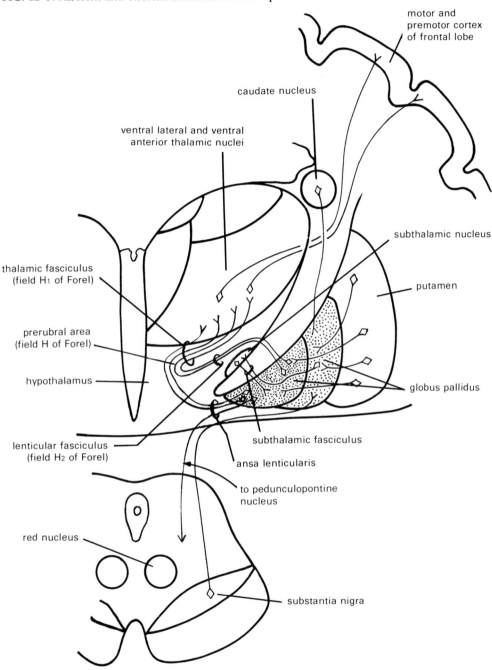

motor and premotor cortex of frontal lobe

caudate nucleus

ventral lateral and ventral anterior thalamic nuclei

subthalamic nucleus

thalamic fasciculus (field H₁ of Forel)

putamen

prerubral area (field H of Forel)

hypothalamus

globus pallidus

lenticular fasciculus (field H₂ of Forel)

subthalamic fasciculus

ansa lenticularis

to pedunculopontine nucleus

red nucleus

substantia nigra

motor and premotor areas of cortex in the frontal lobe, neurons in which are thereby brought under the regulatory influence of the corpus striatum. Only a few fibers of the efferent fasciculi of the globus pallidus turn caudally; these fibers end in a small nucleus, the pedunculopontine nucleus, situated in the tegmentum of the brain stem at the junction of the midbrain and pons. Fibers from the pedunculopontine nucleus end in the medial area of the reticular formation in the pons and medulla, an area from which reticulospinal fibers arise.

The globus pallidus has an important connection with the subthalamic nucleus; it consists of fibers passing in both directions across the internal capsule, these fibers forming the **subthalamic fasciculus.**

Although the corpus striatum is assumed to have motor functions because of the dyskinesias that result if it is involved in a pathologic lesion, the physiology of this part of the brain is one of the least understood aspects of the neurosciences. In addition to the well-documented thalamic projection, a substantial number of fibers from the globus pallidus were thought formerly to terminate in the red nucleus and the reticular formation of the brain stem. Through such connections the corpus striatum would influence lower motor neurons through the rubrospinal tract and reticulospinal fibers, and it was therefore considered as a component of the extrapyramidal motor system. Instead there is only a minor descending projection from the globus pallidus to the brain stem. Although it provides a means of bringing lower motor neurons under the influence of the corpus striatum, the descending pathway appears to be too poorly developed to have an appreciable functional significance. Aside from important connections with the substantia nigra and the subthalamic nucleus, the main relationship of the corpus striatum is with the thalamus and the cerebral cortex. The physiology of the corpus striatum remains a major challenge for research.

DYSKINESIAS AND THE CORPUS STRIATUM

Degenerative lesions which include the corpus striatum cause motor disturbances coming under the general heading of dyskinesias, in which involuntary movements take various forms.

Choreiform movements are brisk, jerky, and purposeless, resembling fragments of voluntary movements. They are most pronounced in the axial and proximal limb musculature; the facial muscles and the tongue are involved at times, and there may be hypotonia of the affected muscles. There are two diseases in which choreiform movements are a cardinal sign. Sydenham's chorea (St. Vitus' dance) is typically a disease of childhood; it occurs more frequently in girls than in boys, and often follows an infectious disease. The pathology of Sydenham's chorea is not well understood, because the disease is seldom fatal. The most common findings are scattered minute hemorrhages and capillary emboli in the corpus striatum. Huntington's chorea is a dominant hereditary disorder, onsetting in middle life, in which there is neuronal degeneration in the corpus striatum, most marked in the neostriatum. Concurrent loss of neurons in the cerebral cortex leads to progressive mental deterioration.

Athetoid movements are slow, sinuous, and aimless, involving the distal musculature of the limbs especially. The movements tend to blend together in a continuous mobile spasm and are usually associated with varying degrees of paresis and spasticity. The muscles of the face, neck, and tongue may be affected, with grimacing, protrusion and writhing of the tongue, and difficulty in speaking and swallowing. Athetosis is often part of a congenital complex of neurologic signs (including those of cerebral palsy) resulting from maldevelopment of the brain, birth injury, or other etiologic factors. Athetoid movements are most frequently associated with pathologic changes in the neostriatum and the cerebral cortex, although lesions are sometimes present as well in the globus pallidus and the thalamus.

Wilson's disease (hepatolenticular degeneration) is a special condition in which the corpus striatum is involved. The disease is caused by a genetically determined error in copper metabolism, and includes cirrhosis of the liver. The signs of Wilson's disease usually appear between the ages of 10–25 years; they include muscular rigidity, tremor, impairment of voluntary movements (including those of speech), and loss of facial expression. There may be uncontrollable laughing or crying without apparent cause. The degenerative changes are most pronounced in the putamen and progress to cavitation of the lenticular nucleus. There may also be cellular degeneration in the cerebral cortex, thalamus, red nucleus, and cerebellum. Dystonia musculorum deformans is a particularly disabling motor disturbance in which degenerative changes involve the corpus striatum along with other parts of the brain. The slow, writhing, involuntary movements of the axial and limb musculature are sustained, which may lead to contracture of muscles.

SUGGESTED READING

Beck E, Bignami A: Some neuro-anatomical observations in cases with stereotaxic lesions for the relief of Parkinsonism. Brain 91:589–618, 1968

Berke JJ: The claustrum, the external capsule and the extreme capsule of Macaca mulatta. J Comp Neurol 115:297–331, 1960

Brodal A: Some data and perspectives on the anatomy of the so-called "extrapyramidal system." Acta Neurol Scand [Supp] 39 (4): 17–38, 1963

Brodal A: Neurological Anatomy in Relation to Clinical Medicine. London, Oxford University Press, 1969

Carpenter MB, Strominger NL: Efferent fibers of the subthalamic nucleus in the monkey. A comparison of the efferent projections of the subthalamic nucleus, substantia nigra and globus pallidus. Am J Anat 121:41–71, 1967

Denny-Brown D: The Basal Ganglia and Their Relation to Disorders of Movement. London, Oxford University Press, 1962

Kemp JM, Powell TPS: The connections of the striatum and globus pallidus: synthesis and speculation. Philos Trans R Soc Lond [Biol] 262:441–457, 1971

Kim R, Nakano K, Jayaraman A, Carpenter MB: Projections of the globus pallidus and adjacent structures: an autoradiographic study in the monkey. J Comp Neurol 169:263–289, 1976

Martin JP: The Basal Ganglia and Posture. Philadelphia, Lippincott, 1967

Martinez A: Fiber connections of the globus pallidus in man. J Comp Neurol 117:37–41, 1961

Nauta WJH, Mehler WR: Projections of the lentiform nucleus in the monkey. Brain Res 1:3–42, 1966

Poirier LJ, Sourkes TL: Influence of the substantia nigra on catecholamine content of the striatum. Brain 88:181–192, 1965

Smith MC: Stereotactic operations for Parkinson's disease: anatomical observations. In Williams D (ed). Modern Trends in Neurology. London, Butterworth, 1967, pp 21–52

Szabo J: Topical distribution of the striatal efferents in the monkey. Exp Neurol 5:21–36, 1962

Szabo J: The efferent projections of the putamen in the monkey. Exp Neurol 19:463–476, 1967

Webster KE: The cortico-striatal projection in the cat. J Anat 99:329–337, 1965

13

Topography of the Cerebral Hemispheres

The complicated folding of the surface of the cerebral hemispheres substantially increases the surface area and therefore the volume of cerebral cortex. The folds or convolutions are called **gyri,** and the intervening grooves are called **sulci.** Two grooves appear early in fetal development and are especially deep in the mature brain; they are known as the lateral and parietooccipital **fissures.** About two-thirds of the cortex forms the walls of the sulci and fissures and is therefore hidden from surface view. Although most gyri are constant features of the cerebral surface, others vary from one brain to another and even between the two hemispheres of the same brain.

MAJOR FISSURES AND SULCI

The lateral and parietooccipital fissures, and the central and calcarine sulci, are boundaries for the division of the cerebral hemisphere into frontal, parietal, temporal, and occipital lobes (Figs. 13–1 and 13–2).

The **lateral fissure** or **fissure of Sylvius** begins as a deep furrow on the inferior surface of the hemisphere. This is the **stem** of the fissure, which extends laterally between the frontal and temporal lobes and divides into three rami on reaching the lateral surface. The **posterior ramus** is the main part of the fissure on the lateral surface of the hemisphere, whereas the **anterior** and **ascending rami** project for only a short distance into the frontal lobe. An area of cortex called the **insula** or **island of Reil** lies at the bottom of the lateral fissure and is hidden from surface view. This cortex appears to have been bound to the underlying corpus striatum

during fetal development, and growth of the surrounding cortex would then produce the deep lateral fissure.

The **central sulcus** or **sulcus of Rolando** is an important landmark for the sensorimotor cortex, because the general sensory area is immediately behind the sulcus and the motor area is immediately in front of it. The central sulcus indents the superior border of the hemisphere about 1 cm behind the midpoint between the frontal and occipital poles. The sulcus slopes downward and forward at an angle of 70 degrees to the vertical, stopping just short of the lateral fissure, and there are usually two bends along its course. The central sulcus is about 2 cm deep, and its walls therefore constitute much of the sensorimotor cortex.

The **calcarine sulcus** on the medial surface of the hemisphere begins under the posterior end of the corpus callosum and follows an arched course to the occipital pole. In some brains the sulcus continues over the pole for a short distance on the lateral surface. The calcarine sulcus is an important landmark for the visual cortex, most of which lies in the walls of the sulcus.

The **parietooccipital fissure,** like the lateral fissure, is a deep groove which appears early in the development of the fetal brain. It extends from the calcarine sulcus to the superior border of the hemisphere, intersects the border about 4 cm from the occipital pole, and continues for a short distance on the lateral surface.

The longitudinal and transverse cerebral fissures are external to the hemispheres and therefore in a different category from the surface markings previously described. The **longitudinal cerebral fissure** separates the

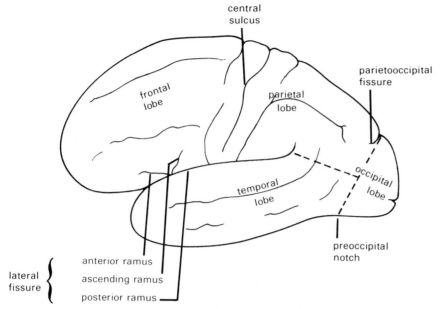

FIG. 13-1. Lobes of the cerebral hemisphere (lateral surface).

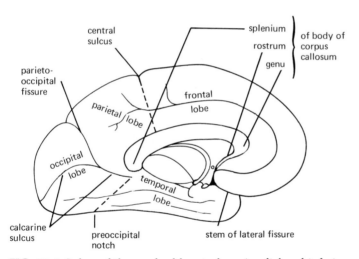

FIG. 13-2. Lobes of the cerebral hemisphere (medial and inferior surfaces).

hemispheres, and a dural partition called the falx cerebri extends into the fissure. The corpus callosum, which constitutes the main cerebral commissure, crosses from one hemisphere to the other at the bottom of the longitudinal fissure. The **transverse cerebral fissure** intervenes between the cerebral hemispheres above and the cerebellum, midbrain, and diencephalon below. The posterior part of the fissure is between the cerebral hemispheres and the cerebellum; it contains a dural partition known as the tentorium cerebelli. The anterior part of the transverse fissure intervenes between the corpus callosum and the diencephalon; it is triangular in outline, tapering anteriorly, and contains the tela choroidea, consisting of vascular connective tissue derived from the pia mater covering the brain. The tela choroidea is continuous with the connective tissue core of the choroid plexuses of the lateral ventricles and the third ventricle, and the plexuses are completed by choroid epithelium derived from the ependymal lining of the ventricles.

LOBES OF THE CEREBRAL HEMISPHERES

Each cerebral hemisphere has lateral, medial, and inferior surfaces, on which the extent of the lobes of the hemisphere needs to be defined (Figs. 13–1 and 13–2).

The **frontal lobe** occupies the entire area in front of the central sulcus and above the lateral fissure on the lateral surface. The medial surface of the frontal lobe envelops the anterior part of the corpus callosum and is bounded posteriorly by an imaginary line drawn between the central sulcus and the corpus callosum. Such lines are used elsewhere; they have no functional significance and can be ignored after serving their initial purpose. The inferior surface of the frontal lobe rests on the orbital plate of the frontal bone.

The natural boundaries of the **parietal lobe** on the lateral surface are the central sulcus and the lateral fissure. The imaginary boundaries consist of two lines; the first of these is drawn between the parietooccipital fissure and the preoccipital notch, and the second line runs from the middle of the one just established to the lateral fissure. (The preoccipital notch is an unsatisfactory landmark, consisting of a shallow indentation of the brain caused by the petrous portion of the temporal bone.) On the medial surface the parietal lobe is bounded by the frontal lobe, corpus callosum, calcarine sulcus, and parietooccipital fissure.

The **temporal lobe** is outlined on the lateral surface by the lateral fissure and the imaginary lines previously noted. The inferior surface of the temporal lobe extends to the temporal pole from a line drawn between the anterior end of the calcarine sulcus and the preoccipital notch. Most of the **occipital lobe** appears on the medial surface of the hemisphere, where it is separated from the temporal lobe as already described and from the parietal lobe by the parietooccipital fissure. On the lateral surface, the occipital lobe consists of the small area posterior to the imaginary line joining the parietooccipital fissure and the preoccipital notch.

The portion of the great cerebral commissure in and near the midline is known as the **body of the corpus callosum,** and the fibers of the commissure spreading out within the medullary centers of the hemispheres constitute the **radiations of the corpus callosum.** Names are assigned to certain regions of the body of the commissure (Fig. 13–2), and these regions are used as reference points further on. The enlarged posterior portion of the body is called the **splenium.** The anterior portion, or **genu,** thins out to form the **rostrum,** which is continuous with the lamina terminalis limiting the third ventricle anteriorly.

GYRI AND SULCI

Some surface markings of the hemisphere are landmarks for important functional areas; the central sulcus for the sensorimotor cortex and the calcarine sulcus for the visual cortex are good examples. For the most part, however, the sulci and gyri serve only as a rough frame of reference for cortical areas whose function may or may not be known. The markings can be identified according to lobes for the lateral surface, but this is not practicable for the medial and inferior surfaces. As already noted, there is considerable variation in detail from one brain to another.

LATERAL SURFACE OF THE HEMISPHERE (Fig. 13–3)

Frontal Lobe

The **precentral sulcus** (often broken into two or more parts) is parallel with the central sulcus; these sulci outline the **precentral gyrus,** which is a landmark for the motor area of the cerebral cortex. The remainder of the lateral surface of the frontal lobe is divided into **superior, middle,** and **inferior frontal gyri** by the **superior** and **inferior frontal sulci.** The superior frontal gyrus extends on the medial surface of the hemi-

sphere. The anterior and ascending rami of the lateral fissure divide the inferior frontal gyrus into **opercular, triangular,** and **orbital portions.** In the frontal lobe, as in the other lobes of the hemisphere, there are secondary gyri and sulci which contribute to the variability in the topography of different brains.

Parietal Lobe

The **postcentral sulcus** is parallel with the central sulcus; these sulci bound the **postcentral gyrus,** which is the landmark for the general sensory area of cortex. The **intraparietal sulcus** extends posteriorly from the postcentral sulcus, and divides that part of the surface not occupied by the postcentral gyrus into **superior** and **inferior parietal lob-**

FIG. 13–3. Gyri and sulci on the lateral surface of the right cerebral hemisphere. **a, b,** and **c** indicate the opercular, triangular, and orbital portions of the inferior frontal gyrus, respectively. (× ⅝)

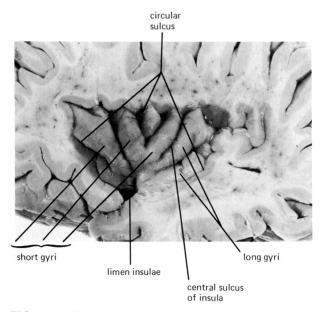

circular
sulcus

short gyri   long gyri

limen insulae

central sulcus
of insula

FIG. 13-4. The insula (island of Reil) of the left cerebral hemisphere, exposed by cutting away the frontal, parietal, and temporal opercula. (× 4/5)

ules. Those portions of the inferior parietal lobule that surround the upturned ends of the lateral fissure and the superior temporal sulcus are called the **supramarginal gyrus** and the **angular gyrus,** respectively.

Temporal Lobe

Superior and **middle temporal sulci** divide the lateral surface of the temporal lobe into **superior, middle,** and **inferior temporal gyri,** the last named continuing on the inferior surface. Among variations in the temporal lobe the middle temporal sulcus may be discontinuous and difficult to identify. The superior temporal gyrus has a large surface that forms the floor of the lateral fissure. On this surface **transverse temporal gyri** (also known as **Heschl's convolutions)** extend to the bottom of the lateral fissure and mark the location of the auditory area of cortex.

Occipital Lobe

In primate brains other than that of man, and in some human brains, the calcarine sulcus continues for a short distance over the occipital pole. There is then a curved **lunate sulcus** around the end of the calcarine sulcus. Ex-

cept for this inconstant marking, the small area of the occipital lobe on the lateral surface has minor grooves and folds of no special significance.

INSULA

It is customary to consider the **insula** or **island of Reil** separately from the four main lobes of the hemisphere. The regions concealing the insula are known as the **frontal, parietal,** and **temporal opercula;** they must be spread apart or cut away in order to expose the insula (Fig. 13-4). The insula is outlined by a circular sulcus and divided into two regions by a central sulcus. Several short gyri lie in front of the central sulcus and one or two long gyri behind it. The inferior part of the insula in the region of the stem of the lateral fissure is known as the **limen insulae.**

MEDIAL AND INFERIOR SURFACES OF THE HEMISPHERE

The **cingulate gyrus** begins beneath the genu of the corpus callosum and continues above the corpus callosum as far back as the splenium (Fig. 13-5). The gyrus is separated from the corpus callosum by the **sulcus of the corpus callosum** (callossal sulcus). The **cingulate sulcus** intervenes between the cingulate gyrus and the extension of the superior fron-

FIG. 13–5. Gyri and sulci on the medial and inferior surfaces of the right cerebral hemisphere. **a.** Uncus. **b.** Isthmus connecting the cingulate and parahippocampal gyri. (× ⅝)

FIG. 13–6. Gyri and sulci on the inferior surface of the right cerebral hemisphere. **a.** Uncus. (× ⅝)

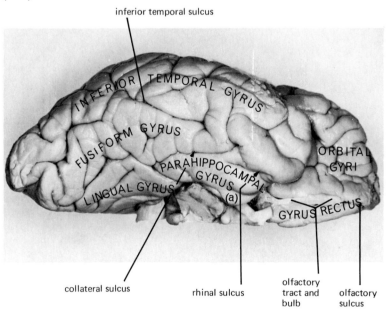

tal gyrus on the medial surface of the hemisphere. The cingulate sulcus gives off a **paracentral sulcus,** then divides into **marginal** and **subparietal sulci** in the parietal lobe. The region bounded by the paracentral and marginal sulci, and surrounding the indentation made by the central sulcus on the superior border, is called the **paracentral lobule.** The anterior and posterior parts of the paracentral lobule are extensions of the precentral and postcentral gyri, respectively, of the lateral surface of the hemisphere. The area above the subparietal sulcus is called the **precuneate gyrus** (precuneus) and is continuous with the superior parietal lobule on the lateral surface. The parietooccipital fissure and the calcarine sulcus bound the **cuneate gyrus** (cuneus) of the occipital lobe.

On the inferior surface of the hemisphere (Figs. 13–5 and 13–6) a convolution extends from the occipital pole almost to the temporal pole. The posterior part of the convolution consists of the **lingual gyrus;** the anterior part forms the **parahippocampal gyrus,** which hooks sharply backward as the **uncus.** The **collateral sulcus** defines the lateral margin of the lingual and parahippocampal gyri, and the short **rhinal sulcus** is situated at the lateral edge of the parahippocampal gyrus anteriorly. The **fusiform gyrus** (occipitotemporal gyrus), which is inconstant in morphology and broken up by irregular sulci, lies along the lateral side of the collateral sulcus. The **inferior temporal sulcus** intervenes between the fusiform gyrus and the extension of the inferior temporal gyrus on the inferior surface of the hemisphere.

On the orbital surface of the frontal lobe (Fig. 13–6), the **olfactory bulb** and **olfactory tract** conceal most of the **olfactory sulcus.** The **gyrus rectus** is medial to the olfactory sulcus, and the large area lateral to the olfactory sulcus consists of irregular **orbital gyri.**

The cingulate and parahippocampal gyri are connected by a narrow **isthmus** beneath the splenium of the corpus callosum, forming the **limbic lobe** of the cerebral hemisphere. This is part of the limbic system of the brain, which also includes the hippocampus, dentate gyrus, and amygdaloid nucleus (all in the temporal lobe), the hypothalamus (especially the mammillary bodies), the anterior nucleus of the thalamus, and connecting fiber tracts. Because of its important specialized functions, the limbic system is discussed separately in Chapter 18.

14

Histology of the Cerebral Cortex

Each cerebral hemisphere has a mantle of gray matter, the cortex or pallium, which makes up about 40% of the weight of the human brain. The cortex has a characteristic structure, consisting of nerve cells and nerve fibers arranged in layers. However, there are several types of cortex on the basis of histology and the sequence of phylogenetic development.

Almost the entire cortex of submammalian vertebrates is olfactory cortex of the rhinencephalon (nosebrain). This cortex becomes the three-layered **paleocortex** and **archicortex** of the mammalian brain. The paleocortex retains an olfactory function, whereas the archicortex is incorporated in the limbic system of the brain, which has a specialized role with respect to the emotions.

Neocortex, in which there are six histologic layers, is an important feature of the mammalian brain. It includes areas for general sensation and the special senses exclusive of smell, and areas from which fibers project to neurons with motor functions at various levels of the central nervous system. The expanse of neocortex increased as higher mammals evolved, mainly because of progressively larger amounts of so-called association cortex. This trend culminated in the condition found in the human brain; 90% of the cerebral cortex of man is neocortex, most of which is association cortex rather than consisting of specific sensory and motor areas. Neocortex is also called **isocortex,** paleocortex and archicortex then being referred to as **allocortex.** Finally the cortex of the cingulate gyrus is known as **mesocortex** because it is intermediate histologically between three-layered and six-layered cortices.

The present chapter deals with the histology or cytoarchitecture of the neocortex. In addition to having important sensory and motor functions, the neocortex merits special attention as the principal contributor to the intellectual capabilities of man. Human society and culture, together with the complexity and individuality of behavior, are largely the consequence of man's possessing a significantly larger volume of neocortex than any other species.

TYPES OF CORTICAL NEURON

Values obtained for the number of nerve cells in the human cerebral cortex vary widely because of technical difficulties in their enumeration. They range from 2.6×10^9 to 14×10^9, and the number of cortical neurons is therefore enormous. Of the morphologic variations among these neurons, five types are especially characteristic. Pyramidal and stellate cells are the most numerous, the others being fusiform cells, cells of Martinotti, and horizontal cells of Cajal. In addition to the arrangement of cells in six layers, the principal characteristic of neocortex is the presence of pyramidal neurons and a large population of small Golgi type II neurons, many of which are stellate cells. As in gray matter elsewhere, there is a large population of neuroglial cells (protoplasmic astrocytes, oligodendrocytes, and microglial cells) and a close capillary network.

Cortical neurons fall into three broad categories according to the nature of their connections. **Projection neurons** transmit impulses to a subcortical center, such as the corpus striatum, the thalamus, a brain stem nucleus, or the spinal cord. **Association neu-**

179

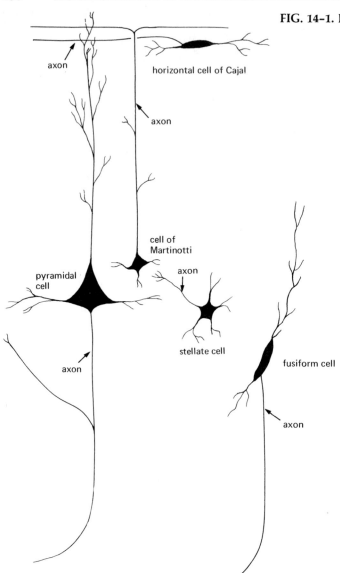

FIG. 14–1. Main types of cortical neuron.

rons establish connections with other cortical nerve cells in the same hemisphere. They include the vast number of Golgi type II cells whose short axons do not leave the cortex, thereby providing for complex intracortical circuits. Axons of the remaining association neurons enter the white matter and terminate in another cortical area of the same hemisphere. Axons of **commissural neurons** proceed to the cortex of the opposite hemisphere. Most of the commissural fibers comprise the corpus callosum; a relatively small number connect cortical areas of the tem-

poral lobes through the anterior commissure.

The five types of neuron present in the cerebral cortex have the following characteristics (Fig. 14–1).

Pyramidal cells derive their name from the shape of the cell bodies, which range in height from 10μ to 50μ for most pyramidal cells. They are classified as small, medium-sized, and large pyramidal neurons, the size increasing with the distance from the surface of the cortex. In addition, there are giant pyramidal cells, also known as **Betz cells,** with cell bodies as large as 100μ in height; these are present in the motor area of the frontal lobe.

The pyramidal cell has an apical dendrite directed toward the surface of the cortex and several basal dendrites. The dendritic branches bear large numbers of spines which make synaptic contact with axons of other neurons. The length of the axon, which arises from the base of the cell body, depends on the size of the cell. In the case of more superficially located, small pyramidal cells, the axon may terminate in a deeper cortical layer. With this exception, the axons of pyramidal neurons enter the white matter as projection, association, or commissural fibers. Collateral branches may arise from the axon while still in the cortex and synapse with neighbouring neurons.

Stellate cells, also known as granule cells, are polygonal or star shaped in outline, and the cell body is about 8μ in diameter. There are several short dendrites and the axon terminates on a neuron nearby.

Of the less numerous cell types, **fusiform cells** are located in the deepest cortical layer and the long axis of the cell body is perpendicular to the surface of the cortex. A dendrite extends from each end of the perikaryon; the deep dendrite is short, whereas the other one reaches into more superficial layers of the cortex. The axon enters the white matter as a projection, association, or commissural fiber. The remaining cell types are intracortical association neurons. **Cells of Martinotti** are present throughout the cortex, except for the most superficial layer. Short dendrites arise from the small, polygonal cell body. The identifying feature of the cell of Martinotti is that the axon is directed toward the surface, ending in any more superficial layer, but preferentially in the external layer. **Horizontal cells of Cajal** are restricted to the surface layer. The cell body is fusiform, with a dendrite extending from each end. The axon, which runs tangentially to the cortical surface, makes synaptic contact with dendritic branches of pyramidal neurons.

CORTICAL HISTOLOGY

The thickness of the cortex varies from 4.5 mm in the motor area of the frontal lobe to 1.5 mm in the visual area of the occipital lobe. The cortex is generally thicker over the crest of a gyrus than in the depths of a sulcus. The six layers, differing in the density of cell population and the size and shape of constituent neurons, can be recognized by about the 7th month of fetal life. The details of the layers differ from one region to another, as will be discussed presently. The names and characteristics of the layers, starting at the surface and omitting regional differences, are as follows (Fig. 14–2A):

1. **Molecular layer.** The superficial layer consists predominantly of delicate neuronal processes, both dendrites and axons, giving it a punctate or "molecular" appearance in sections stained for nerve fibers. Most of the dendritic branches come from pyramidal cells. The axons originate in cortex elsewhere in the same hemisphere, in that of the opposite hemisphere, and in the thalamus. Cells of Martinotti in any deeper layer also contribute axons to layer 1. The infrequent horizontal cells of Cajal and scattered stellate cells intervene between some axons and dendrites. The molecular layer is essentially an important synaptic field of the cortex.

2. **External granular layer.** This layer contains a wealth of small neurons, both small pyramidal cells and stellate cells. The dendrites of many of these cells extend into the molecular layer; most of the axons terminate in deeper layers, and the remainder enter the medullary center. The external granular layer makes an important contribution to the complexity of intracortical circuits.

3. **External pyramidal layer.** The neurons are typical pyramidal cells, increasing in size from the external to the internal borders of the layer. Apical dendrites extend into the synaptic field of layer 1; axons of the pyramidal cells enter the white matter and proceed to their destination as projection, association, or commissural fibers.

4. **Internal granular layer.** The fourth layer consists of closely arranged stellate cells, many of which receive stimuli from fibers originating in the thalamus. The short axons of the stellate cells synapse with dendrites passing through the layer from cells in layers 5 and 6, with other stellate cells, and with cells of Martinotti. As in

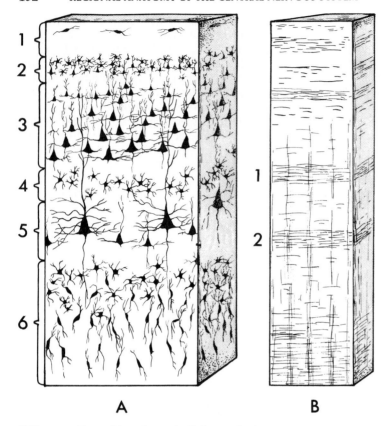

FIG. 14–2. Cortical histology. **A.** Golgi method: **1,** molecular layer; **2,** external granular layer; **3,** external pyramidal layer; **4,** internal granular layer; **5,** internal pyramidal layer; **6,** multiform layer. **B.** Weigert method: **1,** outer line of Baillarger; **2,** inner line of Baillarger.

any nervous tissue that includes large numbers of Golgi type II neurons, the connections and circuits involving the stellate cells of layer 4 are numerous and complex.

5. **Internal pyramidal layer.** This layer contains pyramidal cells intermingled with scattered stellate cells and cells of Martinotti. The giant pyramidal cells (cells of Betz) in the motor area of cortex in the frontal lobe are situated in layer 5.

6. **Multiform layer.** Although fusiform cells predominate, there are also neurons of various shapes. Axons of the neurons in this layer are included among the projection, commissural, and association fibers in the white matter of the hemisphere.

In the paleocortex and the archicortex, there are molecular, pyramidal, and multiform layers. These correspond roughly to layers 1, 5, and 6, respectively, of the neocortex. Layers 2, 3, and 4 of the neocortex are therefore regarded as a more recent acquisition phylogenetically, with a special bearing on higher cortical functions. Layers 1 through 4 of the neocortex, which include patterns for nerve impulse transmission such as are required for particularly complex functions, are sometimes referred to as the supragranular cortex. Layers 5 and 6, which are basically efferent in nature, are then said to compose the infragranular cortex.

The layers described are evident in sections stained by the Nissl and Golgi techniques. When silver methods for axons or the Weigert method for myelin sheaths are used, nerve fibers within the neocortex are seen to accumulate in radial bundles and tangential bands (Fig. 14–2B). The radial bundles are close together; they include

FIG. 14–3. Vertical section through the medial surface of the occipital lobe at the site of the calcarine sulcus. The line of Gennari, extending from **a** to **b,** identifies the visual area of cortex (striate area). (Weigert stain, × 2)

axons of pyramidal and fusiform cells leaving the cortex, together with afferent fibers from the thalamus and from cortex elsewhere. The tangential bands consist largely of collateral and terminal branches of afferent fibers. The branches leave the radial bundles and run parallel to the surface for some distance, making synaptic contact with large numbers of cortical neurons. The most prominent tangential bands are the **outer** and **inner lines of Baillarger,** located in layer 4 and the deep portion of layer 5, respectively. Thalamocortical fibers contribute heavily to the lines of Baillarger, which are therefore especially well developed in sensory areas. In the visual area in the walls of the calcarine sulcus, the outer line of Baillarger is sufficiently thick to be just visible on the cut surface with the unaided eye. In this location, it is known as the **line of Gennari** (Fig. 14–3), having been first described by Francesco Gennari, an eighteenth century Italian medical student. Because of the presence of the line of Gennari, the visual cortex is known alternatively as the striate area.

VARIATIONS IN CYTOARCHITECTURE

The foregoing description of cortical histology is to be regarded only as a general pattern. Six layers can be identified throughout most of the neocortex, which is said to be **homotypical** cortex. In some areas, known as **heterotypical** cortex, it is not possible to identify six layers. For example, in the visual area and part of the auditory and general sensory areas, the stellate cells of layer 4 overflow into adjoining layers. Layers 2 through 5 therefore merge into a single layer of small cells, many of which receive thalamocortical fibers. This type of heterotypical cortex is called **granular cortex** or **koniocortex** (*konis,* dust). The opposite extreme is found in the motor and premotor areas of the frontal lobe. Layers 2 through 5 again appear as a single, well-developed layer consisting mainly of efferent pyramidal cells **(agranular cortex).**

The cerebral cortex has been divided into cytoarchitectural areas, based on differences in the thickness of individual layers, neuronal morphology in the layers, and the details of nerve fiber lamination. Such studies require infinite patience and attention to detail. The few investigators who have undertaken a meticulous analysis of cortical cytoarchitecture hoped to establish a basis for structural and functional correlations. This has been only partially fulfilled because of differing histologic criteria and an incomplete understanding of the functional significance of many parts of the cerebral cortex. Parcelation of the cortex by different investigators varies from 20 to 200 areas, depending on the cytoarchitectural criteria used. Brodmann's map, which was published in 1909 and consists of approximately 50 areas, remains the most widely used map of cortical cytoarchitectural areas.

More recent studies agree that heterotypical areas can be identified without difficulty. For example the anterior portion of the general sensory cortex in the postcentral gyrus is granular heterotypical cortex (area 3 of Brodmann); the visual cortex around the calcarine sulcus (area 17) and the central part of the

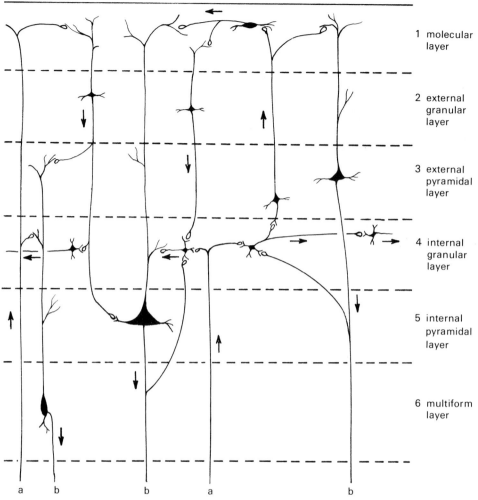

a   b   b   a   b

1 molecular
  layer

2 external
  granular
  layer

3 external
  pyramidal
  layer

4 internal
  granular
  layer

5 internal
  pyramidal
  layer

6 multiform
  layer

FIG. 14-4. A simplified scheme of intracortical circuits. **a.** Afferent cortical fibers. **b.** Efferent cortical fibers.

auditory cortex in the superior temporal gyrus (area 41) also consist of granular cortex. The motor and premotor areas of the frontal lobe (areas 4 and 6) are agranular heterotypical cortex, and are distinguished from one another by the presence of giant pyramidal (Betz) cells in area 4. In view of the obvious difficulties in establishing boundaries between areas with rather subtle histologic differences, it is not surprising that the cytoarchitectural areas described for the large expanse of association cortex have met with some skepticism. However, the concept has considerable appeal, leading to widespread use of the numbering system based on corti-

cal histology. Areas of Brodmann's map that are referred to later in the text are shown in Figures 15-1 and 15-2.

INTRACORTICAL CIRCUITS

Studies of cortical neurons with the Golgi technique, combined with electrical recording from microelectrodes placed in the cortex, have yielded information concerning intrinsic circuits. These are suggested in Figure 14-4; in reality the circuits are much more complex than the figure indicates.

Afferent fibers entering the cortex originate in cortex elsewhere in the same hemisphere and in the opposite hemisphere, or they come from the thalamus. Thalamocortical fibers are either specific afferents, such as those originating in sensory relay nuclei of the thalamus and terminating in sensory areas, or nonspecific afferents from other thalamic nuclei. Specific thalamocortical fibers divide into branches which synapse with cortical neurons mainly in the region of the outer line of Baillarger (line of Gennari in the visual cortex). Nonspecific thalamic afferents and fibers from other regions of cortex terminate in all cortical layers, with an emphasis on layers 1 through 3. Cortical efferent fibers are axons of the larger cells, notably pyramidal and fusiform cells. They enter the white matter for distribution as projection, association, or commissural fibers.

The histology of the neocortex is basically the same in all mammals, but the population of Golgi type II cells with short axons increases, the higher the mammal in the phylogenetic scale. The principal attribute of the neocortex of man is the presence of an especially large population of these small neurons, notably the small pyramidal cells of layer 2 and the stellate cells of layer 4. An afferent fiber may establish synaptic contact directly with an efferent neuron, but usually variable numbers of Golgi type II cells intervene between afferent fibers and efferent neurons. In addition collateral branches of axons of efferent cells establish synaptic contact with Golgi type II neurons, contributing to the reverberating circuits in the cortex.

Recordings from microelectrodes inserted in the cortex have shown that it is organized functionally as minute vertical units which include nerve cells of all layers. This has been demonstrated best in sensory areas. All neurons in the unit are activated selectively by the same peripheral stimulus, whether it originates in a particular type of cutaneous receptor at a particular location or in a specific point on the retina. Adjacent functional units are integrated by means of connections established by small neurons.

SUGGESTED READING

Bailey P, Von Bonin G: The Isocortex of Man. Illinois Monographs in the Medical Sciences, Vol 6. Urbana, University of Illinois Press, 1951

Colonnier M: Synaptic patterns on different cell types in the different laminae of the cat visual cortex: an electron microscope study. Brain Res 9:268–287, 1968

Diamond IT, Hall WC: Evolution of neocortex. Science 164:251–262, 1969

Hubel DH, Wiesel TN: Anatomical demonstration of columns in the monkey striate cortex. Nature 221:747–750, 1969

Powell TPS, Mountcastle VB: Some aspects of the functional organization of the cortex of the postcentral gyrus of the monkey: a correlation of findings obtained in a single unit analysis with cytoarchitecture. Johns Hopkins Med J 105:133–162, 1959

Purpura DP, Carmichael MW, Housepian EM: Physiological and anatomical studies of development of superficial axodendritic synaptic pathways in neocortex. Exp Neurol 2:324–347, 1960

Tower DB, Schadé JP (eds): Structure and Function of the Cerebral Cortex. Amsterdam, Elsevier, 1960

15

Functional Localization in the Cerebral Cortex

Clinicopathologic studies and animal experiments conducted over more than a century have provided information concerning functional specialization in different regions of the cerebral cortex. For example, there are three main sensory areas; they are for general sensation, vision, and hearing, to which may be added gustatory and vestibular areas. There are also motor areas from which contraction of the skeletal musculature can be elicited by electrical stimulation. The remainder of the neocortex falls under the general heading of association cortex, which may be closely related functionally with the sensory areas or have an essential bearing on the even more complex levels of behavior and the intellect. As noted in the preceding chapter, the trend in mammalian evolution has been toward larger areas of so-called association cortex, and the human brain is preeminent in this respect.

DEVELOPMENT OF THE CONCEPT OF CORTICAL LOCALIZATION

The sensory and motor areas are more accessible to investigation than association cortex. In fact our knowledge of cortical function in relation to the higher mental processes is still fragmentary, although regions of association cortex that are of special importance for language have been identified.

The first indications of functional localization came from clinical observations. Broca (1861) examined postmortem the brain of an individual who had suffered from a speech defect (motor aphasia). A lesion was found in the inferior frontal gyrus, and the region is still known as Broca's motor speech area. On

the basis of clinicopathologic studies, Hughlings Jackson (1864) concluded that a form of localized epilepsy (now known as jacksonian epilepsy) is caused by focal irritation of the precentral gyrus. This work drew attention to the probability of a motor area; experimentalists then proceeded to demonstrate such an area by electrical stimulation of the cortex in animals. An area from which motor responses were elicited on weak stimulation was demonstrated by Fritsch and Hitzig (1870) in the dog, and by Ferrier (1875), Horsley and Beevor (1894), and Sherrington and Grünbaum (1901) in the monkey and chimpanzee.

The identification of sensory areas had a somewhat parallel history. In 1870, Gudden showed that removal of the eyes from young animals interfered with full development of the occipital lobes. Ferrier (1873) found that an animal's ears would rise on stimulation of a particular region of the temporal lobe. The region included the auditory area, and stimulation produced the animal's normal response to a sound. Similarly Dusser de Barenne (1916) showed that application of strychnine to a small area of the monkey's postcentral gyrus resulted in scratching of the skin in one place or another, depending on the precise point at which cortical neurons were stimulated. He was able with this technique to map the somesthetic cortex of the monkey. Head's meticulous study of patients with brain injuries received during World War I added greatly to an understanding of the sensory areas of the human cerebral cortex.

The studies on subhuman primates were extended to the human brain by neurosurgeons, notably Cushing, Foerster, and Penfield. In certain neurosurgical procedures it is essential to identify the motor area, a sensory area, or even a particular region within these areas. Identification of sensory areas requires operating on a conscious patient under local anesthesia, a procedure made possible because the brain itself is insensitive to procedures that are painful elsewhere in the body. Electrical stimulation of the brain under these circumstances has provided information of the first importance with respect to functional localization in the cerebral cortex of man.

It is convenient to consider the neocortex as consisting of the following two main parts: 1) cortex of the parietal, occipital, and temporal lobes, and 2) cortex of the frontal lobe. Simply stated the former is concerned with the reception and conceptual elaboration of sensory data, whereas the latter is concerned with motor responses and the judgments, foresight, and moods associated with behavior. Because of the complex nature of all aspects of the cerebral cortex, descriptions of functional areas and the terminology used vary greatly from one author to another. This is especially true of the association cortex situated adjacent to sensory areas and of areas from which motor responses are elicited by electrical stimulation. The following summary of this highly complicated subject is in accordance with one of several interpretations, especially with respect to the areas for which different modes of treatment are most pronounced.

PARIETO-OCCIPITO-TEMPORAL CORTEX

GENERAL SENSATION

The **somesthetic area** (general sensory area) occupies the postcentral gyrus on the lateral surface of the hemisphere and the posterior part of the paracentral lobule on the medial surface (Figs. 15–1 and 15–2). It consists of areas 3, 1, and 2 of the Brodmann cytoarchitectural map. Area 3, most of which is in the posterior wall of the central sulcus, is granular heterotypical cortex. Areas 1 and 2 are homotypical cortex, slightly thicker than area 3. It is possible to elict motor responses by stimulating the somesthetic area, as well as sensory responses from the motor area in the

precentral gyrus. The connections and functions of the two areas therefore overlap to some extent and they should be considered as a sensorimotor strip surrounding the central sulcus.

The ventral posterior nucleus of the thalamus is the main source of afferent fibers for the general sensory area, the larger proportion of these fibers terminating in area 3. The fibers traverse the internal capsule and medullary center, conveying data for the various modalities of general sensation. Fibers for cutaneous sensibility end preferentially in the anterior part of the area, and those for deep sensibility in the posterior part. The contralateral half of the body is represented as inverted. The pharyngeal region, tongue, and jaws are represented in the most ventral part of the somesthetic area, followed by the face, hand, arm, trunk, and thigh. The area for the remainder of the leg and the perineum is in the extension of the somesthetic cortex on the medial surface of the hemisphere, i.e., the posterior part of the paracentral lobule. The size of the cortical area for a particular part of the body is determined by the functional importance of the part and its need for sensitivity. Thus the area for the face, especially the lips, is disproportionately large, and a large area is assigned to the hand, particularly the thumb and index finger. There is some ipsilateral representation of the face for touch, in addition to the main contralateral representation. In fact, single cell recordings from the cortex indicate that there is more ipsilateral conduction of sensory data to the sensorimotor strip than is traditionally recognized.

When the somesthetic cortex is the site of a destructive lesion, a crude form of awareness persists at the thalamic level for the nociceptive sensations of pain, heat, and cold. There is poor localization of the stimulus, for which qualitative and quantitative interpretations are diminished or absent. There may also be minimal awareness of light touch, pressure, and vibration. However, the somesthetic cortex must be intact for any appreciation of the more discriminative sensations of fine touch and position and movement of the body parts. The sensory deficit subsequent to a lesion in the somesthetic area is contralateral and in the part of the body represented in the affected region of the area. Electrical stimulation of this area in a conscious patient elicits modified forms of

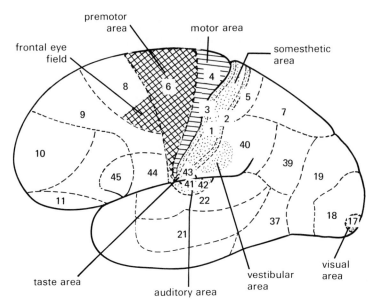

FIG. 15–1. Areas of functional localization on the lateral surface of the cerebral hemisphere. Areas of the Brodmann cytoarchitectural map shown in this figure and in Figure 15–2 are those referred to in the text.

FIG. 15–2. Areas of functional localization on the medial surface of the cerebral hemisphere.

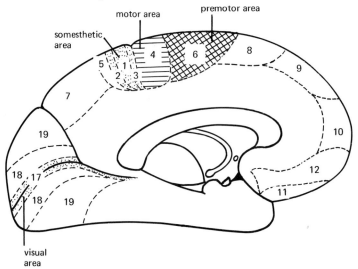

the tactile sense, such as tingling or a feeling of numbness.

In addition to the main or primary somesthetic area already discussed, the existence of a **secondary somesthetic area** has been demonstrated in primates, including man. This small area is situated in the dorsal wall of the lateral fissure in line with the postcentral gyrus, and it may extend onto the insula. The parts of the body are represented bilaterally, although contralateral representation predominates. The slight ipsilateral conduction for general sensory stimuli to both the primary and the secondary somesthetic areas may contribute to such awareness as persists following a destructive lesion that includes the postcentral gyrus or thalamocortical fibers proceeding to the gyrus.

The **somesthetic association cortex** is situated mainly in the superior parietal lobule on the lateral surface of the hemisphere and the precuneate gyrus on the medial surface. Much of it coincides with areas 5 and 7 of the Brodmann cytoarchitectural map. This association cortex receives fibers from the somesthetic area and has reciprocal connections with the dorsal tier of nuclei in the lateral mass of the thalamus. Data pertaining to the general senses are integrated, permitting, for example, a comprehensive assessment of the characteristics of an object held in the hand and its identification without visual aid. When there is a lesion in the somesthetic association cortex, leaving the somesthetic area itself intact, awareness of the general senses persists but the significance of the information received on the basis of previous experience is elusive. A defect in understanding the significance of sensory information is called **agnosia,** of which there are several types, depending on the sense that is most affected. A lesion causing destruction of a large portion of the somesthetic association area causes tactile agnosia and astereognosis, which are closely related. They combine when a person is unable to identify a common object, such as a pair of scissors, held in the hand while the eyes are closed. It is impossible to correlate the surface texture, shape, size, and weight of the object or to compare the sensations with previous experience. Astereognosis includes a loss of awareness of the "body scheme" or "body image" (the spatial relations of parts of the body).

VISION

The **visual area** surrounds the calcarine sulcus on the medial surface of the occipital lobe, extending over the occipital pole in some brains (Fig. 15–2). The area is more extensive than the illustration suggests because most of it is in the walls of the deep calcarine sulcus, on which there are secondary folds. The visual cortex is thinner than cortex elsewhere, being only about 1.5 mm in thickness. It is granular heterotypical cortex, corresponding to area 17 of the Brodmann map. The visual area is also called the **striate area** because the cortex here contains the line of Gennari, which is just visible to the unaided eye.

The chief source of afferent fibers to area 17 is the lateral geniculate nucleus of the thalamus by way of the geniculocalcarine tract. Part of this tract passes forward in the medullary center of the temporal lobe, then swings back (Meyer's loop) to the striate area. A cerebral lesion causing a defect in the visual field may therefore be located in the temporal lobe, far removed from the visual area of cortex.

Through a synaptic relay in the lateral geniculate nucleus, the visual cortex receives data from the temporal half of the ipsilateral retina and the nasal half of the contralateral retina. The dividing line runs vertically through the macula lutea, a specialized region of the retina at the posterior pole of the eye. The left half of the field of vision is therefore represented in the visual area of the right hemisphere and vice versa. There are spatial patterns within the striate area. The lower retinal quadrants (upper field of vision) project on the lower wall of the calcarine sulcus, and the upper retinal quadrants (lower field of vision) project on the upper wall of the sulcus. Another pattern is related to central and peripheral vision. The macula lutea is represented in the posterior part of area 17; proceeding from the macula to the ora serrata (anterior limit of the functional retina), the retina is represented progressively more anteriorly. The macula contains a concentration of cone photoreceptors, accounts for a disproportionately large number of fibers in the optic nerve and optic tract, and is responsible for central vision of maximal discrimination. Consistent with the foregoing, the part of area 17 receiving data for central vision accounts for one-third of the visual cortex.

A lesion that includes the visual cortex of a hemisphere causes an area of blindness in the opposite visual field, the size and location of which is determined by the extent and location of the lesion. However, central vision may be intact on field examination following a unilateral lesion in the occipital lobe, *e.g.,* an infarction caused by a thrombus in the posterior cerebral artery. This clinical observation is known as "macular sparing," for which there is no anatomic explanation on the basis of bilateral cortical representation of the macula. A possible explanation is that collateral circulation from branches of the middle cerebral artery partially maintains the large part of area 17 concerned with central vision following occlusion of the posterior cerebral artery. It has been suggested as well that macular sparing may at times be an artifact of testing, caused by the patient shifting his fixation point a few degrees during examination of the visual field.

The **visual association cortex** is described as corresponding with areas 18 and 19 of Brodmann, which surround the visual area on the medial and lateral surfaces of the hemisphere. These areas receive fibers from area 17 and have reciprocal connections with other cortical areas and the pulvinar of the thalamus. The role of this association cortex includes, among other complex aspects of vision, the relating of present to past visual experience, with recognition of what is seen and appreciation of its significance. A lesion involving a substantial portion of areas 18 and 19 therefore results in visual agnosia, in which there is inability to recognize objects in the opposite field of vision. (Specific cortical areas can be ablated with some precision in experimental animals, such as the monkey and chimpanzee. It will be appreciated that naturally-occurring lesions such as an infarction or a tumor include various functional areas and the subjacent white matter.)

Corticotectal fibers connect the visual association cortex with the superior colliculus of the midbrain, which in turn sends fibers to the oculomotor, trochlear, and abducens nuclei. This is part of a reflex pathway originating in the retina for automatic scanning movements in response to visual stimuli. The corticotectal fibers and the subsequent connection with the nuclei supplying ocular muscles probably function as well in the accommodation–convergence reaction on directing attention to a near object.

HEARING

Most of the **auditory area** (acoustic area) is concealed because it is in the ventral wall of the lateral fissure (Figs. 15–1 and 15–3). The surface of the superior temporal gyrus forming the floor of the fissure is marked by transverse temporal gyri. The two most anterior of these, called **Heschl's convolutions,** are landmarks for the auditory area, which corresponds with areas 41 and 42 of Brodmann. Area 41 is granular heterotypical cortex; area 42 is homotypical and may function in part as auditory association cortex.

The medial geniculate nucleus of the thalamus is the principal source of fibers ending in the auditory cortex, these fibers constituting the auditory radiation in the medullary center. There is a spatial representation in the auditory area with respect to the pitch of sounds. Impulses for low frequencies impinge on the anterolateral part of the area and impulses for high frequencies on the posteromedial part. Although the medial geniculate nucleus receives information originating mainly in the organ of Corti of the opposite side, there is a substantial input from the ear of the same side. A unilateral lesion involving the auditory area causes diminution in the acuity of hearing in both ears, the greater loss being in the opposite ear. However, the impairment is slight because of the bilateral projection to the cortex and the deficit is difficult to detect by simple clinical tests. Loss of function of the auditory area in one hemisphere is said to impair one's ability to detect the direction from which a sound originates.

The **auditory association cortex** occupies the floor of the lateral fissure behind the auditory area (the region labeled "planum temporale" in Fig. 15–3) and the posterior part of Brodmann's area 22 on the lateral surface of the superior temporal gyrus. The region of cortex thus defined is also known as **Wernicke's area** and is of major importance in language functions.

TASTE

The **taste area** (gustatory area) is located in the dorsal wall of the lateral fissure, with an extension onto the insula, corresponding

insula

planum temporale

anterior transverse
temporal gyri
(Heschl's convolutions)

FIG. 15-3. The auditory area of cortex after being exposed by removing part of the hemisphere dorsal to the lateral fissure. (× 4/5)

with area 43 of Brodmann (Fig. 15-1). This location is similar to that of the secondary somatic sensory area, and it places the taste area adjacent to the general sensory cortex for the tongue and pharynx. Nerve impulses from taste buds reach the gustatory nucleus in the brain stem, *i.e.*, the rostral portion of the nucleus of the tractus solitarius. Fibers from the gustatory nucleus cross the midline and ascend near the medial lemniscus and the ventral trigeminothalamic tract. They terminate in the medial part of the ventral posterior nucleus of the thalamus, and the pathway is completed by thalamocortical fibers.

VESTIBULAR REPRESENTATION

The best evidence concerning the location of the **vestibular area** comes from experiments using monkeys, in which evoked potentials in the cortex were recorded during electrical stimulation of the vestibular nerve. When the results are transferred to the human brain, the vestibular area is placed in the inferior parietal lobule near the general sensory area for the head (Fig. 15-1). Electrical stimulation of this region in conscious patients has occasionally produced dizziness and vertigo. The cortical projection from the vestibular labyrinth presumably contributes information for motor regulation and awareness of spatial orientation. The ascending fibers from the vestibular nuclei are almost entirely crossed and travel near the medial lemniscus. The thalamic relay is in the ventral posterior nucleus between the regions receiving fibers for general sensation for the head and for the remainder of the body.

The vestibular area was placed previously in the superior temporal gyrus anterior to the auditory area. This was based on the occasional reporting of dizziness and vertigo during electrical stimulation of the temporal lobe, together with the occurrence of these sensations as auras in temporal lobe epilepsy.

The significance of the foregoing observations with respect to the cortical projection from the vestibular nuclei has yet to be determined.

ASSOCIATION CORTEX

After identifying the areas of association cortex adjacent to the sensory areas, and having a special cognitive relationship with them, additional association cortex remains in the inferior parietal lobule and the posterior part of the temporal lobe. Data reaching the sensory areas and analyzed in the adjacent association cortex are correlated in the intervening region to yield a comprehensive assessment of the immediate environment.

The total expanse of association cortex in the parietal, occipital, and temporal lobes is responsible (along with association cortex in the frontal lobe) for many of the unique qualities and the potentialities of the human brain. Engrams or memory traces are laid down over the years, probably as a macromolecular phenomenon in cortical neurons having other functions. These form the basis of learning at an intellectual level. The complex neuronal circuitry of the cortex permits the coalescence of memory traces in the form of ideas and conceptual, abstract thinking. The anterior part of the temporal lobe appears to have special properties related to the highest level of brain function and has been called the "psychic cortex." Electrical stimulation of this region in the conscious patient may elicit recall of objects seen, music heard, or other experiences in the recent or distant past. A patient with a temporal lobe tumor may have auditory or visual hallucinations, sometimes reproducing earlier events. The association cortex of the three "sensory" lobes has abundant connections with cortex of the frontal lobe through fasciculi in the medullary center. Complex and flexible behavioral patterns are formulated on the basis of experience; emotional tones are added; and overt expression may follow through the motor system.

FRONTAL CORTEX

The neocortex of the frontal lobe has a special role in motor activities, in the attributes of judgment and foresight, and in determining one's mood or "feeling tone."

MOTOR AREA

The **motor area** (primary motor area) has been identified on the basis of histology and the elicitation of motor responses at a low threshold of electrical stimulation. The area is located in the precentral gyrus, including the anterior wall of the central sulcus, and the anterior part of the paracentral lobule on the medial surface of the hemisphere (Figs. 15-1 and 15-2). The motor cortex (area 4 of Brodmann) is 4.5 mm in thickness, with the histologic appearance of agranular heterotypical cortex, in which giant pyramidal cells of Betz are present in the internal pyramidal layer or layer 5.

The main sources of input to area 4 are the premotor cortex (area 6), the somesthetic cortex, and the ventral lateral and ventral anterior thalamic nuclei. Although area 4 contributes fibers to extrapyramidal motor pathways, the efferents that give it a special significance are those included in the pyramidal motor system (corticobulbar and corticospinal tracts). About 40% of these fibers arise in area 4; the remainder originate in area 6 of the frontal lobe and in the parietal lobe, including the somesthetic area. There is a good correlation between the number of Betz cells in the region of area 4 contributing fibers to the corticospinal tract and the number of large, thickly myelinated fibers about 10μ in diameter in the tract. The number is of the order of 35,000 in each instance, which accounts for about 3% of the fibers. The giant pyramidal cells of Betz therefore contribute a small population of rapidly-conducting fibers to the pyramidal tract, the remainder being thin fibers with slower conduction rates.

Electrical stimulation of the motor area elicits contraction of muscles predominantly on the opposite side of the body. Although cortical control of the skeletal musculature is mainly contralateral, there is significant ipsilateral control of most of the muscles of the head and of the axial muscles of the body. The body is represented in the motor area as inverted, the pattern being similar to that described for the somesthetic cortex. The sequence from below upward is pharynx, larynx, tongue, and face, the region for muscles of the head constituting about one-third of the whole of area 4. Continuing dorsally, there is a small region for muscles of the neck, followed by a large area for muscles of the hand, this being consistent with the importance of manual dexterity in man. Next in order are areas for the arm, shoulder, trunk, and thigh, continuing with an area on the medial surface of the hemisphere for the remainder of the leg and the anal and vesical sphincters.

The motor area has a low threshold of excitability, compared with other areas from which contraction of voluntary muscles can be elicited by electrical stimulation. Contractions of contralateral muscles are usually elicited, as has been noted, and the muscles responding depend on the particular part of area 4 that is stimulated. The response usually involves muscles that make up a functional group, although there is occasionally contraction of a single muscle. Destructive lesions of area 4 result in voluntary paresis of the affected part of the body. The muscles involved are flaccid; spastic voluntary paralysis characteristically follows lesions spreading beyond area 4 into the premotor area or which interrupt motor projection fibers (including extrapyramidal fibers) in the medullary center or internal capsule. There is considerable recovery with time, the residual deficit being most evident as impairment of movement in the distal part of the limbs. Destruction of part of the motor area without involvement of adjacent cortex or the underlying white matter is rarely encountered clinically. Deficits resulting from damage to area 4 are inferred from experiments on subhuman primates and on isolated instances in which a region of area 4 was removed in man as a therapeutic procedure, usually in the treatment of epilepsy.

A **secondary** and a **supplementary motor area** have been identified by cortical stimulation in primates, including man, although they are not known to be of importance clinically. The secondary motor area is ventral to the sensorimotor strip in the dorsal wall of the lateral fissure, overlapping the secondary somesthetic area; the supplementary motor area is on the medial surface of the hemisphere anterior to the paracentral lobule. In both areas, contraction of muscles in different parts of the body can be elicited by electrical stimulation.

PREMOTOR AREA

The **premotor area,** which coincides with Brodmann's area 6, is situated anterior to the motor area on the lateral and medial surfaces of the hemisphere. The cytoarchitecture of area 6 is like that of area 4, except that Betz cells are absent. In addition to connections with other cortical areas, the premotor cortex receives fibers from the ventral anterior and ventral lateral thalamic nuclei.

Muscular contractions result from stimulation of area 6, although stronger stimulation is required compared with area 4. Stimulation of the posterior part of area 6 produces responses similar to those obtained from area 4, *i.e.,* they involve several muscles of a functional group. In the experimental animal, this type of response no longer occurs following ablation of area 4 or after an incision is made along the border between areas 6 and 4. Movements elicited by stimulation of the anterior part of area 6, or any part of the premotor area if it has been isolated from the motor area, are generalized and directional; these include turning the head, twisting the trunk, or gross movements of the limbs. These observations suggest that the functions of the premotor area are mediated in part through the motor area and in part through independent motor projection fibers, both pyramidal and extrapyramidal.

Area 6 may be concerned in part with learned motor activity of a complex and sequential nature. The term **apraxia** refers to the result of a cerebral lesion, characterized by impairment in the performance of learned movements even though there is no voluntary motor paralysis. One form of apraxia follows a lesion involving the premotor area; another is caused by a lesion in the superior parietal lobule, proprioception being a necessary background for motor proficiency. When the disability is in writing, it is called **agraphia.** The **frontal eye field** is in the lower part of area 8 on the lateral surface of the hemisphere, extending slightly beyond that area. It controls voluntary scanning movements of the eyes, and electrical stimulation of the frontal eye field produces conjugate deviation of the eyes to the opposite side.

PREFRONTAL CORTEX

The large expanse of cortex in the frontal lobe from which motor responses are not elicited on stimulation falls under the heading of association cortex. The region enveloping the frontal pole is called **prefrontal cortex;** corresponding to areas 9, 10, 11, and

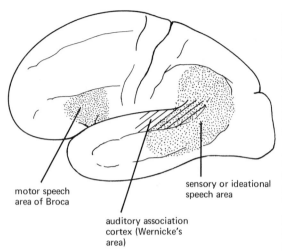

motor speech
area of Broca

sensory or ideational
speech area

auditory association
cortex (Wernicke's
area)

FIG. 15-4. Sensory and motor language areas.

12 in Brodmann's cytoarchitectural map, the prefrontal area is well developed only in primates and especially so in man. It has extensive connections through fasciculi in the medullary center with the parietal, temporal, and occipital lobes, thus gaining access to contemporary sensory experience and the repository of data derived from past experience. There are also reciprocal connections with the dorsomedial thalamic nucleus, forming a system which determines affective reactions to situations presently encountered on a background of past experience. The prefrontal cortices also monitor behavior and exercise control based on such higher mental faculties as judgement and foresight.

LANGUAGE AREAS

The use of language is a peculiarly human accomplishment, requiring special neural mechanisms in association areas of the cerebral cortex. Areas of cortex that have particular roles with respect to language have been identified by the study of patients in whom these areas were damaged by occlusion of blood vessels. The most reliable information is based on long-term studies of patients with deficits in the use of language, and whose brains were subjected to careful postmortem examination. Two cortical areas of special importance in language have been demonstrated; one such area in the temporal and parietal lobes is concerned with sensory as-

pects of language, and a second area in the inferior frontal gyrus functions in motor aspects of language (speech). The two areas are in communication through the superior longitudinal (arcuate) fasciculus in the medullary center. They are situated in the left hemisphere, with few exceptions, and this hemisphere is therefore the **dominant hemisphere** as a rule with respect to language.

Observations made during cortical stimulation in conscious patients led to the concept of a sensory or "ideational" language area in the temporal and parietal lobes (Fig. 15-4). This area has a considerable extent, occupying the posterior part of the superior and middle temporal gyri and most of the inferior parietal lobule. In relation to the Brodmann map, it includes portions of areas 21, 22, and 37 in the temporal lobe, and most of areas 39 and 40 in the inferior parietal lobule (Fig. 15-1). However, clinicopathologic studies of patients with speech disorders have shown quite clearly that the lesion responsible for a sensory or receptive type of language defect typically involves the auditory association cortex or Wernicke's area. A child first experiences language by hearing others talk and only later learns to read and write; it is perhaps for this reason that Wernicke's area has a special role in sensory aspects of language. In any case, association cortex in and around Wernicke's area receives data pertinent to language from the sensory areas and synthesizes these data into a comprehensive totality of the sensory aspects of language.

Broca's area or the **motor speech area** occupies the opercular and triangular portions of the inferior frontal gyrus, corresponding with areas 44 and 45 of Brodmann. Its influence on the lower one-third of the motor cortex for muscles of the head is essential for the appropriate and coordinated action of the diverse muscles used in speech.

A lesion involving the language areas or their connections results in **aphasia,** of which there are several types, depending on the location of the lesion. **Sensory aphasia** (Wernicke's aphasia), in which comprehension of language, naming of objects, and repetition of a sentence spoken by the examiner are all defective, is caused by a lesion in the sensory language area, more specifically in Wernicke's area. A lesion involving Wernicke's area and the superior longitudinal or arcuate fasciculus results in **jargon aphasia,** with fluent but unintelligible jargon. Interruption of the arcuate fasciculus connecting Wernicke's and Broca's areas causes **conduction aphasia,** in which there is poor repetition but relatively good comprehension and spontaneous speech. Infarcts which isolate the sensory language area from surrounding parietal and temporal cortex may cause **anomic aphasia,** characterized by fluent but circumlocutory speech due to word-finding difficulties. **Alexia** refers to loss of ability to read and occurs with or without other aspects of aphasia. "Pure alexia" may result from a lesion involving the occipital lobe of the dominant hemisphere and the splenium of the corpus callosum. **Motor aphasia** (Broca's aphasia), caused by a lesion in Broca's area of the frontal lobe, is characterized by hesitant and distorted speech with relatively good comprehension. The term **global aphasia** refers to complete loss of verbal communication, except perhaps for stereotyped utterances.

CEREBRAL DOMINANCE

Memory traces established in one hemisphere, *e.g.,* in the cortex of the right hemisphere as a result of some particular activity involving the left hand, are in general transferred to the cortex of the other hemisphere through the corpus callosum. There are therefore bilateral cortical memory patterns for one's previous experience. This does not pertain to language, for which there is no fully adequate explanation. In right-handed persons and a proportion of those who are left handed, language is a function of the left hemisphere. The "talking" hemisphere is said to be dominant, relative to the "nontalking" hemisphere. A left-sided cerebral lesion is therefore more serious than one in the right hemisphere because aphasia may be added to other neurologic deficits. The reverse is true for the few individuals whose right hemisphere is the dominant one.

Factors determining cerebral dominance and handedness (these are not always related to one another) are not well known, although heredity is almost certainly involved to some extent. The planum temporale posterior to the auditory area on the dorsal surface of the superior temporal gyrus (Fig. 15-3) is reported as being larger in the left than the right hemisphere in 65% of brains, and larger on the right side in only 11% of brains. This is an indication that the dominance with respect to language may be reflected in cerebral asymmetry because the planum temporale constitutes a large part of Wernicke's area. There is evidence that the nondominant hemisphere is superior in some nonlanguage aspects of cortical function, notably in activities requiring three-dimensional or spatial perception. The evidence is derived from the study of patients whose corpus callosum was sectioned as a therapeutic measure in severe epilepsy. Following commissurotomy these persons are able to execute drawings and place blocks in a desired position better with the left hand than with the right hand. The right hemisphere is therefore better equipped to perform such acts, even though it is called the nondominant hemisphere.

SUGGESTED READING

Brain WR: The physiological basis of consciousness: a critical review. Brain 81:426–455, 1958

Brain WR: Speech Disorders: Aphasia, Apraxia, and Agnosia. London, Butterworth, 1961

Carpenter MB: Human Neuroanatomy, 7th ed. Baltimore, Williams & Wilkins, 1976

Celesia GG: Organization of auditory cortical areas in man. Brain 99:403–414, 1976

Crosby EC, Humphrey T, Lauer EW: Correlative Anatomy of the Nervous System. New York, Macmillan, 1962

Deeke L, Schwarz DWF, Fredrickson JM: Nucleus ventroposterior inferior (VPI) as the vestibular thalamic relay in the Rhesus monkey. I. Field potential investigations. Exp Brain Res 20:88–100, 1974

De Reuck AVS, O'Connor M (eds): Disorders of Language. London, Churchill, 1964

Eccles JC (ed): Brain and Conscious Experience. New York, Springer. 1966

Fessard A, Gerard RW, Konorski J, Delafresnaye JF (eds): Brain Mechanisms and Learning. Springfield, IL, Thomas, 1961

Fredrickson JM, Figge U, Sheid P, Kornhuber HH: Vestibular nerve projection to the cerebral cortex of the Rhesus monkey. Exp Brain Res 2:318–327, 1966

Geschwind N: The organization of language and the brain. Science 170:940–944, 1970

Geschwind N: Language and the brain. Sci Am 226/4:76–83, 1972

Geschwind N, Levitsky W: Human brain: left-right asymmetries in temporal speech region. Science 161:186–187, 1968

Millikan CH, Darley FL (eds): Brain Mechanisms Underlying Speech and Language. New York, Grune & Stratton, 1967

Mountcastle VB (ed): Interhemispheric Relations and Cerebral Dominance. Baltimore, Johns Hopkins Press, 1962

Penfield W, Jasper H: Epilepsy and the Functional Anatomy of the Human Brain. Boston, Little, Brown, 1954

Penfield W, Rasmussen T: The Cerebral Cortex of Man: A Clinical Study of Localization of Function. New York, Macmillan, 1950

Russell WR: Brain, Memory, Learning: A Neurologist's View. Oxford, Clarendon Press, 1959

Wada JA, Clarke R, Hamm A: Cerebral hemisphere asymmetry in humans. Arch Neurol 32:239–246, 1975

Wada JA, Davis AE: Fundamental nature of human infant's brain asymmetry. Can J Neurol Sci 4:203–207, 1977

Williams PL, Warwick R: Functional Neuroanatomy of Man. Philadelphia, Saunders, 1975

Zangwill OL: Cerebral Dominance and Its Relation to Psychological Function. Springfield, IL, Thomas, 1960

16

Medullary Center, Internal Capsule, and Lateral Ventricles

Each cerebral hemisphere includes a large volume of white matter constituting the medullary center in order to accommodate the vast number of fibers running to and from all parts of the cortex. The medullary center is bounded by the cortex, the lateral ventricle, and the corpus striatum. Nerve fibers that establish connections between the cortex and subcortical gray matter continue from the medullary center into the internal capsule. The lateral ventricles, one in each hemisphere, are the largest of the four ventricles of the brain and have a prominent role in the dynamics of the cerebrospinal fluid system.

MEDULLARY CENTER

The nerve fibers of the medullary center are of three types, depending on the nature of their connections (Fig. 16–1). **Association fibers** are confined to a hemisphere, connecting one cortical area with another. Many of these fibers accumulate in longitudinally running bundles which can be displayed by dissection and have been assigned names. **Commissural fibers** connect the cortices of the two hemispheres; most of the neocortical commissural fibers constitute the corpus callosum, the remainder being included in the anterior commissure. **Projection fibers** establish connections between the cortex and such subcortical structures as the corpus striatum, thalamus, nuclei of the brain stem, and spinal cord. As previously noted, these fibers of the

medullary center become concentrated in the internal capsule toward the base of the hemisphere. The projection fibers are afferent (corticipetal) or efferent (corticofugal) with respect to the cortex, the former originating in the thalamus.

ASSOCIATION FASCICULI

Of the three types of fibers noted, association fibers are the most numerous. Operative procedures, vascular accidents, or other lesions involving the fasciculi may lead to dysfunction by disconnecting functionally related regions of the cerebral cortex.

The **cingulum** (Figs. 16–2 and 16–3) is an association bundle of the limbic lobe. Many of its fibers originate in the parahippocampal gyrus in the temporal lobe and reach the medullary core of the cingulate gyrus by means of the isthmus connecting these gyri adjacent to the splenium of the corpus callosum. These fibers terminate in the cortex of the cingulate gyrus and in the medial olfactory (septal) area below the genu of the corpus callosum. Other fibers of the cingulum, running in either direction, interconnect regions of the limbic lobe.

The **superior longitudinal fasciculus** (Figs. 16–2 and 16–3), also known as the **arcuate fasciculus,** runs in an anteroposterior direction above the insula, and many of the fibers turn downward into the temporal lobe. In common with other association bundles, this fasciculus consists of fibers of various lengths, which enter or leave the fasciculus at

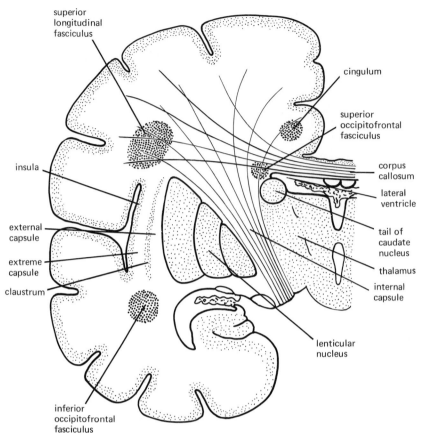

superior
longitudinal
fasciculus

cingulum

superior
occipitofrontal
fasciculus

corpus
callosum

lateral
ventricle

insula

external
capsule

extreme
capsule

claustrum

tail of
caudate
nucleus

thalamus

internal
capsule

lenticular
nucleus

inferior
occipitofrontal
fasciculus

FIG. 16–1. Coronal section through a cerebral hemisphere, indicating the position of association, commissural, and projection fibers.

any point along its course. The superior longitudinal fasciculus provides an important communication between cortex of the parietal, temporal, and occipital lobes and cortex of the frontal lobe, including the sensory and motor language areas of Wernicke and Broca. An **inferior longitudinal fasciculus** has been described as running superficially beneath the lateral and ventral surfaces of the occipital and temporal lobes. However, this thin sheet of association fibers is difficult to demonstrate by dissection or to distinguish from other fibers at a deeper level, in particular from projection fibers of the geniculocalcarine tract.

The **inferior occipitofrontal fasciculus** and the **uncinate fasciculus** are components of a single association system (Figs. 16–4 and 16–5). The fibers are compressed into a well-defined bundle between the stem of the lat-

eral fissure below and the insula and lenticular nucleus above. The longer part of the fiber system, extending the length of the hemisphere, is the inferior occipitofrontal fasciculus. The uncinate fasciculus is that part which hooks around the lateral fissure to connect the frontal lobe, especially cortex on its orbital surface, with cortex in the region of the temporal pole.

The **superior occipitofrontal fasciculus,** also called the **subcallosal bundle,** is located deep in the hemisphere and is therefore not accessible to dissection from a lateral approach. The fasciculus is compact in the midregion of the hemisphere, where it is bounded by the corpus callosum, internal capsule, tail of the caudate nucleus, and lateral ventricle (Fig. 16–1). The fibers spread out to cortex of the frontal lobe and to cortex in the posterior part of the hemisphere. The fasciculus includes some projection fibers proceeding from the cortex to the caudate nucleus.

body of
corpus callosum

cingulum   superior   radiation of
             longitudinal   corpus callosum
             fasciculus

FIG. 16-2. Dissection of the right cerebral hemisphere, dorsal view. (× ⅔)

FIG. 16-3. Dissection of the right cerebral hemisphere, dorsolateral view. (× ⅔)

cingulum

                                    insula

superior longitudinal
(arcuate) fasciculus

corona radiata

external capsule

inferior
occipitofrontal
fasciculus

uncinate
fasciculus

FIG. 16-4. Medullary center of the right cerebral hemisphere, after removal of the superior longitudinal fasciculus, insula, and underlying structures down to the external capsule. (× ⅔)

FIG. 16-5. Dissection illustrated in Figure 16-4 continued by removal of the external capsule to expose the putamen of the lenticular nucleus. (× ⅔)

corona radiata

putamen of
lenticular nucleus

inferior occipitofrontal
fasciculus

uncinate
fasciculus

Large numbers of **arcuate fibers** connect adjacent gyri. These fibers are oriented at right angles to the gyri, bending sharply under the intervening sulci. Spread of activity along a gyrus is provided by other subcortical association fibers and by the wealth of Golgi type II cells which function as intracortical association neurons.

COMMISSURES

Corpus Callosum

Most of the neocortical commissural fibers constitute the corpus callosum; the remainder are included in the anterior commissure along with fibers of other than neocortical origin. The number of fibers in the corpus callosum is of the order of 300 million; however, the commissure varies considerably in size among normal individuals.

The **body** of the corpus callosum is the compact portion of the commissure in and near the midline (Fig. 16–2). On entering the medullary center, the fibers constitute the **radiation** of the corpus callosum, which intersects association bundles and projection fibers. The interhemispheric connections are predominantly between comparable cytoarchitectural and functional cortical areas.

The body of the corpus callosum is considerably shorter than the hemispheres, accounting for the enlargement at each end. These are the **splenium** posteriorly and the **genu** anteriorly (Fig. 13–2). The splenium and the radiations connecting the occipital lobes constitute the **forceps major** (Fig. 16–6), and the genu and the radiations connecting the frontal lobes form the **forceps minor.** The genu tapers into the **rostrum** of the corpus callosum, which is continuous with the lamina terminalis forming the anterior wall of the third ventricle. Some fibers of the radiation form a thin sheet, called the **tapetum,** over the inferior horn of the lateral ventricle (Fig. 16–6). These fibers contribute to communication between the cortex of the temporal lobes, especially cortex on the ventral surface of these lobes.

Certain relations of the corpus callosum are the result in part of invasion of older parts of the brain by this neocortical commissure. The dorsal surface of the body of the corpus callosum is clothed by the **indusium griseum,** an exceedingly thin layer of gray matter in which are embedded two delicate strands of fibers on each side called the **medial** and **lateral longitudinal striae.** The indusium griseum is an insignificant remnant of rhinencephalic cortex. The longitudinal striae consist of fibers proceeding from the medial olfactory or septal area on the medial surface of the frontal lobe to the hippocampus in the temporal lobe.

With respect to the ventral surface of the corpus callosum, this surface forms the roof of the lateral ventricles and has relations with the fornix and the septum pellucidum in the midline. The **fornix,** consisting of symmetric halves, is a robust fiber system connecting the hippocampus of each temporal lobe with the hypothalamus, especially the mammillary bodies. The crura of the fornix begin at the posterior end of each hippocampus; they curve forward and merge to form the body of the fornix, which is in contact with the undersurface of the body of the corpus callosum. The body of the fornix divides into columns which turn ventrally away from the corpus callosum; they form the anterior boundary of the interventricular foramina and continue to the hypothalamus (Fig. 11–2). The resulting interval between the fornix and the corpus callosum is bridged by the **septum pellucidum,** a thin sheet of tissue containing scattered nerve cells and covered on each side by ependyma. The septum pellucidum separates the anterior horns of the lateral ventricles; it is a double membrane containing a slitlike cavity which does not communicate with the ventricular system or the subarachnoid space.

Anterior Commissure

The anterior commissure is a small bundle of fibers which crosses the midline in the lamina terminalis, traverses the anterior part of the corpus striatum, and provides for additional communication between the temporal lobes (Fig. 16–7). The anterior commissure includes fibers connecting the middle and inferior temporal gyri of the two sides; this is a neocortical component similar to the corpus callosum. Other fibers run between olfactory cortex of the temporal lobes (the lateral olfactory areas), for which the uncus is a landmark. There are also fibers which connect the olfactory bulbs, but these are a minor component of the anterior commissure in man.

FIG. 16-6. Dissection of portions of the corpus callosum in the right hemisphere, dorsolateral view. (× ⅔)

FIG. 16-7. Dissection exposing the anterior commissure, anteroventral view. (× 1⅔)

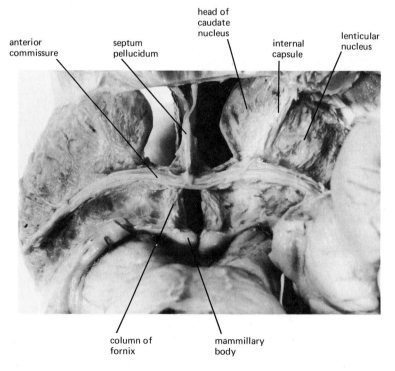

Role of the Cerebral Commissures

The interhemispheric connections provided by the corpus callosum and the anterior commissure contribute to the bilaterality of memory traces. The role of the neocortical commissures in interhemispheric transfer has been studied in recent years by assessing the effect of section of the corpus callosum and the anterior commissure in the monkey and chimpanzee (split-brain preparation). In normal, unoperated animals, a training exercise learned with one hand is performed efficiently by the other hand because of interhemispheric transfer of the neural basis of learning. This is not so in the case of the split-brain monkey or chimpanzee. On the contrary, when a previously unfamiliar task is learned by use of the left hand, for example, that task can not be performed by the right hand unless training in the exercise is repeated with the right hand.

Similar observations, with an extension in the area of language, are available for man. These were made on persons who suffered from severe epilepsy and in whom the corpus callosum was sectioned in order to confine the epileptic discharge to one hemisphere. There are no significant changes in intellect, behavior, or emotional responses that can be attributed to commissurotomy, although there is some impairment of short-term memory. Bimanual skills acquired before operation are not affected. However, an expertise learned postoperatively with one hand is not transferable to the other hand, as is to be expected from the experiments on other primates.

A particularly significant result of commissurotomy in man lies in the area of language. Let us say that the left hemisphere is dominant, as is usually the case. After section of the corpus callosum the patient is unable to describe an object held in the left hand (with the eyes closed) or seen in the left visual field, although the nature of the object is apparently understood. There is no such difficulty when the sensory data reach the left or dominant hemisphere. After commissurotomy the right hemisphere is rendered mute and agraphic because it has no access to memory for language in the left hemisphere. However, there is evidence that the subordinate hemisphere with respect to language is superior in certain activities, such as copying drawings that include perspective or arranging blocks in a prescribed manner. The non-dominant hemisphere therefore appears to be the more proficient side of the brain in functions requiring special competence in three-dimensional perspective.

Developmental anomalies of the brain include agenesis of the corpus callosum, which is not necessarily associated with mental retardation or other obvious neurologic impairment. When such deficits are present, as is frequently the case, study of the patient is seldom informative with respect to the function of the corpus callosum because agenesis of the commissure is likely to be accompanied by developmental anomalies affecting other parts of the brain.

INTERNAL CAPSULE AND PROJECTION FIBERS

The configuration of the projection system of fibers has some resemblance to that of the commissural system. In the latter the fibers are concentrated in the body of the corpus callosum and radiate in the medullary center. Similarly projection fibers are concentrated in the internal capsule and fan out as the **corona radiata** in the medullary center (Fig. 16-5).

The internal capsule consists of an **anterior limb,** a **genu,** and a **posterior limb,** which have topographic relations with adjacent gray masses (Fig. 16-8). The anterior limb is bounded by the lenticular nucleus and the head of the caudate nucleus, and the genu is medial to the apex of the lenticular nucleus. The posterior limb has three portions; this is based on the relation of the fibers to the lenticular nucleus, which does not extend as far posteriorly as does the thalamus. The **lenticulothalamic** portion is between the lenticular nucleus and the thalamus; the **retrolenticular** portion consists of fibers occupying the region behind the lenticular nucleus, and the **sublenticular** portion includes those fibers that pass beneath the posterior part of the lenticular nucleus.

THALAMIC RADIATONS

Many of the projection fibers establish reciprocal connections between the thalamus and the cerebral cortex. The **anterior thalamic ra-**

head of
caudate nucleus

genu

anterior limb

thalamus

retrolenticular
portion of
posterior limb

lenticular nucleus

lenticulothalamic portion
of posterior limb

FIG. 16-8. Horizontal section of the cerebrum, stained by a method which differentiates gray matter and white matter, illustrating the anterior limb, genu, and posterior limb of the internal capsule. (× 1)

diation, which is included in the anterior limb of the internal capsule, consists mainly of fibers connecting the dorsomedial thalamic nucleus and the prefrontal cortex. The **middle thalamic radiation** is a component of the lenticulothalamic portion of the posterior limb of the internal capsule. This radiation includes the projection from the ventral posterior thalamic nucleus to the somesthetic area in the parietal lobe; these fibers run in the posterior part of the lenticulothalamic region, where they are partly intermingled with motor projection fibers. Other fibers of the middle thalamic radiation establish reciprocal connections between the dorsal tier of nuclei of the lateral thalamus and association cortex of the parietal lobe. Fibers from the ventral anterior and ventral lateral nuclei of the thalamus reach the motor and premotor

areas of the frontal lobe by traversing the genu and adjacent region of the posterior limb of the internal capsule.

The **posterior thalamic radiation** establishes connections between the thalamus and cortex of the occipital lobe. The geniculocalcarine tract ending in the visual cortex is a particularly important component of this radiation. Originating in the lateral geniculate nucleus, the geniculocalcarine tract first traverses the retrolenticular and sublenticular portions of the internal capsule. The constituent fibers then spread out into a broad band bordering the lateral ventricle and turn backward into the occipital lobe. Some of the fibers, constituting Meyer's loop, proceed forward for a considerable distance into the temporal lobe above the inferior horn of the lateral ventricle before turning back into the occipital lobe. The posterior thalamic radiation also contains fibers establishing reciprocal connections between the pulvinar of the thalamus and association cortex of the occipital lobe. The **inferior thalamic radiation** consists of fibers directed horizontally in the sublenticular portion of the posterior limb of the internal capsule, connecting thalamic nuclei with cortex of the temporal lobe. Most of the fibers are included in the auditory radiation, which originates in the medial geniculate nucleus and terminates in the auditory area, for which Heschl's convolutions are a landmark. The association cortex of the temporal lobe, compared with that of the other lobes, has a relatively meagre communication with the thalamus, this being confined to a minor reciprocal connection with the pulvinar.

MOTOR PROJECTION FIBERS

The remaining projection fibers are corticofugal and incorporated in tracts with motor functions. The **corticobulbar** (corticonuclear) and **corticospinal tracts,** which together constitute the pyramidal motor system, originate in the motor and premotor areas in the frontal lobe and in the parietal lobe. The fibers converge as they traverse the corona radiata and enter the posterior limb of the internal capsule. From the beginning of the present century, it was believed that the corticobulbar tract occupied the genu of the internal capsule and that the corticospinal tract was situated in the posterior limb immediately behind the genu. Evidence accumulated in recent years, both from electrical stimulation of the internal capsule and the tracing of fiber degeneration following lesions of the capsule, shows clearly that the conventional view is incorrect. In the human brain the pyramidal fibers are in fact situated in the posterior one-third of the lenticulothalamic portion of the posterior limb. In the region thus defined corticobulbar fibers are most anterior, followed in sequence by corticospinal fibers related to the upper limb, trunk, and lower limb. However, there is considerable overlapping of fibers for the major regions of the body.

Corticopontine fibers originate in widespread areas of cortex, but in greatest numbers in the frontal and parietal lobes. Fibers of the **frontopontine tract** traverse the anterior limb of the internal capsule, and probably the genu and adjacent part of the posterior limb as well. The **temporopontine tract** is inappropriately named; the majority of the constituent fibers originate in the parietal lobe and traverse the retrolenticular portion of the internal capsule.

Extrapyramidal motor fibers terminate in various subcortical centers; depending on the destination, they are called **corticostriate, corticorubral, corticonigral, corticoreticular,** or **corticoolivary fibers.** These extrapyramidal fibers originate in widespread areas of the cerebral cortex, and they are therefore situated in various parts of the corona radiata and the internal capsule. This is especially true of corticostriate and corticoreticular fibers, and fibers ending in the putamen and the reticular formation are included in the external capsule as well as the internal capsule. Extrapyramidal fibers destined for the red nucleus, substantia nigra, and inferior olivary complex come mainly from the sensorimotor strip and adjoining cortex. Although their passage through the corona radiata and internal capsule has not been traced precisely, many of these fibers are probably closely related to the pyramidal motor fibers topographically. An infarction in the posterior part of the lenticulothalamic portion of the internal capsule, spreading into the retrolenticular portion, results in especially serious neurologic deficits. These include the effects of an "upper motor neuron lesion" because of interruption of pyramidal and extrapyramidal pathways, general sensory deficits due to involvement of the thalamocortical projection to the somesthetic area, and a visual field defect because of interruption of geniculocalcarine fibers. Stated differently, the consequences of such a lesion are voluntary motor paralysis and impairment of general sensation on the opposite side of the body and blindness in the opposite visual field; the details vary according to the size and precise location of the lesion.

Although the composition of the **external capsule** is incompletely known, this thin layer of white matter between the putamen and the claustrum consists mainly of projection fibers. As noted previously these include corticostriate fibers ending in the putamen and corticoreticular fibers.

LATERAL VENTRICLES

The lateral ventricles, one in each cerebral hemisphere, are roughly C-shaped cavities

FIG. 16-9. Dissection of the right cerebral hemisphere, dorsolateral view. The roof of the lateral ventricle has been removed to show structures forming part of the walls of the body and anterior horn. (× 1¼)

FIG. 16-10. Dissection of the right cerebral hemisphere, lateral view, exposing the inferior horn of the lateral ventricle. (× 1¼)

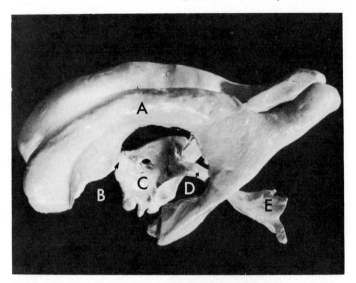

FIG. 16-11. Cast of the ventricular system of the brain. **A,** lateral ventricle, consisting of a body and anterior, inferior, and posterior horns; **B,** interventricular foramen (foramen of Monro); **C,** third ventricle; **D,** cerebral aqueduct (aqueduct of Sylvius); **E,** fourth ventricle. (Prepared by Dr. D. G. Montemurro)

lined by ependymal epithelium and filled with cerebrospinal fluid. Each lateral ventricle consists of a body in the region of the parietal lobe from which anterior, posterior, and inferior horns extend into the frontal, occipital, and temporal lobes. The principal features of the ventricular walls, now to be described, appear in Figures 16-9 and 16-10. The configuration of the entire ventricular system of the brain is illustrated in Figure 16-11.

The **body** or **central part** of the lateral ventricle has a flat roof, formed by the corpus callosum. The floor includes part of the dorsal surface of the thalamus, of which the anterior tubercle is a boundary of the interventricular foramen (foramen of Monro) leading to the third ventricle. The tail of the caudate nucleus forms a ridge along the lateral border of the floor. The stria terminalis, a slender bundle of fibers originating in the amygdaloid nucleus in the temporal lobe, lies in the groove between the tail of the caudate nucleus and the thalamus, along with the vena terminalis. The fornix completes the floor medially, and the choroid plexus is attached to the margins of the choroid fissure separating the fornix and the thalamus.

The **anterior horn** extends forward from the region of the interventricular foramen. The corpus callosum continues as the roof, and the genu of the corpus callosum limits the anterior horn in front. The septum pellucidum bridges the interval between the fornix and the corpus callosum in the midline, separating the anterior horns of the two ventricles. The **posterior horn,** which is variable in length, is surrounded by the medullary center. There are two elevations on the medial wall of the posterior horn. The more dorsal prominence, for which the forceps major is responsible, is referred to as the **bulb of the posterior horn;** the lower prominence, formed by the calcarine sulcus, is called the **calcar avis.**

The **inferior horn** extends to within 3-4 cm of the temporal pole. There is a triangular area, called the **collateral trigone,** in the floor of the ventricle where the posterior and inferior horns diverge from the body of the ventricle. The collateral sulcus on the external surface of the hemisphere is at the site of the trigone and may produce a **collateral eminence.** The tail of the caudate nucleus, now considerably attenuated, extends forward in the roof of the inferior horn as far as the amygdaloid nucleus. This nucleus is situated above the anterior end of the inferior horn, which places it close to the uncus on the external surface. The stria terminalis and the vena terminalis run along the medial side of the tail of the caudate nucleus. The floor of

FIG. 16-12. Pneumoencephalogram for a 9-month-old child, lateral view. The head was in the brow-up position, hence the posterior horn of the lateral ventricle contains cerebrospinal fluid. A, anterior horn of lateral ventricle; B, body of lateral ventricle; C, inferior horn of lateral ventricle; D, interventricular foramen; E, third ventricle; F, cerebral aqueduct; G, fourth ventricle; H, cisterna magna. (Courtesy of Dr. J. M. Allcock)

the inferior horn includes a particularly important structure, the **hippocampus** (Fig. 16-10). The hippocampus may be visualized as an extension of the parahippocampal gyrus on the external surface, which has been "rolled into" the floor of the inferior horn. The slightly enlarged anterior end of the hippocampus is known as the **pes hippocampi** because it resembles an animal's paw. Efferent fibers from the hippocampus form a ridge or **fimbria** along its medial border. The fimbria continues as the **crus of the fornix** after the hippocampus terminates beneath the splenium of the corpus callosum. The choroid plexus of the body of the ventricle continues into the inferior horn, where it is attached to the margins of the choroid fissure above the fimbria of the hippocampus.

The ventricles and the subarachnoid space are not seen in a routine x-ray series, although they can be demonstrated by x-ray when the cerebrospinal fluid is replaced by air. In pneumoencephalography 20-30 ml air is injected into the lumbar subarachnoid space in increments with the patient in a sitting position. The air replaces cerebrospinal fluid in the subarachnoid cisterns and also in the ventricles of the brain by entering the fourth ventricle through its median aperture, the foramen of Magendie (Fig. 16-12). The procedure is dangerous when there is an increase in intracranial pressure because of the risk of herniation of the medial part of the temporal lobe into the tentorial incisura or of the medulla into the foramen magnum. However, when the intracranial pressure is elevated, air can be injected into a lateral ventricle by means of a brain needle inserted through a burr hole in the skull (ventriculography). Visualization of the ventricles is useful in detecting the degree and cause of ventricular dilation (hydrocephalus) as well as the presence of an intracranial space-occupying lesion which alters the normal position or contour of one of the ventricles.

Air studies have been virtually replaced in recent years by computerized tomography (CT scan). This new application of x-ray imaging is based on scanning of the head with a narrow, moving beam of x-rays and measurement of the emerging, attenuated

FIG. 16–13. CT scan at a level showing portions of the ventricular system. **A,** anterior horn of lateral ventricle; **B,** subarachnoid space; **C,** subarachnoid cistern (of the great cerebral vein); **D,** posterior horn of lateral ventricle; **E,** septum pellucidum. (Courtesy of Dr. R. H. Coates and Dr. H. W. K. Barr)

beam by crystal detectors. The density readings from thin "sections" of the head are processed by computer, and the image brightness depending on the absorption value of the tissues is photographed from the picture on a cathode ray tube (Fig. 16–13). The CT scan is so sensitive that the information obtained extends beyond that provided by air studies. In addition to showing the ventricles computerized tomography reveals variations in tissue density in the normal brain, as between gray matter and white matter. The technique is valuable in clinical diagnosis because the density of many cerebral lesions is greater or less than the density of normal brain tissue. Thus CT scanning is capable of showing the presence and location of lesions as diverse as hemorrhage, infarction, tumor, and cyst, as well as such pathologic changes as atrophy, edema, necrosis, and the larger patches of multiple sclerosis.

SUGGESTED READING

Bertrand G: Stimulation during stereotactic operations for dyskinesias. J Neurosurg 24:419–423, 1966

Bertrand G, Blundell J, Musella R: Electrical exploration of the internal capsule and neighbouring structures during stereotaxic procedures. J Neurosurg 22:333–343, 1965

Ettlinger EG, De Reuck AVS, Porter R (eds): Functions of the Corpus Callosum. London, Churchill, 1965

Gawler J, Bull JWD, Du Bourlay GH, Marshall J: Computerized axial tomography: the normal EMI scan. J Neurol Neurosurg Psychiatry 38:935–947, 1975

Gazzaniga MS: The Bisected Brain. New York, Appleton, 1970

Gazzaniga MS, Sperry RW: Language after section of the cerebral commissures. Brain 90:131–148, 1967

Smith MC: Stereotactic operations for Parkinson's disease: anatomical observations. In Williams D (ed): Modern Trends in Neurology. London, Butterworth, 1967, pp 21–52

Sperry RW: The great cerebral commissure. Sci Am 210/1:42–52, 1964

Wilson DH, Reeves A, Gazzaniga M, Culver C: Cerebral commissurotomy for control of intractable seizures. Neurology 27:708–715, 1977

Zaidel D, Sperry RW: Memory impairment after commissurotomy in man. Brain 97:263–272, 1974

17

Olfactory System

The olfactory system consists of the olfactory mucosa, bulbs, and tracts, together with the cerebral cortex having olfactory functions and its projections to other centers. These structures dominate the cerebral hemispheres of lower vertebrates, in which they constitute the rhinencephalon or nosebrain. Two changes greatly altered the significance of the rhinencephalon in mammalian evolution. Firstly the olfactory parts of the brain regressed as nonolfactory neocortex, consisting of six layers rather than three, expanded in size and functional importance. Secondly a portion of the rhinencephalic cortex remained well represented, although it acquired other than olfactory functions, becoming incorporated in the limbic system of the brain. These changes culminated in the situation found in the human brain. In man the olfactory system consists of the olfactory mucosa, small olfactory bulbs and tracts, and a strip of paleocortex extending from the uncus in the temporal lobe, across the anterior perforated substance, to the medial surface of the frontal lobe beneath the genu of the corpus collosum. The remaining rhinencephalic cortex of comparative neurology evolved into the archicortex of the hippocampus and the dentate gyrus in the temporal lobe. These are only indirectly related to the olfactory system, and are included instead in the limbic system.

Lower vertebrates and many mammals rely heavily on the sense of smell for information about the environment. They are said to be "macrosmatic"; in the mammalian class the dog is a familiar example. Man is a "microsmatic" animal, smell being much less important than other senses, especially sight and hearing. However, even in man olfaction is a significant sense which conjures up memories and arouses emotions. Smell also contributes to alimentary pleasures. Persons who have lost their sense of smell complain of impairment of "taste," stating that everything is bland and tastes alike, and they may be unaware of their inability to smell. Most of our enjoyment of "taste" is in fact an appreciation of aromas through the olfactory system. Nevertheless, loss of smell is not a serious disability. There is a technical word, anosmia, for loss of the sense of smell, but there is no word in everyday use comparable to blindness and deafness.

The olfactory system has fewer clinical applications than the other sensory systems; it is therefore discussed here only briefly, with omission of many details. Fiber connections and histologic details of importance in earlier stages of evolution are retained in the human brain; however, some of these are vestigial and not essential to a general understanding of the brain in man. The olfactory system is discussed in the context of the cerebral hemispheres rather than with other neurologic systems because it is an integral part of the telencephalon.

OLFACTORY MUCOSA AND OLFACTORY NERVES

The olfactory mucosa (Fig. 17–1) covers an area of 2.5 cm^2 in the roof of each nasal cavity, extending for a short distance on the lateral wall of the cavity and the nasal septum. The sensory olfactory cells are supported by pseudostratified columnar epithelium, similar to that lining the respiratory passages. Glands of Bowman beneath the epithelium bathe the mucosa with a layer of serous fluid, in which odoriferous substances are dissolved. The functional cells with respect to smell, the **olfactory cells,** are bipolar neurons

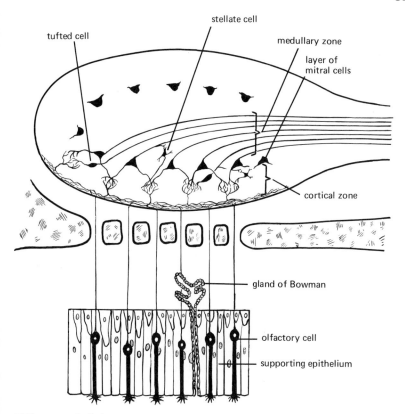

tufted cell

stellate cell

medullary zone

layer of
mitral cells

cortical zone

gland of Bowman

olfactory cell

supporting epithelium

FIG. 17-1. Cellular components of the olfactory mucosa and the olfactory bulb.

which are modified to serve as sensory receptors as well as conducting neurons. The major modification consists of specialization of the dendrite; this process extends to the surface of the epithelium, where it ends as an exposed bulbous enlargement bearing cilia that are exceptional in being up to 100μ in length.

Unmyelinated axons of the olfactory cells constitute the olfactory nerves, which pass through the foramina of the cribriform plate of the ethmoid bone and enter the olfactory bulb. The axons form a superficial fibrous stratum in the olfactory bulb, then continue more deeply and terminate in specialized synaptic configurations, the **glomeruli.** The olfactory cell is a primitive type of receptor, being similar to neuroepithelial cells of invertebrates. This is the only instance in man where the effective stimulus has direct access, without the intervention of nonnervous tissue, to a neuron which is specialized to serve as a receptor cell. In the semidiagram-

matic representation of the olfactory mucosa and the olfactory bulb (Fig. 17-1), the few olfactory cells shown represent some 25 million such cells in each half of the olfactory mucosa. Similarly the axons of olfactory cells represent a corresponding number of fibers incorporated in about 20 olfactory nerve bundles on each side.

The olfactory system is exquisitely sensitive to minute amounts of excitants in the air. Direct stimulation of the receptors, convergence of many olfactory cells on neurons of the olfactory bulb, and facilitation by neuronal circuits in the bulb are among the factors responsible for the low threshold. Smell is a chemical sense, as is taste. In order for a substance to be detected it must have a vapor pressure. An odoriferous substance must also be soluble in both water and lipids for it to be taken up by the serous fluid covering the olfactory mucosa and the lipoprotein plasma membrane of the olfactory cilia. The mechanism of excitation of olfactory cells must be very complex in view of the range of odors and aromas that are appreciated. Sensitivity to particular substances appears to differ from one part of the olfactory mucosa to another, and discrimination between organic odoriferous compounds must eventually be explained at a molecular level. The olfactory system adapts rather quickly to a continuous stimulus, so that the odor becomes unnoticed. Older persons tend to have a reduced acuity of smell, caused in part by degeneration of olfactory sensory cells throughout life.

OLFACTORY BULB, TRACT, AND STRIAE

The olfactory tract extends forward from its point of attachment to the brain in front of the anterior perforated substance (Fig. 17–2). The olfactory bulb appears as a slight terminal expansion of the tract, situated above the cribriform plate of the ethmoid bone.

FIG. 17-2. A portion of the ventral surface of the brain, showing some of the components of the olfactory system. The anterior portion of the right temporal lobe has been cut away. (× 1)

The olfactory bulb has a characteristic cytoarchitecture in animals that rely heavily on the sense of smell. There are three layers or zones: a **cortical zone,** a **layer of mitral cells,** and a **medullary zone** (Fig. 17–1). It is sometimes difficult to demonstrate the typical mammalian histology in the olfactory bulb of adult man, although the layers are obvious in fetal stages of development.

The most prominent cells of the olfactory bulb are the **mitral cells** (shaped like a bishop's miter). The dendrites of these cells terminate in the complex synaptic configurations (glomeruli) in the cortical zone. (The glomeruli are of historical interest because they were among the first synapses to be studied, by Ramón y Cajal, after the introduction of silver staining methods.) There is a tremendous convergence of olfactory receptors on mitral cells; several thousand olfactory cell axons enter a single glomerulus, and a mitral cell contributes dendrites to several glomeruli. There is some evidence that different glomeruli, or perhaps groups of glomeruli, function in relation to specific

olfactory
tract

olfactory
bulb

olfactory
trigone

lateral
olfactory
stria

medial
olfactory
stria

limen
insulae

anterior
perforated
substance

uncus

optic tract

odors. Axons of mitral cells enter the medullary zone and continue to olfactory areas of the brain through the olfactory tract.

There are numerous **stellate cells** (Golgi type II neurons) throughout the olfactory bulb. They are intercalated between collateral branches of mitral cell axons and dendrites of mitral cells, the synapse between the axon of a stellate cell and the dendrite of a mitral cell being in a glomerulus. Intrabulbar circuits are thereby established, which facilitate neuronal activity in the olfactory bulb. The olfactory tract contains a modest number of fibers traveling to the bulb, where they end on stellate cells; these fibers originate in the opposite olfactory bulb or in olfactory cortex. There are neurons known as **tufted cells** in the cortical zone; they are similar to mitral cells in that their dendrites end in glomeruli and their axons proceed centrally in the olfactory tract. A small group of nerve cells, making up the **anterior olfactory nucleus,** is situated at the transition between the olfactory bulb and the olfactory tract. Collateral branches of axons of mitral and tufted cells terminate in this nucleus; fibers originating in the anterior olfactory nucleus comprise the fibers which pass from one olfactory bulb to the other through the anterior commissure.

In macrosmatic animals the well-developed olfactory tract expands posteriorly into a prominent **olfactory trigone,** from which large **lateral** and **medial striae** (gyri) extend to the cortex of the olfactory system. The tract, trigone, and striae of such animals are covered with a layer of paleocortex. Although the basic pattern persists in man, the gray layer is vestigial and the fibers are greatly reduced in number. The olfactory trigone and striae are therefore poorly represented in the human brain and may not be obvious on casual inspection (Fig. 17–2). In any case impulses from the olfactory bulb are conveyed to cortical olfactory areas for subjective appreciation of odors and aromas. These areas also establish connections with other parts of the brain for emotional and visceral responses to olfactory stimuli. The medial olfactory stria includes the fibers which originate in the anterior olfactory nucleus of one side, cross the midline in the anterior commissure, and terminate in the contralateral olfactory bulb.

OLFACTORY CORTICAL AREAS

The anatomy of the olfactory areas and the projections from these areas to other parts of the brain are important topics in the discipline of comparative neurology. The details are many and complex, in view of the dominance of smell in the lives of lower animals. These topics are barely touched on here because of the regression of the olfactory system in primate evolution and the infrequency with which disorders of this system are encountered in clinical neurology. It was noted at the beginning of the chapter that the olfactory paleocortex consists of a strip extending from the uncus in the temporal lobe, across the anterior perforated substance, to the medial surface of the frontal lobe. The strip cannot be considered as a unit, however, because of functional variations in different regions. Three components have therefore to be considered; these are the lateral, intermediate, and medial olfactory areas.

LATERAL OLFACTORY AREA

The lateral olfactory area receives afferents from the olfactory bulb through the lateral olfactory stria. The area consists of the cortex of the uncus in the temporal lobe, extending to include cortex in the region of the limen insulae (Fig. 17–2). Part of the amygdaloid nucleus (amygdala) is also included in the lateral olfactory area; this nucleus is situated above the tip of the inferior horn of the lateral ventricle, immediately beneath the lenticular nucleus (Fig. 18–3). The amygdala is a nuclear complex, consisting of a dorsomedial portion continuous with the cortex of the uncus and a larger ventrolateral portion. The dorsomedial portion receives olfactory fibers, whereas the ventromedial portion is a component of the limbic system. The lateral olfactory area is the principal region for awareness of olfactory stimuli and is therefore called the **primary olfactory area.** The three-layered cortex of the uncus merges into six-layered cortex of the parahippocampal gyrus. This anterior part of the parahippocampal gyrus is called the **entorhinal area** and functions as olfactory association cortex. Association fibers provide connections between the entorhinal area and other cortical areas of the temporal lobe. The uncus, limen insulae, and entorhinal area are known as the **pyriform area** (or lobe) because they have a pear-shaped outline in animals with a well-developed olfactory system.

INTERMEDIATE OLFACTORY AREA

The anterior perforated substance, situated between the olfactory trigone and the optic tract (Fig. 17-2), derives its name from the penetration of many small blood vessels into the brain in this region. The thin paleocortex at this site receives fibers from the olfactory trigone and is designated the intermediate olfactory area. A zone of gray matter interposed between this area and the lenticular nucleus is known as the **innominate substance.** The **diagonal band of Broca** consists of subcortical fibers immediately in front of the optic tract, connecting the three areas of olfactory cortex.

MEDIAL OLFACTORY AREA

The medial olfactory area is on the medial surface of the frontal lobe, ventral to the genu and rostrum of the corpus callosum and anterior to the lamina terminalis. Groups of neurons, called **septal nuclei,** lie beneath the cortex and extend as scattered cells into the septum pellucidum. The medial olfactory area, known alternatively as the **septal area,** receives olfactory fibers through the medial olfactory stria and is connected with the other olfactory areas by means of the diagonal band of Broca. It is doubtful, however, that the septal area makes a significant subjective contribution to the sense of smell. Instead the septal area is more closely related to the limbic system, contributing to the function of this system with respect to emotions. In support of this interpretation, the septal area has been shown to be a "pleasure zone" in the rat. Animals with electrodes implanted in the area self-stimulate by pressing on a lever until they are exhausted, preferring the effect of stimulation to pleasurable activities such as consuming food.

PROJECTIONS FROM THE OLFACTORY AREAS

Olfactory stimuli readily produce visceral responses through the autonomic nervous system; examples are salivation when there are pleasing aromas from the preparation of food

FIG. 17-3. Some of the connections of the olfactory cortex.

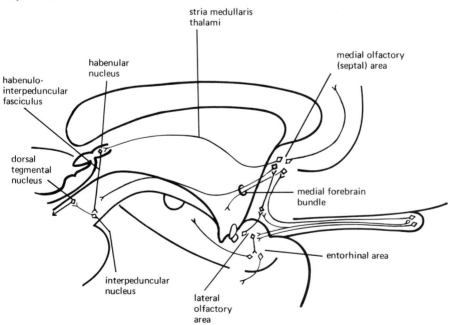

stria medullaris thalami

habenular nucleus

medial olfactory (septal) area

habenulo-interpeduncular fasciculus

dorsal tegmental nucleus

medial forebrain bundle

entorhinal area

interpeduncular nucleus

lateral olfactory area

and responses associated with nausea when an odor is very unpleasant. In view of the prominence of the olfactory system in ancestral forms, it is not surprising that even in man the projections to autonomic centers are multiple and complex. The main projections involve the medial forebrain bundle and the stria medullaris thalami. The three olfactory areas contribute to these fasciculi; however, most of the fibers originate in the medial olfactory or septal area, and these are represented in Figure 17–3.

The **medial forebrain bundle,** a small fasciculus in man, gives off fibers to hypothalamic nuclei as it traverses the lateral area of the hypothalamus. Olfactotegmental fibers of the bundle continue into the midbrain; they terminate in the mesencephalic reticular nucleus, from which impulses spread to autonomic nuclei in the brain stem and spinal cord. The **stria medullaris thalami** runs along the dorsomedial border of the thalamus and ends in the habenular nucleus in the epithalamus. The pathway continues as the habenulointerpeduncular fasciculus to the interpeduncular nucleus in the midbrain, then to the dorsal tegmental nucleus, and finally to autonomic nuclei in the brain stem and spinal cord through the dorsal longitudinal fasciculus and relays in the reticular formation.

The sense of smell is powerful in arousing emotions, for which spread of activity to the limbic system is responsible. The hippocampal formation in the temporal lobe has an input from the olfactory association cortex (entorhinal area), and fibers from the medial olfactory or septal area reach the hippocampus by way of delicate **longitudinal striae** which partially encircle the corpus callosum. Activity in the septal area also spreads to the cingulate gyrus.

Neurologic signs caused by dysfunction of the olfactory system may have considerable diagnostic importance. A tumor, usually a meningioma, in the floor of the anterior cranial fossa may interfere with the sense of smell because of pressure on the olfactory bulb or olfactory tract. It is necessary to test in each nostril separately because the olfactory loss is likely to be unilateral. A lesion affecting the uncus and amygdaloid nucleus may cause "uncinate fits," characterized by an imaginary disagreeable odor, by movements of the lips and tongue, and often by a "dreamy state."

SUGGESTED READING

Amoore JE: Molecular Basis of Odor. Springfield, IL, Thomas, 1970

Amoore JE, Johnston JW Jr, Rubin M: The stereo-chemical theory of odor. Sci Am 210/2:42–49, 1964

Bargmann W, Schadé JP (eds): The rhinencephalon and related structures. Prog Brain Res 3:1–253, 1963

Moulton DG, Beidler LM: Structure and function in the peripheral olfactory system. Physiol Rev 47:1–52, 1967

Mozell MM: Olfactory discrimination: electro-physiological spatiotemporal basis. Science 143:1336–1337, 1964

Zotterman Y (ed): Olfaction and Taste. New York, Macmillan, 1963

18

Limbic System

Certain components of the cerebral hemispheres and the diencephalon are brought together under the heading of the limbic system of the brain. The concept of such a system with special functions developed from comparative neuroanatomic studies and neurophysiologic investigations. The following regions of gray matter are included in the limbic system: the limbic lobe, consisting of the cingulate and parahippocampal gyri, the hippocampal formation, part of the amygdaloid nucleus, the hypothalamus (especially the mammillary bodies), and the anterior nucleus of the thalamus. The fornix, mammillothalamic fasciculus, and stria terminalis are fiber bundles of the limbic system.

The limbic system is concerned with 1) emotions of importance to survival of the individual and the species, together with visceral responses to these emotions, and with 2) processes involved in memory. The limbic system is also known as the **visceral brain** because of its substantial influence on visceral functions through the autonomic nervous system.

HIPPOCAMPAL FORMATION

The hippocampal formation consists of the hippocampus, the dentate gyrus, and a strip of the parahippocampal gyrus in direct continuity with the hippocampus.

The **hippocampus** develops in the fetal brain by a process of continuing expansion of the medial edge of the temporal lobe, in such a way that the hippocampus comes to occupy the floor of the inferior horn of the lateral ventricle (Fig. 16–10). In the mature brain, therefore, the parahippocampal gyrus on the external surface is continuous with the hippocampus along the medial edge of the temporal lobe. The hippocampus is C-shaped in

coronal section (Fig. 18–1). The outline bears some resemblance to a ram's horn, and the hippocampus is sometimes called Ammon's horn, Ammon being the name of an Egyptian diety with a ram's head. The ventricular surface of the hippocampus consists of a thin layer of white matter called the **alveus,** which consists of fibers originating in the hippocampal cortex. The fibers are directed toward the medial border of the hippocampus, along which they proceed posteriorly as the **fimbria of the hippocampus.** The fimbria constitutes the crus of the fornix after the hippocampus terminates beneath the splenium of the corpus callosum.

Continued growth of the cortical tissue comprising the hippocampus is responsible for the **dentate gyrus** (Fig. 18–1.) This gyrus occupies the interval between the fimbria of the hippocampus and the parahippocampal gyrus; its surface is toothed or beaded, hence the name "dentate gyrus." The **hippocampal sulcus** is a groove between the parahippocampal and dentate gyri, and the **choroid fissure** in this location is dorsal to the fimbria of the hippocampus.

Most of the parahippocampal gyrus consists of six-layered neocortex. In the region of the gyrus known as the **subiculum** (Fig. 18–1) there is a gradual transition between neocortex and the archicortex of the hippocampus, in which there are the following three layers: 1) The **molecular layer,** consisting of delicate nerve fibers and scattered small neurons, is continuous with the outermost layer of neocortex. 2) The prominent **pyramidal cell layer** is composed of large neurons, many of them having a pyramidal outline. Dendrites of cells in this layer extend into the molecular layer, and their axons comprise the alveus while en route to the fornix. 3) The **polymorphic cell layer** is similar to the innermost layer of the neocortex.

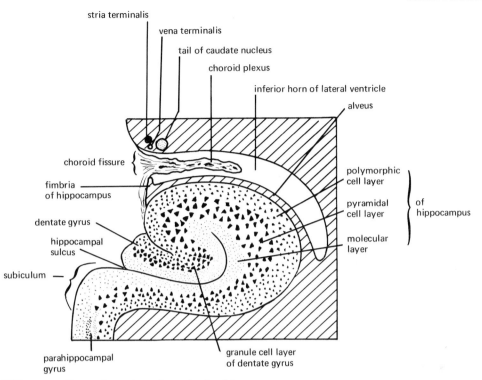

stria terminalis
vena terminalis
tail of caudate nucleus
choroid plexus
inferior horn of lateral ventricle
alveus
choroid fissure
fimbria
of hippocampus
dentate gyrus
hippocampal
sulcus
subiculum
polymorphic
cell layer
pyramidal
cell layer
molecular
layer
of
hippocampus
parahippocampal
gyrus
granule cell layer
of dentate gyrus

FIG. 18-1. Coronal section through the hippo-campal formation (medial surface at the left).

This layer includes neurons which contribute fibers to the fornix; other neurons are comparable to the cells of Martinotti of neocortex because the axons of these cells extend into the molecular layer.

The dentate gyrus likewise has three layers. The cytoarchitecture differs from that of the hippocampus in that the pyramidal cell layer is replaced by a **granule cell layer** of small neurons. Efferent fibers from the gyrus terminate in the hippocampus; very few enter the fornix. The cytoarchitecture and connections of the dentate gyrus suggest that it is a reinforcing and regulating part of the hippocampal formation.

AFFERENT CONNECTIONS OF THE HIPPOCAMPAL FORMATION

Although direct connections between the lateral olfactory area and the hippocampal formation are few or lacking, the entorhinal area or olfactory association cortex is a source of afferent fibers. Fibers reaching the hippocampus from the medial olfactory or septal area constitute the delicate **longitudinal**

striae embedded in the indusium griseum, an attenuated layer of gray matter covering the dorsal surface of the body of the corpus callosum. In addition the fornix, although primarily an efferent tract of the hippocampus, includes a few fibers proceeding from the septal area to the hippocampus. These afferents provide for emotional responses to odors and aromas. There is no good evidence that the hippocampal formation contributes to subjective awareness of olfactory stimuli, this being a function mainly of the lateral olfactory area.

The hippocampal formation receives fibers from the cortex of the parahippocampal gyrus, which is in communication with widespread areas of the cerebral cortex through association fibers of the medullary center. These include fibers in the cingulum, the association bundle of the limbic lobe through which the cortex of the parahippocampal and cingulate gyri are in communication.

EFFERENT CONNECTIONS OF THE HIPPOCAMPAL FORMATION

The connections through which the cortex of the hippocampal formation is influenced by

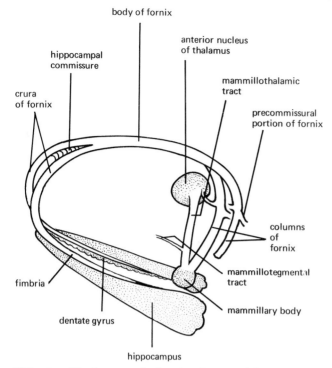

FIG. 18-2. The fornix and related pathways of the limbic system.

the cerebral cortex generally are paralleled by connections providing for spread of activity from the hippocampal formation to other regions of the cerebral cortex. In addition to these avenues of communication, the fornix constitutes a large and discrete efferent pathway of the hippocampus.

The **fornix,** which contains in excess of a million fibers in man, consists of myelinated axons of cells in the pyramidal and polymorphic cell layers of the hippocampus. As described previously, the fibers traverse the alveus on the ventricular surface of the hippocampus en route to the fimbria of the hippocampus (Fig. 18-1). The fimbria continues as the **crus** of the fornix, which begins at the posterior limit of the hippocampus beneath the splenium of the corpus callosum (Fig. 18-2). The crus curves around the posterior end of the thalamus and joins its partner to form the **body** of the fornix. A small **hippocampal commissure** at the convergence of the crura consists of decussating fibers joining the hippocampi of the two sides. The body of the fornix separates into **columns,** each of which curves ventrally in front of the

interventricular foramen. The column of the fornix continues through the hypothalamus, where it is the landmark for dividing the hypothalamus into medial and lateral areas. Most of the fibers terminate in the mammillary body, and the remainder end in the ventromedial nucleus of the hypothalamus. A bundle of fibers leaves the column of the fornix immediately below the interventricular foramen and ends in the anterior nucleus of the thalamus. Other fibers separate from the column of the fornix just above the anterior commissure; these constitute the **precommissural portion** of the fornix and are distributed to the medial olfactory (septal) area and the anterior part of the hypothalamus. The septal area sends fibers to hypothalamic nuclei by means of the medial forebrain bundle.

There are reciprocal connections between the mammillary body and the anterior nucleus of the thalamus through the **mammillothalamic fasciculus** (bundle of Vicq d'Azyr), which is readily demonstrable by gross dissection (Fig. 11-14). The anterior thalamic nucleus and the cingulate gyrus are in reciprocal communication by means of fibers which travel around the lateral side of the lateral ventricle. The structures compos-

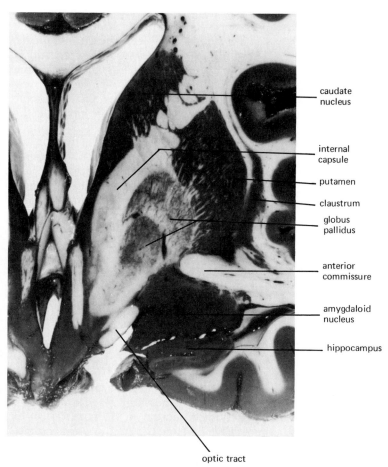

caudate
nucleus

internal
capsule

putamen

claustrum

globus
pallidus

anterior
commissure

amygdaloid
nucleus

hippocampus

optic tract

FIG. 18-3. Coronal section through the region of the brain that includes the amygdaloid nucleus. (This is a portion of the section shown in Figure 12-3.) Stained by a method which differentiates gray matter and white matter. (× 2)

ing the limbic system are therefore closely integrated, with abundant provision for feedback within the system.

AMYGDALOID NUCLEUS (Amygdala)

The amygdaloid nucleus is situated between the anterior end of the inferior horn of the lateral ventricle and the ventral surface of the lenticular nucleus (Fig. 18-3). The dorsomedial portion of the amygdaloid nucleus, which blends with the cortex of the uncus, receives fibers from the olfactory bulb and is part of the lateral olfactory area. The larger, ventrolateral portion has no direct input from the olfactory bulb, although it connects with

the dorsomedial portion and the olfactory association cortex in the entorhinal area. The ventrolateral part of the amygdaloid nucleus is included in the limbic system on the basis of experiments involving stimulation and ablation in laboratory animals and clinical observations in man.

The amygdaloid nucleus, especially the ventrolateral portion, has widespread connections, most of which are not in the form of discrete and well-defined fiber bundles. Afferent fibers converge on the nucleus from neocortical areas, thalamic nuclei, and the hypothalamus. Many of the efferent fibers take the shortest ventral routes to cortex of the temporal and frontal lobes, the thalamus (especially its dorsomedial nucleus), the hypothalamus, and the reticular formation of the brain stem. The most discrete efferent bundle of the amygdala is the **stria terminalis.** This slender fasciculus follows the curvature of the tail of the caudate nucleus, continuing along the groove between the caudate nucleus and the thalamus in the floor of the body of the lateral ventricle. The constituent fibers diverge in the region of the interventricular foramen; the majority terminate in the medial olfactory or septal area and the anterior part of the hypothalamus, whereas the remainder join the stria medullaris thalami and end in the habenular nucleus of the epithalamus. The projections of the amygdala through the stria terminalis are similar in some respects to those of the hippocampus through the fornix.

SOME FUNCTIONAL CONSIDERATIONS

Ablation or stimulation of portions of the limbic system in monkeys and other experimental animals gives some indication of its function. Bilateral removal of the temporal lobes, which include the hippocampal formation and the amygdala, is followed by docility and lack of emotional responses such as fear or anger to situations that normally arouse those responses. The animals exhibit increased sexual activity, and the sexual drive may be perverted, being directed toward either sex, a member of another species, or even inanimate objects. Lesions confined to the amygdala produce comparable changes in behavior, although sexual behavior is less affected.

In man, removal of both temporal lobes results in the Klüver–Bucy syndrome, which is characterized by a voracious appetite, increased (sometimes perverse) sexual activity, and docility. There is also loss of recognition of people and a memory defect. It has been reported that electrical stimulation of the amygdala in man induces feelings of fear or anger.

Studies of the type just indicated led to the view that the limbic system represents a phylogenetically old part of the brain and that it is responsible for emotions having a broad biologic importance with respect to preservation of the individual and the species. These include such strong affective reactions as fear, anger, and emotions associated with sexual behavior. Changes in visceral function are a natural result of these emotions, and electrical stimulation of the hippocampus, amygdala, or cingulate gyrus has

been shown to produce a wide range of visceral responses in experimental animals. These include changes in respiration and in gastrointestinal movements and secretion, piloarrection, and pupillary dilation. The visceral responses to activity within the limbic system are mediated mainly through the hypothalamus.

The assignment of a role in memory to the limbic system, in particular the hippocampus, is an interesting development of recent years. Impairment of memory is most evident following bilateral temporal lobectomy, or when arterial occlusion, having caused an infarction in the hippocampal formation of one side, is followed at a later time by a similar infarction in the other hemisphere. Interruption of the major circuit within the limbic system, such as occurs when the mammillary bodies are involved in a lesion, may also result in a memory defect. Persons with such lesions forget information obtained recently and are unable to commit anything to memory. It is not implied that memory traces are stored in the hippocampus. Although there are only hypotheses at this point, one possibility is that memory is a function of neurons of the cerebral cortex generally, perhaps depending on macromolecular changes in these neurons superimposed on their other activities. It is further proposed that there is a tendency for these macromolecular changes to decay with time; there would therefore be no memory beyond a short interval in the absence of a mechanism that promotes retention of memory traces in neuronal macromolecules. It is envisaged that the hippocampus may provide a bias against "forgetting" through its diversified connections, direct and indirect, with the cerebral cortex generally. When the hippocampi are no longer functional, memories of earlier events are retained, these having already been established. But there is amnesia for events occurring subsequent to the lesion because the mechanism for retention or consolidation of memory is no longer in operation. Amnesia may also follow bilateral lesions in the dorsomedial nuclei of the thalamus, as in Korsakoff's syndrome. It may not be a coincidence that the hippocampus and the dorsomedial thalamic nucleus both contribute to affective aspects of brain function and are involved in processes for memory.

SUGGESTED READING

Douglas RJ: The hippocampus and behavior. Psychol Bull 67:416–442, 1967

Green JD: The hippocampus. Physiol Rev 44:561–608, 1964

Livingston KE, Escobar A: Anatomical bias of the limbic system concept: a proposed reorientation. Arch Neurol 24:17–21, 1971

MacLean PD: The limbic system with respect to self-preservation and the preservation of the species. J Nerv Ment Dis 127:1–11, 1958

Penfield W, Milner B: Memory deficit produced by bilateral lesions in the hippocampal zone. Arch Neurol Psychiatry 79:475–497, 1958

Raisman J, Cowan WM, Powell TPS: The extrinsic efferent, commissural and association fibres of the hippocampus. Brain 88:963–996, 1965

Symonds C: Disorders of memory. Brain 89:625–644, 1966

Terzian H, Dalle Ore G: Syndrome of Klüver and Bucy: reproduced in man by bilateral removal of the temporal lobes. Neurology (Minneap) 5:373–380, 1955

Victor M: The amnesic syndrome and its anatomical basis. Can Med Assoc J 100:1115–1125, 1969

Young JZ: What can we know about memory? Br Med J 1:647–652, 1970

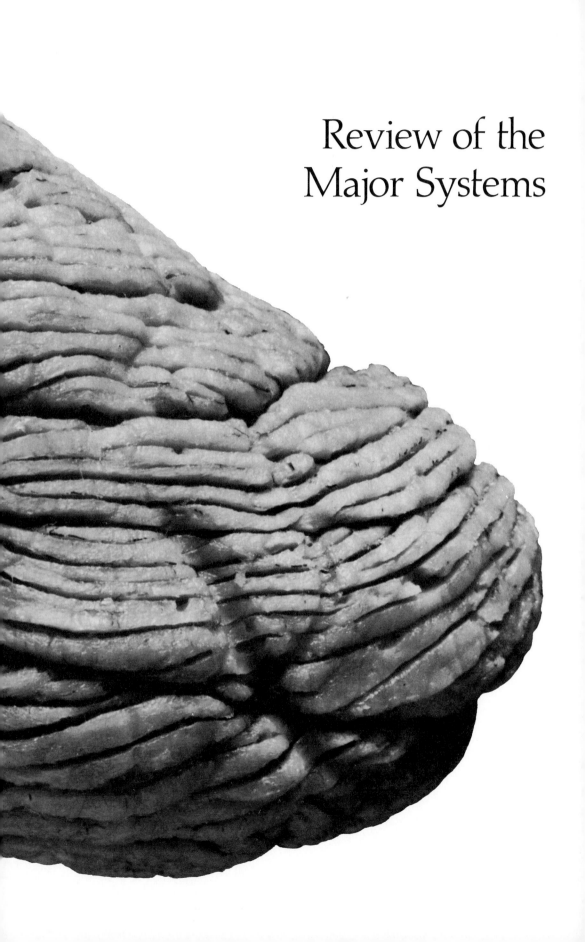

Review of the Major Systems

19

General Sensory Systems

Impulses originating in general sensory receptors initiate reflex responses through pathways in the spinal cord and the brain stem, and impulses from certain of these receptors reach the cerebellum. The various circuits are of the first importance in the physiology of the nervous system, and their interruption by a disease process usually results in some form of motor dysfunction. However, the present chapter deals with the pathways from the general sensory receptors to the thalamus and thence to the cerebral cortex, where the sensations are appreciated subjectively. With an understanding of the anatomy of these pathways, an appraisal of sensory deficits gives valuable information concerning the location of a lesion in the central nervous system. (An additional avenue of transmission to the cerebral cortex is provided by the ascending reticular activating system, discussed in Chapter 9.)

Sensory fibers entering the spinal cord in dorsal roots of spinal nerves segregate in such a way that there are two main general sensory systems. The phylogenetically older system includes a synaptic relay in the dorsal gray horn to the crossed spinothalamic tracts in the lateral and ventral white columns. This system is for pain and temperature (lateral spinothalamic tract) and light touch and pressure (ventral spinothalamic tract). The spinothalamic system is partly protective in function, especially with respect to pain, and emotional responses to stimuli are easily aroused. In the more phylogenetically recent pathway, fibers entering the spinal cord in dorsal roots ascend in the ipsilateral dorsal white column and end in the nuclei gracilis and cuneatus in the medulla. Fibers from these nuclei constitute the crossed medial

lemniscus, which terminates in the thalamus. This system is for proprioception (position and movement of body parts), fine touch, and vibration. The sensations are discriminative and closely related to mental processes; emotional responses are minimal or lacking.

The pathways from receptors to the cerebral cortex consist of a series of three neurons, called primary, secondary, and tertiary neurons, or neurons of the first, second, and third order. The cell bodies of **primary sensory neurons** are in dorsal root ganglia and sensory ganglia of cranial nerves (mainly the trigeminal ganglion); their peripheral processes reach out to receptors, and their central processes enter the spinal cord or the brain stem. The cell bodies of **secondary sensory neurons** are in the gray matter of the spinal cord (for spinothalamic tracts), in the nuclei gracilis and cuneatus in the medulla (for the medial lemniscus), and in sensory trigeminal nuclei (for the trigeminothalamic tract). **Tertiary sensory neurons** in the ventral posterior nucleus of the thalamus project to the somesthetic area of cortex in the parietal lobe. However, the concept of a simple relay involving only three neurons does not reflect the true situation, because small neurons with short axons may be interposed between the major neurons of the pathways. In addition the secondary sensory neurons of a pathway are excited or inhibited by impulses from various sources, including the cerebral cortex. Further the ventral posterior nucleus of the thalamus has connections with other thalamic nuclei; the thalamic organization is such that there is awareness of some aspects of general sensation at the thalamic level and emotional overtones are added.

PATHWAY FOR PAIN AND TEMPERATURE

RECEPTORS

The receptors for pain consist of nonencapsulated endings of peripheral nerve fibers; these fibers are the smaller components of group A, with thin myelin sheaths, and unmyelinated group C fibers. These simple endings are phylogenetically old receptors; although not concerned with pain exclusively, they appear to be the only type of receptor that responds to painful stimuli. Pain may be felt as two waves, separated by a very short interval. The first wave is sharp and localized, with conduction by group A fibers. The second wave, which is rather diffuse and still more disagreeable, depends on group C fibers with a slower speed of conduction.

The identity of receptors for temperature is still not resolved. The view that specific encapsulated endings, in particular the endbulbs of Krause and Ruffini, are sensors for coolness and warmth, respectively, appears to be untenable. In the absence of firm evidence concerning the nature of temperature receptors, nonencapsulated endings similar to those for pain, together with some form of end bulb yet to be identified, are regarded as sensors of temperature differences between body surfaces and the immediate environment. The nerve fibers are of similar caliber to those conducting impulses for pain.

PATHWAY FOR THE BODY

The cell bodies in dorsal root ganglia are small and of intermediate size. Their central processes traverse the dorsal roots and enter the **dorsolateral fasciculus** (zone of Lissauer) of the spinal cord, in which ascending and descending branches travel for a length corresponding to one segment or two segments at the most. These fibers, which give off many collateral branches in their short course, terminate in the **substantia gelatinosa** (of Rolando) in the dorsal gray horn.

The substantia gelatinosa consists of Golgi type II neurons whose axons are confined to the nucleus or run for short distances in the dorsolateral fasciculus, connecting adjacent regions of the substantia gelatinosa. The nucleus does not include "tract cells," *i.e.*, the cell bodies of secondary sensory neurons, which are situated instead in the nucleus proprius of the dorsal gray horn. Dendrites of tract cells ramify in the substantia gelatinosa, where they receive stimuli from the incoming sensory fibers, with the small cells composing the nucleus usually intervening. The transmission of messages from pain and temperature receptors is apparently subject to alteration in the substantia gelatinosa. Excitation of second order neurons with dendritic ramifications in the nucleus may be inhibited or facilitated by nerve impulses reaching the substantia gelatinosa by means of collateral branches of fibers for other modalities of general sensation in the dorsal white column. There is inhibition, for example, when one shakes the hand vigorously in an attempt to diminish the pain from a bruised or burned finger. In addition transmission for pain and temperature in the substantia gelatinosa appears to be altered by nerve impulses coming from the cerebral cortex. The fibers responsible for this inhibition or facilitation originate in the sensorimotor strip (especially the somesthetic area) and accompany the corticospinal tract. Inhibition may be exemplified by the diminished awareness of pain at the time of injury in combat and in contact sports.

Axons of tract cells in the nucleus proprius of the dorsal horn cross the midline in the ventral gray and white commissures. Continuing through the ventral horn of gray matter, the fibers ascend in the **lateral spinothalamic tract,** which is situated in the ventral part of the lateral white column and separated from the surface of the cord by the ventral spinocerebellar tract. Proceeding in a cephalad direction, fibers are continually being added to the ventromedial aspect of the lateral spinothalamic tract. At upper cervical levels, therefore, fibers from sacral segments are dorsolateral, followed by fibers from lumbar and thoracic segments, and those from cervical segments are in a ventromedial position.

The ascending tracts of the spinal cord continue into the medulla without appreciable change of position. At the level of the inferior olivary nucleus, the lateral spinothalamic tract traverses the lateral medullary zone (Monakow's area) between the inferior olivary nucleus and the nucleus of the spinal tract of the trigeminal nerve, where it is close to the lateral surface of the medulla. The lateral and ventral spinothalamic tracts and the spinotectal tract are closely associated at this level and throughout the remainder of the brain stem; together they constitute the **spinal lemniscus.** The spinal lemniscus continues through the ventrolateral region of the dorsal pons and close to the surface of the tegmentum in the midbrain, running along the lateral edge of the medial lemniscus. Spinotectal fibers leave the spinal lemniscus in the midbrain and terminate in the superior colliculus; the spinothalamic tracts then continue to the **ventral posterior nucleus** of the thalamus. This nucleus consists of the following parts: 1) the ventral posterolateral nucleus (VPL), in which the spinothalamic tracts and the medial lemniscus terminate; and 2) the ventral posteromedial nucleus (VPM), sometimes called the arcuate or semilunar nucleus, which receives trigeminothalamic fibers. The somatotopic representation is such that the contralateral lower limb is represented dorsolaterally and the contralateral upper limb ventromedially in the ventral posterolateral nucleus; the opposite side of the head is represented in the ventral posteromedial nucleus.

The ventral posterior nucleus has connections with other thalamic nuclei, especially those composing the dorsal tier of the lateral mass of the thalamus, the intralaminar nuclei, and the medial nucleus. There is subjective awareness of pain, heat, and cold at the thalamic level, and emotional responses are elicited. Neural processes in the cortex are required for precise recognition of the source, severity, and quality of painful and thermal stimuli. Tertiary neurons in the ventral posterior nucleus project to the **somesthetic area** in the parietal lobe, the fibers traversing the lenticulothalamic portion of the posterior limb of the internal capsule and the corona radiata. The contralateral half of the body, exclusive of the head, is represented as inverted in the dorsal two-thirds of the somesthetic area. Beginning ventrally the sequence is therefore hand, arm, and trunk, followed by representation of the leg, foot, and anogenital region on the medial surface of the hemisphere. The cortical area for the hand is disproportionately large, providing for maximal sensory discrimination. The somatotopic arrangement at various levels of the sensory pathways forms the basis for recognition of the site of stimulation.

PATHWAY FOR THE HEAD

The cell bodies of primary sensory neurons of the trigeminal nerve (with the exception of those in the mesencephalic nucleus) are in the trigeminal ganglion. The peripheral processes have a wide distribution through the ophthalmic, maxillary, and mandibular divisions of the nerve. The central processes enter the pons in the sensory root, and those for pain and temperature turn caudally in the **spinal tract of the trigeminal nerve.** There is a spatial arrangement of fibers in the sensory root and the spinal tract corresponding to the divisions of the trigeminal nerve. In the sensory root ophthalmic fibers are dorsal, mandibular fibers ventral, and maxillary fibers in between. Because of a rotation of the fibers as they enter the pons, the mandibular fibers are dorsal and the ophthalmic fibers ventral in the trigeminal spinal tract. The fibers for pain and temperature terminate in the pars caudalis of the **nucleus of the trigeminal spinal tract,** the pars caudalis being in the lower medulla and upper three cervical segments of the spinal cord. The portion of the pars caudalis in the cervical cord receives sensory data from areas of distribution of both the trigeminal nerve and the upper cervical spinal nerves. The cellular characteristics of the pars caudalis are like those of the dorsal gray horn of the spinal cord. A layer of small cells, identical with the substantia gelatinosa, lies external to a layer which includes larger neurons similar to those of the nucleus proprius of the dorsal horn.

The dorsal part of the trigeminal spinal tract includes a small bundle of fibers for pain and temperature from the facial, glossopharyngeal, and vagus nerves. The cell bodies of the primary sensory neurons are in the geniculate ganglion of the facial nerve and the superior ganglia of the glossopharyngeal and vagus nerves. Fibers in the facial and vagus nerves, and the glossopharyngeal nerve inconstantly, supply the external ear, the acoustic canal, and the tympanic membrane. The glossopharyngeal and vagus nerves also supply the mucosa of the back of the tongue, pharynx, esophagus, larynx, auditory (eustachian) tube, and middle ear.

The second order neurons consist of cells in the pars caudalis of the nucleus of the spinal trigeminal tract, whose axons cross to the

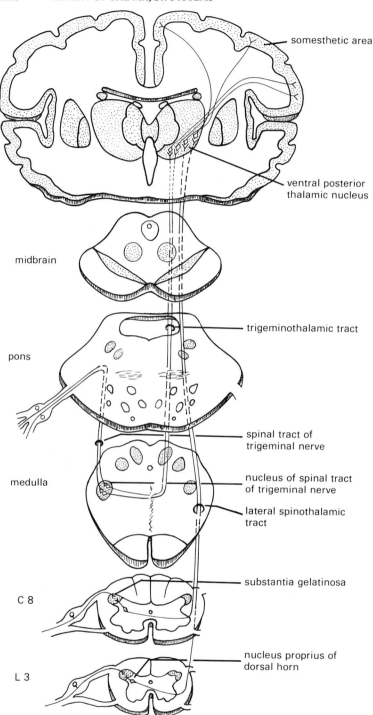

FIG. 19-1. Pathways for pain and temperature.

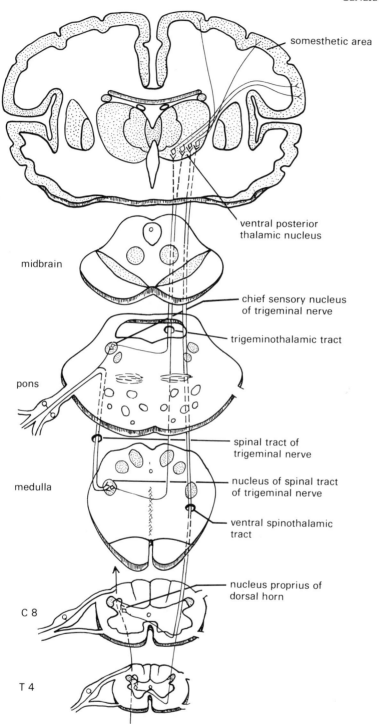

somesthetic area

ventral posterior
thalamic nucleus

midbrain

chief sensory nucleus
of trigeminal nerve

trigeminothalamic tract

pons

spinal tract of
trigeminal nerve

nucleus of spinal tract
of trigeminal nerve

medulla

ventral spinothalamic
tract

nucleus proprius of
dorsal horn

C 8

T 4

FIG. 19-2. Pathways for light touch and pressure.

opposite side of the medulla and continue rostrally in the **trigeminothalamic tract.** The tract terminates in the ventral posterior nucleus of the thalamus, and tertiary neurons complete the pathway to the ventral one-third of the somesthetic area of cortex. (There are, in fact, two trigeminothalamic tracts. The ventral one is a contralateral pathway from all parts of the nucleus of the spinal tract and the chief sensory nucleus to the thalamus. The smaller dorsal trigeminothalamic tract, which includes a few ipsilateral fibers, originates in the chief sensory nuclei and also conveys data from the mesencephalic nucleus. The tracts are close to one another in the rostral pons and the midbrain; it is permissible to consider them as a single trigeminothalamic tract, or trigeminal lemniscus, conveying impulses from all the sensory trigeminal nuclei to the thalamus.)

SOME CLINICAL COMMENTS

The pathways just described are important clinically. Inflammatory reactions in dorsal roots of spinal nerves or in peripheral nerves and pressure on spinal nerve roots by a herniated intervertebral disk stimulate pain and temperature fibers, causing painful and burning sensations in the area supplied by the affected roots or nerves. Degenerative changes in the region of the central canal of the spinal cord interrupt pain and temperature fibers as they decussate in the ventral gray and white commissures. The best example is syringomyelia, which is characterized by central cavitation of the spinal cord. When the disease process is most marked in the cervical enlargement, as is frequently the case, the area of anesthesia includes the hands, arms, and shoulders (yokelike anesthesia).

A lesion that includes the ventrolateral part of the spinal cord on one side results in loss of pain and temperature sensibility below the level of the lesion and on the opposite side of the body. If, for example, the lateral spinothalamic tract is interrupted on the right side at the level of the first thoracic segment, the area of anesthesia includes the left leg and the left side of the trunk. Careful testing of the upper margin of sensory impairment will show that cutaneous areas supplied by the first and second thoracic nerves are spared. Some impulses from these areas reach the opposite spinothalamic tract above its interruption because of the short ascending branches of dorsal root fibers in the dorsolateral fasciculus. Surgical section of the pathway for pain (tractotomy or chordotomy) may be required for relief of intractable pain. The section must extend deeply in the ventral quadrant of the spinal cord to be effective because pain and temperature fibers mingle with fibers in fasciculi adjoining the lateral spinothalamic tract as it is conventionally illustrated. Also visceral pain is conducted partly by fibers deep in the white matter, including spinospinalis relays. Tractotomy is most likely to be considered in later stages of malignant disease of a pelvic viscus; interruption of the tract may be unilateral or bilateral depending on circumstances prevailing in the individual patient. Even though the operation interrupts the generally accepted pathway for pain, the results are occasionally disappointing. This suggests, among other possible explanations, that there are pathways in addition to those traditionally recognized for conduction of pain and other sensations in the spinal cord. The spinocervical tract, which is described further on, is one such possible route.

The spinal lemniscus may be included in an area of infarction in the brain stem. An example is provided by the lateral medullary or Wallenberg's syndrome; the area of infarction usually includes the spinal lemniscus and the spinal tract of the trigeminal nerve and its associated nucleus. The principal sensory deficit is loss of pain and temperature sensibility on the side of the body opposite the lesion, but on the same side for the face. A lesion in or near the thalamus may result in the thalamic syndrome, in which there are exaggerated and exceptionally disagreeable responses to cutaneous stimulation.

The standard method of testing for integrity of the pain and temperature pathway is to stimulate the skin with a pin and ask the patient whether it feels sharp or dull. Temperature perception need not be tested separately as a rule; if such testing is required, the method used is touching the skin with test tubes containing hot or cold water.

PATHWAY FOR LIGHT (SIMPLE) TOUCH AND PRESSURE

Central transmission for the sense of touch is not restricted to a single pathway. The quality of touch sensation conveyed by the dorsal column system is discriminative, *i.e.*, two points on the skin touched simultaneously are both felt, even though they are close together. The alternative touch (and pressure) pathway now to be described involves ipsilateral transmission in the dorsal white column of the spinal cord and contralateral transmission in the ventral white column. Localization of the source of a stimulus is less refined compared with the dorsal column system, although there is a high level of sensitivity. The clinical test is light touching of the skin with a wisp of cotton.

RECEPTORS

Several types of receptor in the skin and at other sites such as the cornea and some mucous membranes respond to light touch. They include undifferentiated nerve terminals, Merkel's disks, hair follicle plexuses, Meissner's corpuscles, and probably end bulbs which have not yet been identified specifically. Pacinian corpuscles respond to the slightest deformity, and these sensors in the dermis and subcutaneous tissue serve as pressure receptors.

PATHWAY FOR THE BODY

The cell bodies in dorsal root ganglia are of intermediate size; their processes are group A fibers of medium diameter with moderately thick myelin sheaths. The central processes bifurcate on entering the dorsal white column of the spinal cord, the short descending branches giving off collaterals to the gray matter. Most of the ascending branches, which also give off collaterals to the gray matter, travel in the lateral part of the dorsal white column for six to eight segments, and some are even longer. The fibers for light touch and pressure are therefore spread out over many segments, effecting synaptic contact in the dorsal gray horn and intermediate zone with tract cells and with internuncial neurons for spinal reflexes. Axons of the tract cells cross the midline in the ventral gray and

white commissures and form the **ventral spinothalamic tract** in the ventral white column. Because of the overlapping of fibers from several spinal nerves in the dorsal column at any particular level some tract cells receive afferents from a number of dorsal roots. This convergence and the consequent summation of excitation of second order neurons reduce the discriminative quality of light touch and pressure, but they ensure a low threshold of excitation. The ventral spinothalamic tract is included in the spinal lemniscus in the brain stem and terminates in the ventral posterior nucleus of the thalamus. Although there may be minimal awareness of light touch and pressure at the thalamic level, subjective appreciation depends almost entirely on the tertiary relay to the somesthetic area of cortex in the parietal lobe.

The ascending pathway for light touch and pressure in the spinal cord is ipsilateral for some distance in the dorsal white column as well as contralateral in the ventral spinothalamic tract. Moreover the pathway for discriminative touch is ipsilateral in the dorsal white column as far as the nuclei gracilis and cuneatus in the medulla. Conduction for touch to the thalamus is therefore not entirely contralateral until mediated by the spinal and medial lemnisci in the brain stem. For this reason impairment of the sense of touch is most readily demonstrable as part of the sensory deficit caused by interruption of the spinal and medial lemnisci or, more commonly, the tertiary component of the sensory pathway in the internal capsule, medullary center, or somesthetic cortex.

The **spinocervical tract** provides an additional pathway to the brain for impulses originating in receptors for pain, temperature, touch and pressure. Although most of the information comes from animal experiments, there appears to be a spinocervical tract of significant size in man. The cells of origin are in the dorsal gray horn throughout the spinal cord, and the tract ascends ipsilaterally in the dorsal part of the lateral white column. The constituent fibers terminate in the **lateral cervical nucleus,** situated in the gray matter of the first two cervical segments of the spinal cord and continuing for a short distance in the medulla. Axons from the nucleus cross the midline and proceed to the ventral posterior nucleus of the thalamus.

PATHWAY FOR THE HEAD

As for pain and temperature, the cell bodies of primary sensory neurons for light touch and pressure are in the trigeminal ganglion, together with a small complement in the geniculate ganglion of the facial nerve and the superior ganglia of the glossopharyngeal and vagus nerves. Most of the central processes of the trigeminal neurons terminate in the pars rostralis and pars interpolaris of the **nucleus of the trigeminal spinal tract,** only a few of them ending in the pars caudalis along with fibers for pain and temperature. In addition to the foregoing fibers, others for light touch and pressure bifurcate on entering the pons. One branch joins the fibers descending in the spinal tract, and the other branch ends in the **chief sensory nucleus.** The pathway continues through the **trigeminothalamic tract** to the ventral posterior nucleus of the thalamus and the tertiary projection to the somesthetic area of cortex in the parietal lobe.

The facial and vagus nerves, and the glossopharyngeal nerve inconstantly, include fibers for touch and pressure for the external ear and the external acoustic meatus. The glossopharyngeal and vagus nerves include fibers for touch for the mucosa of the back of the tongue, the pharynx, and the larynx. The central connections of primary sensory neurons supplying cutaneous areas correspond to those of trigeminal neurons for light touch and pressure, and this is probably true as well for neurons supplying mucous membranes.

PATHWAY FOR PROPRIOCEPTION, FINE TOUCH, AND VIBRATION

RECEPTORS

The dorsal column system for proprioception, fine or discriminative touch, and vibration developed later than the other general sensory systems in evolution. This system is especially important in man because of the discriminative quality of the sensations as perceived subjectively and their value in the learning process. With respect to proprioception, the pathway provides information

concerning the precise position of parts of the body, the shape, size, and weight of an object held in the hand, and the range and direction of movements. The proprioceptors are neuromuscular spindles, neurotendinous spindles or Golgi tendon organs, nonencapsulated endings in the capsules and ligaments of joints, and pacinian corpuscles adjacent to joints. All of them function in pathways through various parts of the nervous system that affect muscle action, but the endings associated with joints appear to figure more prominently than the others in subjective proprioception.

The characteristics of fine or discriminative touch are that one can recognize the location of the stimulated point with precision and is aware that two points are touched simultaneously, even though they are close together (two-point discrimination). Of the receptors responding to touch, Meissner's corpuscles, which have been found only in primates, have a special significance in discriminative touch. They are most abundant in hairless skin, such as that of the volar surface of the hand, and in the borders of the lips; preferential sites for Meissner's corpuscles correspond to those areas in which two-point discrimination is best developed. Nonencapsulated endings and pacinian corpuscles in or close to periosteum are regarded as sensors for vibration.

PATHWAY FOR THE BODY

Primary sensory neurons for the discriminative senses are represented by the largest cells in the dorsal root ganglia; their peripheral and central processes are large group A fibers with thick myelin sheaths. The central processes bifurcate on entering the **dorsal white column.** The short descending branches tend to accumulate in the fasciculus septomarginalis in the lower half of the spinal cord, and in the fasciculus interfascicularis in the upper half of the cord. These fibers, including their collateral branches, form the afferent limbs of spinal reflex arcs and some of them synapse with cells such as those giving rise to the spinocerebellar tracts. The ascending branches, from which collaterals to the spinal gray matter also arise, proceed in the ipsilateral dorsal white column to the medulla. Above the midthoracic level the dorsal column consists of a medial **fasciculus**

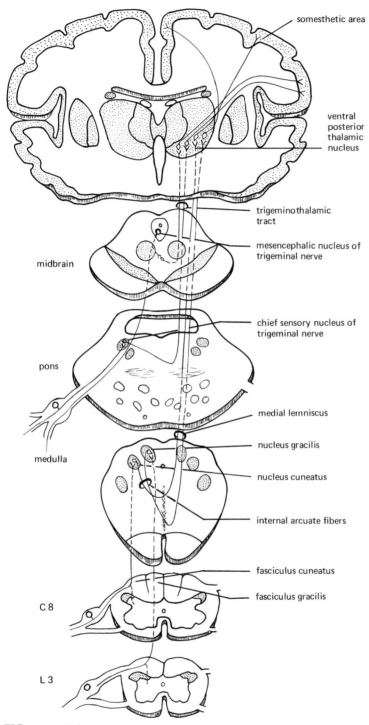

somesthetic area

ventral
posterior
thalamic
nucleus

trigeminothalamic
tract

mesencephalic nucleus of
trigeminal nerve

midbrain

chief sensory nucleus of
trigeminal nerve

pons

medial lemniscus

nucleus gracilis

medulla

nucleus cuneatus

internal arcuate fibers

fasciculus cuneatus

fasciculus gracilis

C 8

L 3

FIG. 19-3. Pathways for proprioception, fine touch, and vibration.

gracilis and a lateral **fasciculus cuneatus.** The fibers of the fasciculus gracilis, which entered the spinal cord below the midthoracic level, terminate in the **nucleus gracilis;** fibers of the fasciculus cuneatus, coming from the upper thoracic and cervical spinal nerves, end in the **nucleus cuneatus.** More precisely there is a lamination of the dorsal column according to segments. Fibers that entered the spinal cord in lower sacral segments are most medial, and fibers from successively higher segments ascend in an orderly manner along the lateral side of those already present. (Animal experiments and clinical studies indicate that conduction for proprioception and vibration to the thalamus and cerebral cortex may not be entirely by way of the dorsal column system.)

Axons of second order neurons in the nuclei gracilis and cuneatus curve ventrally as **internal arcuate fibers,** cross the midline of the medulla in the decussation of the medial lemniscus, and continue to the thalamus as the **medial lemniscus.** This substantial tract is situated between the midline and the inferior olivary nucleus in the medulla, in the most ventral portion of the tegmentum of the pons, and lateral to the red nucleus in the tegmentum of the midbrain. The medial lemniscus and the spinothalamic tracts intermingle in the dorsal region of the subthalamus before entering the ventral posterior nucleus of the thalamus. A topographic arrangement of fibers is maintained throughout the medial lemniscus. In the medulla the larger dimension of the lemniscus is vertical as seen in cross section; fibers for the lower limb are most ventral (adjacent to the pyramid), and fibers for the upper part of the body are most dorsal. On entering the pons the medial lemniscus rotates through 90 degrees; from here to the thalamus fibers for the lower limb are in the lateral part of the lemniscus, and those for the upper part of the body are in its medial portion. This pattern conforms with the representation of the body in the ventral posterior nucleus of the thalamus. The projection from this nucleus to the somesthetic area of cortex is required for any subjective appreciation of proprioceptive and fine tactile stimuli; there may be some slight awareness of vibration at the thalamic level.

There is considerable convergence from one order of neuron to the next in the pathways for pain, temperature, light touch, and pressure, establishing limits on the discriminative quality of these sensations. In the dorsal column system the number of primary, secondary, and tertiary neurons approaches a 1:1:1 ratio. This makes possible a detailed transmission of information with respect to somatotopic localization and the type of receptor involved. Transmission through the nuclei gracilis and cuneatus may be facilitated or inhibited by impulses from the cerebral cortex. The neurons responsible are in the sensorimotor cortex (especially the sensory strip), and their axons accompany the corticospinal tract as far as the medulla.

PATHWAY FOR THE HEAD

Separate nuclei in the brain stem are involved in tactile and proprioceptive sensations. The cell bodies of primary sensory neurons for discriminative touch, which is well developed in the face, are large cells in the trigeminal ganglion. The central processes terminate in the **chief sensory nucleus** of the trigeminal nerve, from which impulses reach the somesthetic cortex by way of the trigeminothalamic tract and the thalamocortical projection.

The primary sensory neurons for proprioception (and presumably for vibration) are unique in that most of the cell bodies of these neurons are in a nucleus in the brain stem instead of a sensory ganglion. Composing the **mesencephalic nucleus** of the trigeminal nerve, they are unipolar neurons like most primary sensory neurons elsewhere. The peripheral branch of the single process proceeds through the trigeminal nerve without interruption; these fibers supply proprioceptors in the trigeminal area of distribution, such as those related to the temporomandibular joint and the muscles of mastication. The other branch of the single process synapses with a cell in the reticular formation, the axon of which joins the trigeminothalamic tract or terminates in the trigeminal motor nucleus for reflex action. The innervation of proprioceptors in muscles receiving their motor supply from other than the trigeminal nerve was discussed in Chapter 8.

SOME CLINICAL COMMENTS

Sensory deficits involving proprioception, fine touch, and vibration result from interruption of the pathway anywhere along its course. For example the dorsal and lateral white columns are sites of symmetrical demyelination in subacute combined degeneration of the spinal cord, and conduction may be interrupted at any level by trauma, infarction, or the plaques of disseminated sclerosis. One test of the integrity of the pathway is to move the patient's finger or toe, asking him to say when the movement begins and describe the direction of movement. In the Romberg test any abnormal unsteadiness is noted when the patient stands with the feet together and the eyes closed, thereby evaluating proprioception in the lower limbs. Another useful test is to ask the patient to identify an object held in the hand with the eyes closed. Proprioception is especially helpful in recognizing the object on the basis of shape and size (stereognosis) as well as its weight. This is a sensitive test which the patient may perform unsuccessfully when there is a lesion in the parietal association cortex, even though the pathway to the somesthetic area is intact.

Another test of the integrity of the dorsal column system is to ask the patient if vibration as well as touch or pressure is felt when a tuning fork, preferably with a frequency of 128 Hz, is placed against a bony prominence such as the medial malleolus at the ankle or a finger joint. The sense of vibration is often reduced in elderly persons, but even slight vibration should be felt in the young. Routine testing of fine touch is not necessary, because the other tests are sufficient to detect an interruption of the pathway. If testing of two-point touch discrimination is required, two pointed objects are applied lightly to the skin simultaneously. A suitable test object can be devised from a paper clip. A normal person is able to detect simultaneous stimuli in the tip of a finger when they are 3–4 mm apart, or even less.

SUGGESTED READING

Calne DB, Pallis CA: Vibratory sense: a critical review. Brain 89:723–746, 1966

Dubrovsky B, Davelaar E, Garcia-Rill E: The role of dorsal columns in serial order acts. Exp Neurol 33:93–102, 1971

Dykes RW: Nociception. Brain Res 99:229–245, 1975

Gordon G, Jukes MGM: Descending influences on the exteroceptive organizations of the cat's gracile nucleus. J Physiol (Lond) 173:291–319, 1964

Kuypers HGJM: Some projections from the pericentral cortex to the pons and lower brain stem in monkey and chimpanzee. J Comp Neurol 110:221–255, 1958

Melzak R, Bridges JA: Dorsal column contributions to motor behavior. Exp Neurol 33:53–68, 1971

Rasmussen AT: The Principal Nervous Pathways. New York, Macmillan, 1957

Schwartzman RJ, Semmes J: The sensory cortex and tactile sensitivity. Exp Neurol 33:147–158, 1971

Sinclair D: Cutaneous Sensation. London, Oxford University Press, 1967

Walberg F: Corticofugal fibers to the nuclei of the dorsal columns: an experimental study in the cat. Brain 80:273–287, 1957

Wall PD: The sensory and motor role of impulses travelling in the dorsal columns towards cerebral cortex. Brain 93:505–524, 1970

20

Visual System

The visual pathway begins with photoreceptors in the retina from which nerve impulses reach the visual cortex in the occipital lobe through a series of neurons. There are two types of photoreceptor cell: rod cells have a special role in peripheral vision and vision under conditions of low illumination, whereas cone cells are responsible for central, discriminative vision and the detection of colors. Action potentials generated in the photoreceptors are transmitted by bipolar cells to ganglion cells within the retina, and axons of ganglion cells reach the lateral geniculate nucleus of the thalamus through the optic nerve and optic tract. The final relay is from the lateral geniculate nucleus to the visual cortex by way of the geniculocalcarine tract. Some fibers from the retina terminate in the midbrain for reflex responses to visual stimuli.

The following account of the visual system is restricted to nervous elements and presupposes a general understanding of the structure of the eye.

RETINA

Optic vesicles evaginate from the prosencephalon at an early stage of embryonic development. Each optic vesicle "caves in" to form the optic cup, consisting of two layers and connected to the developing brain by the optic stalk. The outer layer of the optic cup becomes the pigment epithelium of the retina, and the inner layer differentiates into the complex neural layer of the retina. In addition to photoreceptors, bipolar cells, and ganglion cells, the neural layer contains association neurons and neuroglial cells. The complex neuronal pattern of the retina resembles the gray matter of the brain. Similarly the optic nerve corresponds histo-

logically to white matter of the brain rather than a peripheral nerve. The retina and the optic nerve may therefore be viewed as outgrowths of the brain which are specialized for sensitivity to light, some modification of the sensory data, and transmission of the resulting information to the thalamus and the cerebral cortex.

RETINAL LANDMARKS

Certain specialized regions serve as landmarks which need to be identified before the cellular components of the retina are described.

The basic cell layers of the retina, listed from the choroid to the vitreous body, are the pigment epithelium, rod and cone cells, bipolar cells, and ganglion cells (Fig. 20–1). Axons of ganglion cells run toward the posterior pole of the eye and enter the optic nerve at the **optic papilla** or **optic disk.** The papilla is slightly medial to the posterior pole, about 1.5 mm in diameter, and pale pink in color. The nerve fibers are heaped up as they converge at the margin of the optic papilla, then pass through the fibrous tunic (sclera) of the eyeball into the optic nerve. The optic papilla is a blind spot because it contains only nerve fibers.

The **macula lutea,** the central area of the retina in line with the visual axis, is a specialized region 6 mm in diameter and abutting on the lateral edge of the optic papilla. The name macula lutea or "yellow spot" is derived from the presence of a diffuse yellow pigment (xanthophyll) among the neural elements in this location. However, the yellow color is apparent only when the retina is examined with red-free light, and the macula is therefore not ordinarily seen when the ocular fundus is inspected with an ophthalmoscope. The macula is specialized for acuity of vision;

the function of the yellow pigment is probably to screen out some of the blue part of the visible spectrum, thereby protecting the photoreceptors from the dazzling effect of strong light.

The **fovea** (or fovea centralis) is a depression in the center of the macula; the fovea is about 1.5 mm in diameter and separated from the edge of the optic disk by a distance of about 2 mm. Visual acuity is greatest at the fovea, the center of which contains only cone receptors. The capillary network present elsewhere in the retina is absent from the center of the fovea. When the retina is viewed with an ophthalmoscope the fovea appears darker than the reddish hue of the retina generally because the black melanin pigment in the choroid and the pigment epithelium is not screened by capillary blood. The visible fovea is frequently re-

ferred to as the "macula" in an ophthalmoscopic examination of the retina.

The functional retina terminates anteriorly along an irregular border, the **ora serrata.** Forward of this line the ciliary portion of the retina consists of a double layer of columnar epithelium, the outer layer being pigmented.

PIGMENT EPITHELIUM

Consisting of a single layer of cells, the pigment epithelium reinforces the light-absorbing property of the choroid in reducing the scattering of light within the eye (Fig. 20–1). Each pigment cell has a flat hexagonal base which is adherent to Bruch's membrane of the choroid. The basal portion of the cell contains the nucleus and a few pigment granules. Processes extending from the free surface of the cell interdigitate with the outer, photosensitive regions of rod and cone cells. The processes, which are filled with granules of melanin pigment, isolate individual pho-

FIG. 20–1. Schematic representation of the cellular components of the retina.

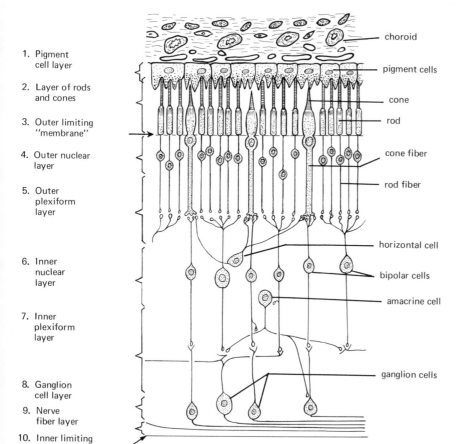

1. Pigment cell layer

2. Layer of rods and cones

3. Outer limiting "membrane"

4. Outer nuclear layer

5. Outer plexiform layer

6. Inner nuclear layer

7. Inner plexiform layer

8. Ganglion cell layer

9. Nerve fiber layer

10. Inner limiting membrane

choroid

pigment cells

cone

rod

cone fiber

rod fiber

horizontal cell

bipolar cells

amacrine cell

ganglion cells

toreceptors and enhance visual acuity. In lower vertebrates there is a flow of pigment granules toward the tips of the processes in response to bright light; such a response has not been described in mammals, including man.

The pigment epithelium is fixed to the choroid, but it is not so firmly attached to the neural part of the retina. Detachment of the retina, such as may follow a blow to the eye, consists of separation of the neural layers from the pigment epithelium, *i.e.*, at the junction of parts of the retina derived from the two layers of the optic cup.

PHOTORECEPTORS

The light-sensitive part of the photoreceptor cell is the outer portion adjacent to the pigment epithelium. The inverted retina is characteristic of vertebrates, whereas in some invertebrates light reaches the photoreceptors without traversing the retina. The inverted retina does not introduce a significant barrier to light, because the retina is transparent and at no point more than 0.4 mm in thickness.

Rod Cells

The number of rod cells in the human retina is of the order of 130 million, outnumbering cone cells by nearly 20:1. Rod cells are lacking in the central part of the fovea and become progressively more numerous from that point to the ora serrata. The distribution is such that rod cells are important for peripheral vision. Each rod cell consists of an outer portion, the **rod** (or rod proper), and an inner portion, the **rod fiber.** Rods are about 2μ in thickness and vary in length from 60μ near the fovea to 40μ at the periphery of the retina. The unspecialized rod fiber consists of a slender filament which includes the nucleus in an expanded region and terminates as an end bulb in synaptic contact with bipolar and association neurons.

The rod consists of outer and inner segments, of which the former is light sensitive. In electron micrographs most of the **outer segment** is occupied by about 700 double-layered membranous disks or flattened saccules (Figs. 20–2 and 20–3). The membranous disks contain the pigment **rhodopsin (visual purple),** which gives the retina a purplish-red

FIG. 20–2. Ultrastructural components of rod and cone cells. (Modified from Missotten L: The Ultrastructure of the Human Retina. Brussels, Belgium. Copyright by Editions ARSCIA, 1965)

color when removed from the eye and viewed under dim light. Rhodopsin consists of retinine (an aldehyde form of vitamin A) combined with a protein named opsin. The compound is broken down into its major constituents by light, causing the retina to bleach, and is restored in the dark. Studies of the photochemical reactions show that there are primary and secondary steps in the transduction of light energy to that of a nerve impulse. The primary step is absorption of a

FIG. 20-3. Electron micrograph of a rod from the human retina, showing a portion of the outer segment and the adjoining region of the inner segment. **A.** membranous disks; **B.** mitochondria in the ellipsoid; **C.** centrioles; **D.** cilium (× 36,000) (Courtesy of Dr. M. J. Hogan)

quantum of light by rhodopsin and a change in configuration of the pigment molecule. The secondary step consists of a series of reactions, still poorly understood, resulting in a change in the ionic polarization of the surface membrane of the rod cell.

The photochemical properties of rhodopsin and the summation of excitation in the visual pathway through the retina are responsible for the sensitivity of the rod system to low illumination (twilight or night vision). The rod-free area of the fovea is night blind, and a faint point of light such as a star of low magnitude is best detected by looking slightly away from it.

The **inner segment** of a rod is less differentiated than the outer segment and includes organelles found in cells generally. A region adjacent to the outer segment, known as the **ellipsoid,** contains numerous elongated mitochondria. A cilium extends into the outer segment from one of two centrioles situated at the junction of the outer and inner segments (Fig. 20–3). The remainder of the inner segment contains neurofibrils and vesicles with round or oval profiles, some of which are covered with ribosomes (granular endoplasmic reticulum). This region is known as the **myoid** because it is contractile in lower vertebrates and responds to changes in light intensity. A contractile property has not been established for the corresponding region in higher vertebrates, including man.

Cone Cells

The cone photoreceptors, although less numerous than rod photoreceptors, are especially important because of their role in visual acuity and color vision. Like the rod cell the cone cell consists of an outer portion, the **cone** (or cone proper), and an inner portion, the **cone fiber;** the cone likewise has outer and inner segments, the former being light sensitive.

The tapering **outer segment** of a cone consists principally of double-layered disks, varying in number from 1000 in cones at the fovea to several hundred at the periphery of the retina (Fig. 20–2). There are differences in detail between the disks of cones and rods, including somewhat closer stacking of the disks in cones. They contain a substance called **iodopsin,** which is related chemically to rhodopsin. However, the chemistry of the

disks has to account for the sensitivity of the cones to colors, and one theory proposes that separate cones contain one of three photosensitive substances, providing differential sensitivity to red, green, and blue light. The **inner segment** of a cone is thicker than the inner segment of a rod, and it contains a larger ellipsoid and a larger amount of granular endoplasmic reticulum. Cone cells contain a cilium like that of rod cells.

The **cone fiber** is thicker than a rod fiber, and the nucleus is in an expansion adjacent to the cone. The fiber expands again terminally, establishing synaptic contact with bipolar and association neurons.

The human retina contains about 7 million cone cells. The central part of the fovea, or the foveola, contains about 35,000 cone cells and no rod cells; there are some 100,000 cone cells in the whole of the fovea. The proportion of cone cells to rod cells remains high through the macular area for central vision, but it steadily decreases from the macula to the periphery of the retina. The fovea is specialized in other ways for visual acuity. In this region the cones are longer and more slender than elsewhere (75 by $1.0–1.5\mu$ at the fovea and 40 by 6μ at the periphery). The cone fibers and bipolar cells diverge from the center of the fovea, producing a slight concavity and eliminating any slight impediment to light passing through the retina. Such scattering of light as may be caused by capillary blood flow is eliminated by absence of a retinal capillary network in the center of the fovea.

Photoreceptor cells in the retina of the monkey are shown in Figure 20–4 as they appear in a scanning electron micrograph.

BIPOLAR CELLS

Bipolar cells are true neurons interposed between photoreceptor cells and ganglion cells (Fig. 20–1). One bipolar cell receives stimuli from numerous rod cells (10 near the macula to 100 at the periphery); the summation of excitation is an important factor in the sensitivity of the rod system to small amounts of light. The ratio between cone cells and bipolar cells is 1:1 at the fovea, as required for maximal visual acuity. Elsewhere variable numbers of cone cells converge on a bipolar cell, and some bipolar cells receive stimuli from both rod and cone cells.

FIG. 20-4. Scanning electron micrograph (freeze-fracture preparation) showing photoreceptor cells in the retina of the monkey. **OS,** outer segments of rods and cones; **R,** inner segment of a rod; **C,** inner segment of a cone; **ONL,** nuclei of rod and cone cells, composing the outer nuclear layer of the retina. (× 3,800) (Courtesy of Dr. D. H. Dickson)

GANGLION CELLS

Ganglion cells are rather large neurons with clumps of Nissl material, forming the last retinal link in the visual pathway (Fig. 20-1). Impulses are received from bipolar cells through axodendritic and axosomatic syn-apses. A ganglion cell receives impulses from one bipolar cell in the foveal region in order to maintain the discrete relay from cone photoreceptors that is required for maximal acuity of vision. Outside the fovea the number of bipolar cells converging on a ganglion cell increases toward the periphery of the retina. Axons of ganglion cells form a layer of nerve fibers adjacent to the vitreous body. The fibers converge on the optic papilla from all directions, those from the lateral part of the retina curving above and below the macula. On reaching the papilla, bundles of fibers pass through foramina in the sclera and then constitute the optic nerve. The axons acquire myelin sheaths only after traversing the sclera.

ASSOCIATION NEURONS

Impulse transmission in the retina is subject to modification by association neurons (Fig. 20-1). **Horizontal cells** are in the outer part of the zone occupied by the cell bodies of bipolar cells. The processes of horizontal cells, which are essentially dendrites, establish synaptic contact with either cone cells or rod cells, so that in this respect there are two classes of horizontal cells. These cells have no axon in the conventional sense; instead, small protuberances from the cell processes make synaptic contact with the dendrites of bipolar cells. **Amacrine cells** are in the inner part of the layer occupied by the cell bodies of bipolar cells. Each amacrine cell has a single process, whose branches end in the synaptic complexes between bipolar and ganglion cells or on the cell bodies of ganglion cells. Axon collaterals of bipolar cells are in synaptic contact with the cell body of an amacrine cell or with branches of its single process.

The impulses received by association neurons and the influence of these neurons on other cells may be excitatory or inhibitory. The effect is to modify, in transit through the retina, visual data originating in photoreceptors. An example of such modification is the enhancement of information passed to the brain about borders and contours, with an increase in contrast. Another example relates to the activation of ganglion cells. Most ganglion cells discharge throughout photic stimulation, the number of impulses per second being determined by the intensity of stimulation. However, through the influence of association neurons, some ganglion cells are activated only at the beginning of photic stimulation and others only when stimulation ceases.

NEUROGLIAL CELLS

The retina, in particular the innermost layers, contains neuroglial cells similar to those present in the gray matter of the brain. There are also large numbers of modified neuroglial cells called **cells of Müller.** These extend from the interface between the nerve fiber layer of the retina and the vitreous body to the junction of the rod and rod fiber, and the cone and cone fiber. Microvilli project from the outer end of a Müller's cell, and the cell is connected to photoreceptor cells by desmosomes (Fig. 20-2). Müller's cells therefore extend through most of the retina; lateral processes are given off which intervene between the neuronal elements of the retina and give these modified neuroglial cells a supporting role among other possible functions.

HISTOLOGIC LAYERS OF THE RETINA

When studied in sections stained with hematoxylin and eosin rather than by the Golgi method the retina is described as consisting of ten layers (Fig. 20-5). These layers can now be defined in relation to the cells which constitute the retina (Fig. 20-1). Layer 1 is the **pigment epithelium,** and layer 2 consists of **rods** and **cones.** Layer 3 is called the **outer limiting membrane** because it appears as a delicate line in histologic sections. In fact it is not a membrane but rather the row of desmosomes where the outer ends of Müller's cells make contact with photoreceptor cells. Layer 4, the **outer nuclear layer,** consists of nuclei of rod and cone cells. Layer 5, the **outer plexiform layer,** includes principally rod and cone fibers and dendrites of bipolar cells. Layer 6 is called the **inner nuclear layer;** it is made up of nuclei of bipolar cells together with nuclei of horizontal cells, amacrine cells, and cells of Müller. Layer 7, the **inner plexiform layer,** consists mainly of axons of bipolar cells and dendrites of ganglion cells. The cell bodies of **ganglion cells** are in layer 8, and the axons of these cells constitute layer 9, the **nerve fiber layer.** Layer 10 is the **inner limiting membrane** formed by the inner ends of Müller's cells.

BLOOD SUPPLY OF THE RETINA

The retina receives nourishment from two sources. The central artery of the retina enters the eye through the optic disk and its branches spread out over the inner surface of the retina. Fine branches penetrate the retina and form a capillary network extending to the outer border of the inner nuclear layer. The capillary bed drains into retinal veins which converge on the optic papilla to form the central vein of the retina. The other

choroid

1. pigment cell layer

2. layer of rods and cones

3. outer limiting membrane

4. outer nuclear layer

5. outer plexiform layer

6. inner nuclear layer

7. inner plexiform layer

8. ganglion cell layer

9. nerve fiber layer

10. inner limiting membrane
vitreous body

FIG. 20–5. Section of human retina. (Hematoxylin and eosin stain, × 350)

source of nourishment is from the capillary layer of the choroid, which is separated from the retina by the semipermeable Bruch's membrane. The outer part of the retina, extending from the pigment epithelium to the outer border of the inner nuclear layer, is devoid of capillaries.

PATHWAY TO THE VISUAL CORTEX

There is a point-to-point projection from the retina to the lateral geniculate nucleus of the thalamus and from this nucleus to the visual cortex of the occipital lobe. There is therefore a spatial pattern of cortical excitation according to the retinal image of the visual field. Before discussing the components of the visual pathway, certain general rules concerning the projection from the retina to the cortex may usefully be established.

For the purpose of describing the retinal projection, each retina is divided into nasal and temporal halves by a vertical line passing through the fovea. A horizontal line, also passing through the fovea, divides each half of the retina into upper and lower quadrants.

The macular area for most acute vision is represented separately from the remainder of the retina. Figure 20–6 illustrates the following rules with respect to the central projection of retinal areas. 1) Fibers from the right halves of the two retinae terminate in the right lateral geniculate nucleus, and the visual information is then relayed to the visual cortex of the right hemisphere. The converse holds true, of course, for the contralateral projection. 2) Fibers from the upper quadrants peripheral to the macula end in the medial part of the lateral geniculate nucleus, and impulses are relayed to the anterior two-thirds of the visual cortex above the calcarine sulcus. 3) Fibers from the lower quadrants peripheral to the macula end in the lateral portion of the geniculate nucleus, with a relay to the anterior two-thirds of the visual cortex below the calcarine sulcus. 4) The macula projects to a relatively large posterior region of the lateral geniculate nucleus, which in turn sends fibers to the posterior one-third of the visual cortex in the region of the occipital pole. The portions of the lateral geniculate nucleus and the visual cortex receiving fibers from the macula (which is only 6 mm in diameter) are disproportionately large because of the role of the macula in central vision with maximal discrimination.

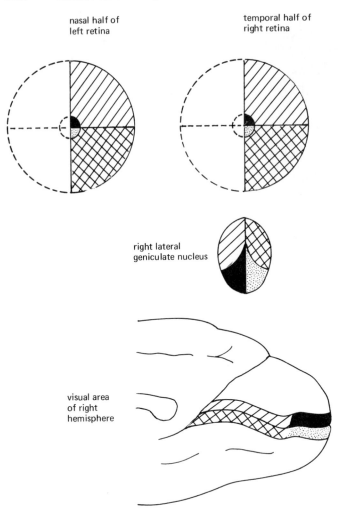

nasal half of
left retina

temporal half of
right retina

right lateral
geniculate nucleus

visual area
of right
hemisphere

FIG. 20-6. Projection of the retina on the lateral geniculate nucleus and the visual cortex.

Visual defects, which result from interruption of the pathway at any point from the retina itself to the visual cortex, are described in terms of the visual field rather than the retina. The retinal image of an object in the visual field is inverted and reversed from right to left, just as an image on the film in a camera is inverted and reversed. The following rules therefore apply to the nuclear and cortical representation of regions of the visual field. 1) The left visual field is represented in the right lateral geniculate nucleus and the visual cortex of the right hemisphere. 2) The upper half of the visual field is represented in the lateral portion of the lateral geniculate nucleus and the visual cortex below the calcarine sulcus. 3) The lower half of the visual field is projected on the medial portion of the lateral geniculate nucleus and the visual cortex above the calcarine sulcus.

OPTIC NERVE, OPTIC CHIASMA, AND OPTIC TRACT

Each optic nerve in man contains about 1 million fibers, all of them myelinated; the large number of fibers is indicative of the importance of human vision. The optic nerve is surrounded by extensions of the meninges; the pia mater adheres to the nerve and is separated from the arachnoid by an extension of the subarachnoid space. The dura mater forms an outer sheath, and the meningeal extensions around the nerve fuse with the fibrous scleral coat of the eyeball. The nerve fibers are arranged in fasciculi which are separated by connective tissue septa continuous with the sheath of pia mater. Each fasciculus is further divided into small bundles by neuroglial cells, whose processes penetrate between individual fibers. The myelin sheaths are formed by oligodendrocytes rather than Schwann cells because the optic nerve is comparable to a tract within the central nervous system.

The central artery and the central vein of the retina traverse the meningeal sheaths and are included in the anterior part of the optic nerve. An increase in pressure of cerebrospinal fluid around the nerve impedes the return of venous blood. Edema or swelling of the optic disk (papilledema) results; this is a valuable indication of an increase in intracranial pressure.

The partial crossing of optic nerve fibers in the optic chiasma is a requirement for binocular vision. Fibers from the nasal or medial half of each retina decussate in the chiasma and join uncrossed fibers from the temporal or lateral half of the retina to form the optic tract. Impulses conducted to the right cerebral hemisphere by the right optic tract therefore represent the left half of the field of vision, whereas the right visual field is represented in the left hemisphere. Immediately

after crossing in the chiasma fibers from the nasal half of the retina loop forward for a short distance in the optic nerve. A lesion affecting the optic nerve adjacent to the chiasma may therefore cause a temporal field defect with respect to the opposite eye, in addition to blindness in the eye whose optic nerve has been interrupted. The optic tract curves around the rostral end of the midbrain and ends in the lateral geniculate nucleus of the thalamus.

A few fibers from the retina leave the optic tract adjacent to the chiasma and terminate in the supraoptic nucleus of the hypothalamus and the reticular formation of the brain stem. One possible function of these fibers is that, through a reticulospinal relay to the intermediolateral cell column of the spinal cord, they constitute part of a pathway by which ambient illumination influences the antigonadotropic activity of the pineal gland.

LATERAL GENICULATE NUCLEUS, GENICULOCALCARINE TRACT, AND VISUAL CORTEX

The lateral geniculate nucleus is responsible for a small swelling, the lateral geniculate body, beneath the posterior projection of the

FIG. 20–7. The geniculocalcarine projection.

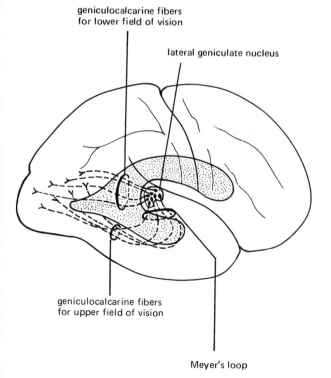

geniculocalcarine fibers
for lower field of vision

lateral geniculate nucleus

geniculocalcarine fibers
for upper field of vision

Meyer's loop

pulvinar of the thalamus. The nucleus is the terminus of all fibers in the optic tract except the few which serve as afferent limbs of reflex arcs. The lateral geniculate nucleus consists of six layers of cells, numbered consecutively from its ventral surface. Within the general pattern shown in Figure 20–6 and described previously, crossed fibers of the optic tract terminate in layers 1, 4, and 6, whereas uncrossed fibers end in layers 2, 3, and 5.

The geniculocalcarine tract originating in the lateral geniculate nucleus first traverses the retrolenticular and sublenticular portions of the posterior limb of the internal capsule. Its fibers then pass around the lateral ventricle, curving posteriorly toward their termination in the visual cortex (Fig. 20–7). Some of the geniculocalcarine fibers travel far forward over the inferior horn of the lateral ventricle. These fibers, which constitute the temporal or Meyer's loop of the geniculocalcarine tract, terminate in the visual cortex below the calcarine sulcus. It is evident from the retinal projection shown in Figure 20–6 that a temporal lobe lesion involving Meyer's loop causes a defect in the upper visual field on the side opposite the lesion. A lesion in the parietal lobe, on the other hand, may involve geniculocalcarine fibers proceeding to the visual cortex above the calcarine sulcus; the result is then a defect in the lower visual field on the side opposite the lesion.

The visual cortex occupies the upper and lower lips of the calcarine sulcus on the medial surface of the cerebral hemisphere. The area is much larger than suggested by the usual cortical maps because of the depth of the calcarine sulcus. The visual cortex is thin, heterotypical cortex of the granular type (area 17 of Brodmann); it is marked by the line of Gennari and known alternatively as the **striate area.** There is a detailed point-to-point projection of the retina on the lateral geniculate nucleus and the visual cortex. The size of the retinal point is reduced to the diameter of a single cone for most acute vision in the central part of the fovea. Precise coordination of movements of the eyes ensures that the retinal patterns of excitation correspond with one another, as required for binocular vision. The visual association cortex, corresponding to areas 18 and 19 of Brodmann, is involved in recognition of objects, perception of color and depth, and other complex aspects of vision.

VISUAL DEFECTS CAUSED BY INTERRUPTION OF THE PATHWAY

Certain general rules governing defects in the visual field as a result of a lesion involving the visual pathway are indicated in Figure 20–8. The first example is an obvious one; severe degenerative disease or trauma involving an optic nerve results in blindness in the corresponding eye. Example 2 refers to interruption of decussating fibers in the optic chiasma, which causes bitemporal hemianopsia if the full thickness of the chiasma is interrupted. The most common lesion affecting the optic chiasma is a pituitary tumor pressing on it from below, which first interrupts fibers from the inferior nasal quadrants of both retinae. The visual defect begins as a scotoma in each upper temporal quadrant of the visual field, and spreads throughout the temporal fields as the chiasma is increasingly affected. Pressure on the lateral edge of the optic chiasma (example 3) happens infrequently, but may occur when there is an aneurysm of the internal carotid artery in this location. The field defect, in the case of pressure on the right edge of the chiasma, is nasal hemianopsia for the right eye. Interruption of the right optic tract (example 4) causes left homonymous hemianopsia.

Example 5 refers to a lesion involving the geniculocalcarine tract or the visual cortex. An extensive right-sided lesion results in left homonymous hemianopsia, except that central vision may remain intact (macular sparing). Decussating fibers that would provide bilateral cortical representation of the macula have not been found. When the lesion is an infarction caused by occlusion of the posterior cerebral artery or one of its branches, collateral circulation from branches of the middle cerebral artery may partially maintain the large region of visual cortex and subjacent white matter concerned with central vision. A slight shifting of the patient's fixation of gaze during examination of the visual fields may explain some instances of "macular sparing." Lesions affecting only a portion of the geniculocalcarine tract or the visual cortex cause field defects of lesser proportions than hemianopsia. An example is provided by the upper quadrantic defect in the opposite visual field following interruption of fibers composing Meyer's loop in the white matter of the temporal lobe.

VISUAL REFLEXES

A small bundle of fibers from the optic tract bypasses the lateral geniculate nucleus and enters the superior brachium. These fibers, which constitute the afferent limb of reflex arcs, terminate in the pretectal nucleus and the superior colliculus.

The **pupillary light reflex** is tested in the routine neurologic examination; the response consists of constriction of the pupil when light, as from a pen flashlight, is directed into the eye. Impulses from the retina impinge on the pretectal nucleus, a small group of cells immediately rostral to the superior collic-

ulus. Impulses are relayed to the Edinger–Westphal nucleus of the oculomotor complex, then to the ciliary ganglion in the orbit, and finally to the sphincter pupillae muscle in the iris. Both pupils constrict in response to light entering one eye because the pretectal nucleus sends fibers to parasympathetic neurons for the sphincter pupillae muscles of both eyes.

Visual impulses reaching the superior colliculus are concerned with reflex responses through tectobulbar and tectospinal connections. These responses include directing the gaze toward the source of a visual stimulus, together with closing the eyes and perhaps

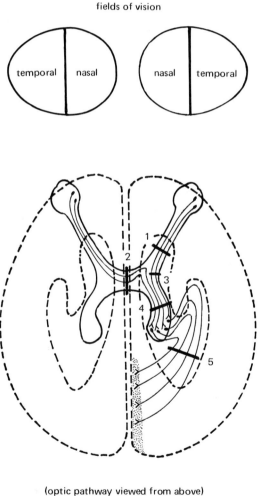

fields of vision

temporal | nasal   nasal | temporal

(optic pathway viewed from above)

FIG. 20-8. Visual field defects caused by lesions affecting different parts of the visual pathway.

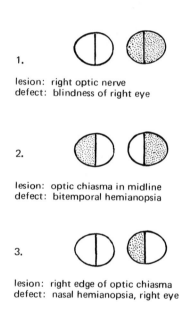

1.

lesion: right optic nerve
defect: blindness of right eye

2.

lesion: optic chiasma in midline
defect: bitemporal hemianopsia

3.

lesion: right edge of optic chiasma
defect: nasal hemianopsia, right eye

4.

lesion: right optic tract
defect: left homonymous hemianopsia

5.

lesion: right geniculocalcarine
    tract or visual cortex
defect: left homonymous hemianopsia
    with sparing of macular
    vision

raising the arms for protection against a rapidly approaching object. However, the number of afferent fibers to the superior colliculus from the retina is small in man, the largest single component of the superior brachium being corticotectal fibers. They originate in the visual association cortex and end in the superior colliculus, from which impulses are relayed to the oculomotor, trochlear, and abducens nuclei. The connections thereby established provide for automatic scanning movements of the eyes, such as occur when reading. Corticotectal fibers probably function as well in the accommodation reflex, to be discussed next.

The **accommodation reflex** or **accommodation–convergence reaction** consists of ocular convergence, pupillary constriction, and thickening of the lens when attention is directed to a near object. The reflex is tested in the routine neurologic examination by asking the patient to examine an object held about a foot from the eyes after looking into the distance, and noting whether there is pupillary constriction. When attention is directed to a near object the medial recti muscles contract for convergence of the eyes. At the same time contraction of the ciliary muscle allows the lens to thicken, increasing its refractive power, and pupillary constriction sharpens the image on the retina.

The pathway for accommodation to near objects, which includes the cerebral cortex, is not fully understood. Impulses from the visual association cortex may reach the midbrain through fibers traversing the superior brachium, probably being relayed to the oculomotor nucleus through the superior colliculus. Alternatively, although less likely, impulses from the visual association cortex may be conveyed by association fibers of the hemisphere to the motor cortex, from which corticobulbar fibers reach the oculomotor nucleus. The pathways for the light and accommodation reflexes are known to be different because they may be dissociated by

disease. This occurs, for example, in central nervous system syphilis, in which there is loss of pupillary constriction in response to light but not to accommodation (the Argyll Robertson pupil). The lesion may involve the pretectal nucleus or its immediate connections, but this is at present uncertain.

There is dilation of the pupils in response to severe pain or strong emotional states. The pathway begins with fibers from the thalamus and hippocampal formation to the hypothalamus, from which impulses reach the intermediolateral cell column of the spinal cord through a relay in the reticular formation. The pathway continues to the superior cervical ganglion of the sympathetic trunk, and it is completed by postganglionic fibers in the carotid plexus to the dilator pupillae muscle in the iris.

SUGGESTED READING

Dowling JE: Foveal receptors of the monkey retina: fine structure. Science 147:57–59, 1965

Dowling JE: Organization of vertebrate retinas. Invest Ophthalmol 9:655–680, 1970

Hollenberg MJ, Bernstein MH: Fine structure of the photoreceptor cells of the ground squirrel (Citellus tridecemlineatus tridecemlineatus.) Am J Anat 118:359–373, 1966

Michael CR: Retinal processing of visual images. Sci Am 220/5:105–114, 1969

Missotten L: The Ultrastructure of the Human Retina. Brussels, Editions ARSCIA, 1965

Moses RA: Adler's Physiology of the Eye, 5th ed. St Louis, Mosby, 1970

Polyak SL: The Vertebrate Visual System. Chicago, University of Chicago Press, 1957

Rushton WAH: Visual pigments and color blindness. Sci Am 232(3):64–74, 1975

Straatsma BR, Hall MO, Allen RA, Crescitelli F (eds): The Retina: Morphology, Function and Clinical Characteristics. Los Angeles, University of California Press, 1969

Werblin FS: The control of sensitivity in the retina. Sci Am 228(1):70–79, 1973

21

Auditory System

Hearing is second in importance among the special senses of man, yielding first place only to sight. Their role in language accounts to a large extent for the reliance placed on these special senses.

The auditory system consists of the external ear, the middle ear, the cochlea of the internal ear, the cochlear nerve, and pathways in the central nervous system. The external ear consists of the auricle or pinna and the external acoustic meatus, the latter being separated from the middle ear by the tympanic membrane. The function of the external ear is to collect sound waves, which cause a resonant vibration of the tympanic membrane. The vibration is transmitted across the middle ear cavity by a chain of three ossicles, the malleus, incus, and stapes. The malleus is attached to the tympanic membrane and articulates with the incus, which articulates in turn with the stirrup-shaped stapes. The foot plate of the stapes occupies the fenestra vestibuli in the wall between the middle and internal ears; the rim of the foot plate is attached to the margin of the fenestra vestibuli by the annular ligament, composed of elastic connective tissue. The ossicles constitute a bent lever with the longer of the two arms attached to the tympanic membrane, and the area of the foot plate of the stapes is considerably smaller than the area of the tympanic membrane. The vibratory force of the tympanic membrane is therefore magnified about 15 times at the fenestra vestibuli; the substantial increase in force is important because the sound waves are transferred from air to a fluid medium. Protection against the effect of sudden, excessive noise is provided by reflex contraction of the tensor tympani and stapedius muscles, which are inserted on the malleus and the stapes, respectively.

The internal ear, which has a dual func-

tion, consists of a membranous labyrinth encased in a bony labyrinth. Certain parts of the internal ear contain sensory areas for the vestibular system, which is discussed in Chapter 22. The cochlear portion of the internal ear contains the organ of Corti (spiral organ), from which nerve impulses arise as a result of the sound waves produced in the fluid in the cochlea by vibration of the stapes. The nerve impulses are conducted to the brain stem by the cochlear division of the vestibulocochlear nerve, reaching the auditory area of the cerebral cortex through several synaptic relays or causing reflex responses through connections in the brain stem. Although the present chapter is concerned primarily with the organ of Corti and the central pathways, the main features of the bony and membranous labyrinths are reviewed as an aid in understanding how vibration of the stapes results in stimulation of sensory cells in the organ of Corti and initiation of nerve impulses traveling to the brain.

BONY AND MEMBRANOUS LABYRINTHS

The bony labyrinth (Fig. 21–1) is in the petrous portion of the temporal bone, which forms a prominent oblique ridge between the middle and posterior cranial fossae. The **fenestra vestibuli** (oval window) in which the foot plate of the stapes fits is in the wall of the **vestibule,** the middle part of the bony labyrinth. The **fenestra cochleae** (round window) is situated below the fenestra vestibuli; it is closed by a thin membrane which makes pressure waves possible in the fluid in the internal ear. The fluid would otherwise be enclosed completely in a rigid "box," except for the source of the waves at the fenestra vestibuli. Three **semicircular canals** extend posterolaterally from the vestibule, and the **cochlea** constitutes the anteromedial portion of the bony labyrinth. The cochlea has the shape of a snail shell; its base abuts against the deep end of the internal acoustic meatus, which opens into the posterior cranial fossa. Cochlear nerve fibers emerge from the base of the cochlea, where they are joined by fibers of the vestibular nerve. The two divisions of the vestibulocochlear nerve leave the internal acoustic meatus and are attached to the brain stem at the junction of the medulla and pons.

The delicate membranous labyrinth conforms, for the most part, to the contours of the bony labyrinth (Fig. 21–2). However, there are two dilations, the **utricle** and the **saccule,** in the vestibule of the bony labyrinth. Three **semicircular ducts** arise from the utricle. There is a patch of sensory epithelium supplied by the vestibular nerve on the inner surface of the utricle, the saccule, and each semicircular duct. The saccule is continuous with the **cochlear duct** through a narrow channel known as the ductus reuniens. The cochlear duct contains a highly specialized strip of sensory epithelium along its entire length; this is the organ of Corti (spiral organ), the end organ for hearing.

The lumen of the membranous labyrinth is continuous throughout and filled with **endolymph,** whereas the interval between the membranous and bony labyrinths is filled with **perilymph.** The vestibular portion of the membranous labyrinth is suspended within the bony labyrinth by trabeculae of connective tissue. However, the cochlear duct is firmly attached along two sides to the wall of the cochlear canal.

COCHLEA

The **cochlear canal** makes two and a half turns around a bony pillar or core, the **modiolus,** in which there are channels for nerve fibers and blood vessels. The cochlea is most conveniently described as if it were resting on its base (Fig. 21–3), although its base in fact faces posteromedially.

The cochlear canal, the cavity of this portion of the bony labyrinth, is divided by two partitions into three spiral spaces. The middle of these is the **cochlear duct** (scala media), *i.e.,* the portion of the membranous labyrinth within the cochlea. The cochlear duct is firmly fixed to the inner and outer walls of the cochlear canal. The remaining spiral spaces are the **scala vestibuli** and the **scala tympani.** The unspecialized wall of the cochlear duct apposing the scala vestibuli is called the **vestibular** or **Reissner's membrane,** whereas the wall apposing the scala tympani constitutes the specialized **basilar membrane,** on which the organ of Corti rests.

The basilar membrane is of special importance in the physiology of hearing because it responds to vibration of the stapes in the following manner. As shown in Figure 21–4, vibration of the foot plate of the stapes produces corresponding waves in the perilymph, beginning with that of the vestibule. The vestibule opens into the scala vestibuli, which communicates with the scala tympani through a small aperture, the **helicotrema,** at the apex of the cochlea. The sound waves could be thought of as passing along the scala vestibuli and into the scala tympani through the helicotrema, causing vibration of the basilar membrane from the scale tympani. However, the helicotrema is a minute orifice, and it is more likely that the basilar membrane vibrates in response to sound waves transmitted through the endolymph in the cochlear duct from the scala vestibuli to the scala tympani. These same waves create a vibration of the membrane closing the fenestra cochleae at the base of the scala tympani, this being essential in order to eliminate the dampening effect of bone-encased fluid that would occur otherwise.

The scala vestibuli and the scala tympani are lined by a single layer of squamous cells of mesenchymal origin, this layer resting on periosteum where the scalae are bounded by the bony labyrinth. The perilymph filling the scala vestibuli and scala tympani is a watery fluid, similar in composition to cerebrospinal fluid. In fact there is a communication between the perilymph-filled spaces of the bony labyrinth and the subarachnoid space. It consists of a narrow channel in the petrous portion of the temporal bone, extending from the scala tympani in the basal turn of the cochlea to an extension of the subarachnoid space around the ninth, tenth, and eleventh cranial nerves as they traverse the jugular foramen.

The **cochlear** or **spiral ganglion** consists of cells in a spiral configuration at the periphery

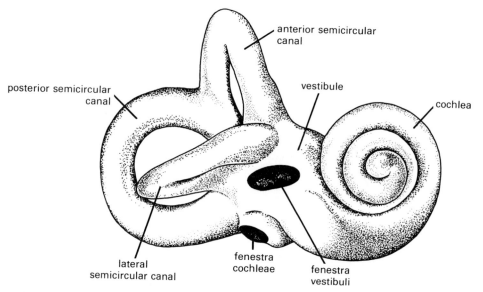

FIG. 21-1. Anterolateral view of the right bony labyrinth.

FIG. 21-2. Anterolateral view of the right membranous labyrinth.

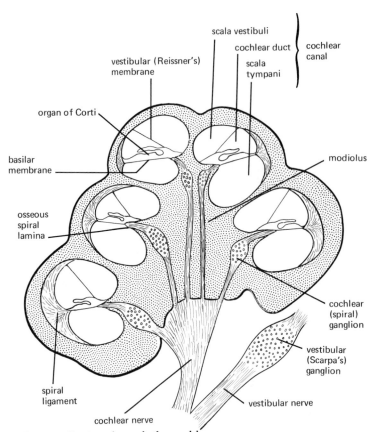

FIG. 21-3. Section through the cochlea.

FIG. 21-4. Schematic representation of the manner in which sound waves in the perilymph and endolymph cause vibration of the basilar membrane.

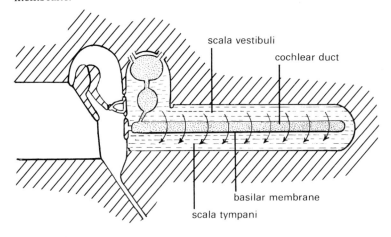

of the modiolus (Fig. 21-3). The primary sensory neurons of both divisions of the vestibulocochlear nerve are bipolar, rather than unipolar as in other cerebrospinal nerves, retaining this embryonal characteristic of primary sensory neurons. The peripheral processes (dendrites) reach the organ of Corti by traversing openings in the osseous spiral lamina projecting from the modiolus, where the myelin sheaths terminate. The central processes (axons) traverse channels in the modiolus, enter the internal acoustic meatus from the base of the cochlea, and continue in the cochlear division of the vestibulocochlear nerve.

COCHLEAR DUCT

Certain specialized regions in the wall of the cochlear duct need to be described (Fig. 21-5). The organ of Corti is considered separately because of its complex structure and importance as the receptor of acoustic stimuli.

Vibration of the **basilar membrane** is essential in the transduction of a mechanical stimulus (sound waves) to the electrical potential of a nerve impulse in the organ of Corti. The inner edge of the basilar membrane is attached to the **osseous spiral lamina,** which projects from the modiolus like the thread on a screw. The outer edge of the membrane is attached to the **spiral ligament,** consisting of a thickening of the periosteum along the outer wall of the cochlear canal. The basilar membrane consists of collagen fibers and sparse elastic fibers embedded in a ground substance, most of the fibers being directed across the membrane. The surface presenting to the scala tympani is covered by a thin layer of vascular connective tissue and a single layer of squamous cells. The width of the basilar membrane increases steadily from the beginning of the basal turn of the cochlea to the apex, this being made possible by a progressive narrowing of the osseous spiral lamina and the spiral ligament in the same direction. The width of the membrane at any point determines the pitch of sound to which it responds maximally. High tones therefore cause maximal vibration in the basal turn of the cochlea and low tones near the apex. The range of audible frequencies in the human ear is from 20–20,000 Hz. (With advancing age there is a gradual decrease in perception of high frequencies.) The range extends over 11 octaves, of which 7 are used in musical instruments such as the piano. Ordinary conversation falls within the range of 300–3000 Hz.

The **vestibular** or **Reissner's membrane** consists of two layers of simple squamous epithelium separated by a trace of connective tissue. The outer wall of the cochlear duct is specialized as the **stria vascularis** for production of endolymph. The epithelium here consists principally of cuboidal cells containing numerous mitochondria; capillaries extend into the epithelium from the vascular connective tissue beneath it. Endolymph is similar to intracellular fluid in respect to its high concentration of potassium ions and low concentration of sodium ions. Endolymph produced by the stria vascularis fills the membranous labyrinth; absorption takes place into venules surrounding the endolymphatic sac in the dura mater on the posterior surface of the petrous portion of the temporal bone. This sac is an expansion of the endolymphatic duct arising from the communication between the saccule and the utricle (Fig. 21-2).

The epithelial lining of the membranous labyrinth, including the specialized sensory areas for the auditory and vestibular systems, is ectodermal in origin. The epithelium differentiates from the cells lining the otic vesicle, formed by an invagination of ectoderm at the level of the hindbrain of the early embryo.

ORGAN OF CORTI

The **organ of Corti** or **spiral organ** (Fig. 21-5) consists of cells specialized for a supporting role and sensory cells for conversion of a mechanical stimulus into the ionic and electrical events which constitute a nerve impulse.

Supporting cells containing bundles of tonofibrils are of two types, pillar cells and phalangeal cells. There are two rows of **pillar cells,** inner and outer, on each side of the **tunnel of Corti.** The number in each row is of the order of 5000, although the inner pillar cells are rather more numerous than the outer pillar cells. Each cell consists mainly of a compact bundle of tonofibrils (the pillar), extending from the basilar membrane to the surface of the organ of Corti. The tonofibrils

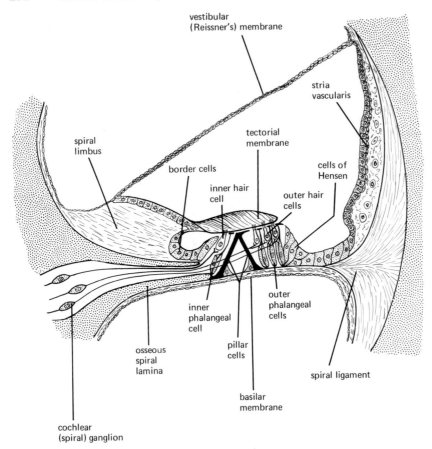

FIG. 21-5. Structure of the cochlear duct and the organ of Corti.

appear in electron micrographs as compact arrays of microtubules. The inner and outer pillars converge, and each pillar ends in a flange directed outward. The nucleus of the pillar cell is in a cytoplasmic region in the acute angle between the pillar and the basilar membrane.

The **phalangeal cells** afford intimate support for the sensory cells; they are arranged as a single row of inner phalangeal cells and three to five rows of outer phalangeal cells, the number of rows increasing from the base to the apex of the cochlea. The base of the slender, flask-shaped phalangeal cell rests on the basilar membrane, and a bundle of tonofibrils extends the length of the cell. Some of the tonofibrils form a supporting shelf for the base of a sensory cell, and the remainder continue alongside a sensory cell. At the surface of the organ of Corti, the tonofibrils of phalangeal and pillar cells form a thin reticular plate in which holes accommodate the

ends of sensory cells. The organ of Corti is completed on the inner side by **border cells** and on the outer side by **cells of Hensen.**

The sensory cells are called **hair cells** because of the hairlike projections from their free ends. There is a single row of inner hair cells, numbering about 7000; the outer hair cells, of which there are some 25,000, are arranged in three rows in the basal turn of the cochlea, increasing to five rows at the apex. The hairs project from the cell along a V- or W-shaped line, their tips being embedded in the tectorial membrane. The number of hairs per cell varies from 50–150, the largest number being on hair cells at the base of the cochlea and the smallest number on cells at the apex. The hairs are microvilli of an unusual type; there is also a single cilium extending from a centriole, but the cilium disappears in the adult. The inner and outer hair cells differ not only in their position but also in certain details of ultrastructure and innervation. The roles of the inner and outer hair cells are probably different in some respects, although their separate contributions to acoustic input to the brain have yet to be fully determined.

Dendritic terminals of primary sensory neurons are in synaptic contact with the hair cells. For the most part a neuron receives stimuli from a small group of hair cells, which is therefore the smallest sensory unit in the organ of Corti. However, the dendritic fields overlap so that impulses originating in a hair cell may be conducted centrally by more than one neuron. The cochlear nerve includes efferent fibers originating in the superior olivary nucleus in the pons (see Auditory Pathways). These fibers also terminate on hair cells, on which they have an inhibitory effect. The axonal terminals of the efferent fibers can be distinguished from dendritic terminals of cochlear ganglion cells in electron micrographs because only the former contain synaptic vesicles. The fluid in the tunnel of Corti and the interstitial fluid in much of the organ of Corti have a chemical composition similar to that of perilymph rather than endolymph. The high concentration of potassium ions in endolymph would prevent impulse conduction by the nerve fibers crossing the tunnel of Corti to reach the outer hair cells.

The **tectorial membrane** is a ribbonlike structure consisting of a gelatinous type of connective tissue; it is attached to the **spiral limbus,** a thickening of the periosteum on the osseous spiral lamina. The tectorial membrane extends over the organ of Corti, and the tips of the hairs of the sensory cells are embedded in the membrane.

It is basic to the physiology of the cochlea that a particular region of the basilar membrane, depending on the pitch of sound, responds by maximal vibration. Through a complex mechanism of transduction, bending of the hairs produces a change in the ionic polarization of the surface membrane of the hair cells and stimulation of dendritic terminals. Regardless of the pitch of sound, vibration of the basilar membrane begins at the base of the cochlea and travels along the membrane with increasing magnitude to a point determined by the pitch. At this point the vibration suddenly dies away, and impulses reaching the brain from the place of maximal stimulation of the organ of Corti are interpreted as a particular pitch of sound. Tonotopic localization is sharpened by the inhibitory effect of efferent fibers in the

cochlear nerve and feedback circuits in the central pathway to the auditory cortex. Increase in intensity of sound causes maximal vibration in a larger region of the basilar membrane, thereby activating more hair cells and neurons. Persistent exposure to excessively loud sounds causes degenerative changes in the organ of Corti at the base of the cochlea. This results in high tone deafness, which is prone to occur in workers who are exposed to the sound of compression engines or jet engines and in those who work for long hours on farm tractors. High tone deafness was formerly encountered most frequently among workmen in boiler factories and is still sometimes known as "boiler-makers' disease."

AUDITORY PATHWAYS

The **cochlear nerve,** consisting of axons or central processes of cells in the spiral ganglion, traverses the internal acoustic meatus in the petrous portion of the temporal bone as a component of the vestibulocochlear nerve. The internal acoustic meatus also contains the labyrinthine artery (a branch of the basilar artery) and the facial nerve. On emerging from the meatus, the cochlear nerve continues to the junction of the medulla and pons. The constituent fibers then bifurcate, one branch ending in the **dorsal cochlear nucleus** and the other branch in the **ventral cochlear nucleus.** The cochlear nuclei are situated superficially in the rostral end of the medulla adjacent to the base of the inferior cerebellar peduncle (Fig. 21-6). A tonotopic pattern of axonal endings has been demonstrated in both nuclei in experimental animals and probably exists in man. The dorsal and ventral cochlear nuclei differ in cellular organization, and the pattern of axonal endings in the ventral nucleus is more precise than in the dorsal nucleus. It is therefore probable that the nuclei also differ in their contribution to the central pathways and to the overall functioning of the auditory system.

PATHWAY TO THE AUDITORY CORTEX

The pathway to the cerebral cortex is characterized by one or more synaptic relays between the cochlear nuclei and the specific

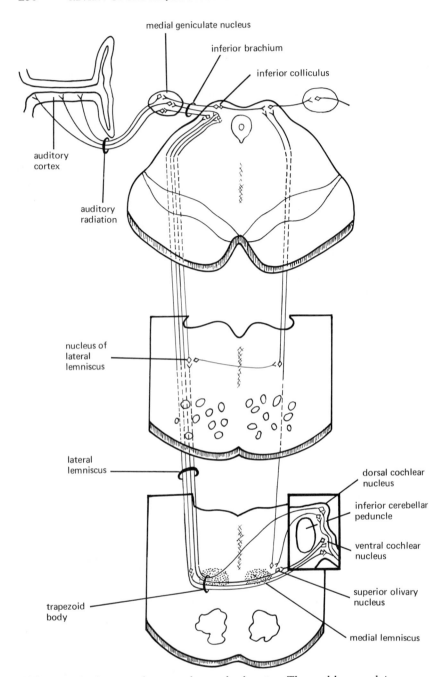

FIG. 21-6. Auditory pathway to the cerebral cortex. The cochlear nuclei are situated at a slightly more caudal level than that shown in the bottommost section in this figure.

thalamic nucleus for hearing, the medial geniculate nucleus (Fig. 21–6). There is a relay in the inferior colliculus, and additional synaptic interruptions may occur in the superior olivary nucleus and the nucleus of the lateral lemniscus. The pathway is also characterized by a significant ipsilateral projection to the cortex. In view of the complicated nature of the pathway the transmission of acoustic data to the cortex can best be described after certain components of the pathway in the brain stem have been identified.

The small **superior olivary nucleus** is situated in the ventrolateral corner of the dorsal portion or tegmentum of the pons at the level of the motor nucleus of the facial nerve (Fig. 7–8). Auditory fibers crossing the pons in the ventral part of the tegmentum constitute the **trapezoid body;** these fibers pass ventral to the ascending fibers of the medial lemniscus or intersect them. Nerve cells situated among the transverse fibers on each side constitute the **nucleus of the trapezoid body,** whose connections are similar to those described below for the superior olivary nucleus. The **lateral lemniscus,** which is the principal ascending auditory tract, extends from the region of the superior olivary nucleus, through the lateral part of the pontine tegmentum, and close to the surface of the brain stem in the isthmus region between the pons and the midbrain. The **nucleus of the lateral lemniscus** consists of cells situated among the fibers of the tract in the pons.

(As noted in the appropriate chapters, the cerebellum receives impulses of both acoustic and optic origin, as does the reticular formation of the brain stem in connection with the ascending reticular activating system.)

The projection from the cochlear nuclei to the inferior colliculus and then to the medial geniculate nucleus, through the components of the pathway just identified, is as follows. Fibers from the **ventral cochlear nucleus** proceed to the region of the ipsilateral superior olivary nucleus, in which some of the fibers terminate. The majority continue across the pons, with a slight forward slope; these fibers, together with others contributed by the superior olivary nucleus, constitute the trapezoid body. On reaching the region of the superior olivary nucleus on the other side of the brain stem the fibers either continue into the lateral lemniscus or terminate in the superior olivary nucleus, from which

fibers are added to the lateral lemniscus. Fibers from the **dorsal cochlear nucleus** pass over the base of the inferior cerebellar peduncle and continue obliquely to the region of the contralateral superior olivary nucleus. Most of the fibers join the lateral lemniscus; the remainder end in the superior olivary nucleus, from which axons are contributed to the lateral lemniscus.

Impulses conveyed by the lateral lemniscus reach the **inferior colliculus** in the midbrain with or without a synaptic relay in the nucleus of the lateral lemniscus. Fibers from the inferior colliculus traverse the inferior brachium and end in the **medial geniculate nucleus.** (A few fibers of the lateral lemniscus have been described as bypassing the inferior colliculus and proceeding directly through the inferior brachium to the medial geniculate nucleus.) The termination of axons in the medial geniculate nucleus of experimental animals is such as to produce a spiral tonotopic pattern corresponding to the spiral of the cochlea, and a similar pattern is probably present in man. Some awareness of sounds appears to occur at the thalamic level in subprimates. However, any subjective appreciation of sounds at the subcortical level is minimal at best in man.

The last link in the auditory pathway consists of the **auditory radiation** in the sublenticular portion of the posterior limb of the internal capsule, through which the medial geniculate nucleus projects on the **auditory cortex** of the temporal lobe. The auditory area, corresponding to areas 41 and 42 of Brodmann, is in the floor of the lateral fissure, extending only slightly on the lateral surface of the hemisphere. A landmark is provided by the two most anterior of the transverse temporal gyri (Heschl's convolutions) on the dorsal surface of the superior temporal gyrus. The tonotopic pattern in the auditory area is such that fibers for sounds of low frequency end in the anterolateral part of the area, whereas fibers for sounds of high frequency terminate in the posteromedial part of the auditory cortex. Analysis of acoustic stimuli at a higher neural level, notably the recognition and interpretation of sounds on the basis of past experience, occurs in the auditory association cortex of the temporal lobe (Wernicke's area). This cortex also makes an important contribution to sensory aspects of language.

The auditory pathway was described as an entirely crossed pathway, yet deafness in the opposite ear does not ensue from unilateral destruction of the auditory cortex. There is, instead, a slight diminution in acuity of hearing in both ears, most noticeably in the opposite ear, together with some difficulty in judging the direction and distance of the source of sounds. The impairment may not be detected unless special audiometric tests are used. These observations are explained in part by a contribution to the lateral lemniscus from the ipsilateral cochlear nuclei, probably with a synapse in the superior olivary nucleus. A bilateral cortical projection from each organ of Corti is also provided by interneurons establishing cross connections between the nuclei of the lateral lemnisci and between the inferior colliculi (Fig. 21–6).

DESCENDING FIBERS IN THE AUDITORY PATHWAY

Parallel with the neurons conducting information from the organ of Corti to the auditory cortex, there are descending and efferent neurons conducting impulses in the reverse direction, thereby providing for feedback circuits. The descending connections consist of 1) fibers from the auditory and adjacent cortex to the medial geniculate nucleus and the inferior colliculus, 2) fibers from the medial geniculate nucleus to the inferior colliculus, and 3) fibers from the inferior colliculus to the cochlear nuclei and the superior olivary nucleus. The **olivocochlear bundle** (of Rasmussen) originates in the superior olivary nuclei, especially the contralateral nucleus. Its fibers leave the brain stem in the vestibular nerve, join the cochlear nerve in the internal acoustic meatus, and terminate as synaptic end bulbs on hair cells of the organ of Corti. The central transmission of data from the sensory hair cells is therefore far more than just a relay to the cortex. In the various cell stations of the pathway there is a complex processing of acoustic data, providing for refinement of such qualities as pitch, timbre, and volume of sound perception. In particular, feedback inhibition sharpens the perception of pitch, especially through the olivocochlear bundle. This is accomplished by inhibition of hair cells in the organ of Corti except for the region in which the basilar membrane is responding by maximal vibration to a particular frequency of sound waves (auditory sharpening). Central inhibition probably suppresses background noise when attention is being concentrated on a particular acoustic stimulus.

AUDITORY REFLEXES

Connections provide for reflex turning of the head and eyes toward the source of a sound, one such pathway being through the tectum of the midbrain. Impulses are relayed from the inferior to the superior colliculus, from which they reach nuclei controlling extraocular muscles and motor neurons in the cervical region of the spinal cord through tectobulbar fibers and the tectospinal tract. A second pathway for ocular movements in response to acoustic stimuli consists of fibers passing from the superior olivary nucleus directly to the abducens nucleus, and to the trochlear and oculomotor nuclei in the medial longitudinal fasciculus. Fibers from the superior olivary nucleus, and probably the nucleus of the lateral lemniscus, terminate in the motor nuclei of the trigeminal and facial nerves for reflex contraction of the tensor tympani and stapedius muscles, respectively. Contraction of these muscles in response to loud sounds reduces the vibration of the tympanic membrane and the stapes.

SUGGESTED READING

Békésky G von: Experiments in Hearing. Wever EG (trans). New York, McGraw-Hill, 1960

Clopton BM, Winfield JA, Flammino FJ: Tonotopic organization: review and analysis. Brain Res 76:1–20, 1974

Dallos P, Billone MC, Durrant JD, Wong C-y, Raynor S: Cochlear inner and outer hair cells: functional differences. Science 177:356–358, 1972

Engström H, Wersäll J: Structure and innervation of the inner ear sensory epithelia. Int Rev Cytol 7:535–585, 1958

Friedmann I: The cytology of the ear. Br Med Bull 18:209–213, 1962

Galambos R: Neural mechanisms of audition. Physiol Rev 34:497–528, 1954

Goldberg JM, Moore RY: Ascending projections of the lateral lemniscus in the cat and monkey. J Comp Neurol 129:143–155, 1967

Hawkins JE Jr, Johnsson L-G: Light microscopic observations in the inner ear in man and monkey. Ann Otol Rhinol Laryngol 77:608–628, 1968

Kimura RS, Schuknecht HF, Sando I: Fine morphology

of the sensory cells in the organ of Corti of man. Acta Otolaryngol (Stockh) 58:390–408, 1965

Klinke R, Galley N: Efferent innervation of vestibular and auditory pathways. Physiol Rev 54:316–357, 1974

Rasmussen GL, Windle WF (eds): Neural Mechanisms of the Auditory and Vestibular Systems. Springfield, IL, Thomas, 1960

Smith CA: Electron microscopy of the inner ear. Ann Otol Rhinol Laryngol 77:629–643, 1968

Smith CA, Rasmussen GL: Recent observations on the olivocochlear bundle. Ann Otol Rhinol Laryngol 72:489–506, 1963

Whitfield IC: The Auditory Pathway. Monographs of the Physiological Society, No. 17. London, Arnold, 1967

22

Vestibular System

Three sources of sensory information are used by the nervous system in the maintenance of equilibrium. These are the eyes, proprioceptive endings throughout the body, and the vestibular portion of the internal ear. The role of the vestibular system, vis-à-vis visual information especially, is illustrated by the individual with congenital atresia of the vestibular apparatus, usually accompanied by cochlear atresia and deaf-mutism. A person so afflicted is able to orient himself satisfactorily by visual guidance but becomes disoriented in the dark or if submerged while swimming. In addition, vestibular impulses caused by motion of the head contribute to appropriate movements of the eyes in order to maintain fixation on an object in the visual field. These functions require the distribution of nerve impulses from the vestibular labyrinth to motor neurons through pathways in the spinal cord, brain stem, and cerebellum, and there is also a projection to the cerebral cortex.

The static labyrinth represented by the utricle and the saccule detects the position of the head with respect to gravity, whereas the kinetic labyrinth represented by the semicircular ducts detects movement of the head. Both parts of the membranous labyrinth function in the maintenance of equilibrium, and the kinetic labyrinth has a special role in coordination of movement of the eyes with movement of the head.

STATIC LABYRINTH

The **utricle** and **saccule** are endolymph-containing dilations of the membranous labyrinth, enclosed by the vestibule of the bony labyrinth (Figs. 21-1 and 21-2). Except at the maculae or specialized sensory areas, the utricle and saccule are lined by simple cuboidal epithelium derived from the otic vesicle of the embryo and supported by a thin layer of connective tissue. The utricle and saccule are suspended from the wall of the vestibule by connective tissue trabeculae, and they are surrounded by a perilymphatic space lined by a single layer of squamous cells of mesenchymal origin.

Each dilation includes a specialized area of sensory epithelium, the macula, about 2 by 3 mm in size. The **macula utriculi** is in the floor of the utricle and parallel with the base of the skull, whereas the **macula sacculi** is vertically disposed on the medial wall of the saccule. The two maculae are identical in histologic structure (Fig. 22-1).

The columnar **supporting cells** of the maculae are continuous with the cuboidal epithelium lining the utricle and saccule elsewhere. The sensory **hair cells,** of which two types have been identified in electron micrographs, are basically similar to hair cells in the organ of Corti. Type I hair cells are flask shaped, whereas type 2 hair cells are cylindrical. From 40-80 hairs (stereocilia) project from each cell, together with a cilium (kinocilium) arising from a centriole (Fig. 22-2A). The hairs are microvilli of an unusual type, like those of hair cells in the organ of Corti except for their greater length, which may be as much as 100μ. The tips of the hairs and the cilium are embedded in the **otolithic membrane,** consisting of gelatinous, noncellular connective tissue in which there are crystals of protein and calcium carbonate (otoliths).

The cell bodies of the primary sensory neurons are in the **vestibular ganglion** (Scarpa's ganglion), situated at the bottom of the internal acoustic meatus. The peripheral processes or dendrites enter the maculae with loss of myelin sheaths and end on the hair cells. The dendritic terminals on type 1 hair cells take the form of chalicelike branches surrounding the cells, whereas minute terminal swellings of dendrites make the synaptic contact with type 2 hair cells. In addition efferent fibers in the vestibular nerve terminate as synaptic end bulbs on the hair cells.

The otoliths give the otolithic membrane a higher specific gravity than the endolymph, thereby causing bending of the hairs in one or another direction except when the macula is in a strictly horizontal plane. The detailed sensory output of the macula is, however, quite complicated. In each hair cell the cilium is situated at one side of the tuft of hairs, and the position of the cilium at the periphery of the hairs differs from one region of the macula to another. The hair cells are excited when the hairs and the cilium are bent in the direction of the cilium, and they are inhibited when the deflection is in the opposite direction (Fig. 22–2A). The pattern of afferent impulses conducted by the fibers of the vestibular nerve to the vestibular nuclei and the cerebellum differs, therefore, according to the orientation of the macula to the direction of gravitational pull (Fig. 22–2B). The appropriate changes in muscle tonus follow, as required to maintain equilibrium.

Although the macula is predominantly a static organ, the higher specific gravity of the otolithic membrane with respect to the endolymph allows the macula to respond to quick tilting movements of the head and to rapid linear acceleration and deceleration. Motion sickness is caused predominantly by prolonged, fluctuating stimulation of the maculae. The utricle and saccule are not as efficient sensors of orientation in man as they are in lower animals. This is illustrated by the pilot of a small aircraft, flying without the aid of instruments, whose intended level flight through clouds may be altered considerably without the pilot being aware of it.

KINETIC LABYRINTH

The three semicircular ducts are attached to the utricle and enclosed in the semicircular canals of the bony labyrinth (Figs. 21–1 and 21–2). The **anterior** and **posterior semicircular ducts** are in vertical planes, the former being transverse to and the latter parallel with, the long axis of the petrous portion of the temporal bone. The **lateral semicircular duct** slopes downward and backward at an angle of 30 degrees to the horizontal plane. The semicircular ducts of the two sides form spatial pairs; the lateral ducts are in the same plane, and the anterior vertical duct of one side and the posterior vertical duct of the opposite side are in the same plane. The sensory areas of the semicircular ducts respond only to movement, the response being maximal when movement is in the plane of the duct.

Each semicircular duct has an expansion or **ampulla** at one end, in which the **crista ampullaris** or sensory epithelium is supported by a transverse septum of connective tissue (Fig. 22–3). Among the columnar supporting cells are situated the sensory **hair cells,** whose structural details conform to those already described for hair cells of the static labyrinth. The hairs and the cilium of each hair cell are embedded in gelatinous material forming the **cupula,** in which otoliths are lacking.

The cristae are sensors of movement of the head, as has been indicated. More specifically they respond to rotary movement, sometimes called angular movement, especially when accompanied by acceleration or deceleration. At the beginning of movement in or near the plane of a semicircular duct, the endolymph lags because of inertia, and the cupula swings like a door in a direction opposite to that of movement of the head. The momentum of the endolymph causes the cupula to swing momentarily in the opposite direction when the movement ceases. The hairs and the cilium of the sensory cells bend accordingly, initiating a process of transduction which alters the ionic polarization of the surface membrane of the hair cells.

The cilium is consistently on the side of the tuft of hairs nearest the opening of the ampulla into the utricle. Excitation of the hair cells therefore occurs when the flow of endolymph is from the ampulla into the adjacent utricle, whereas there is inhibition of the hair cells when the flow is in the opposite direction. (There is a slight tonic discharge from the hair cells of both the maculae and the cristae even in the absence of bending of the hairs.) The hair cells of the cristae, like those of the maculae, are supplied by primary sensory neurons whose bipolar cell bodies are in the **vestibular ganglion.** The pattern of nerve fiber conduction, *i.e.,* the

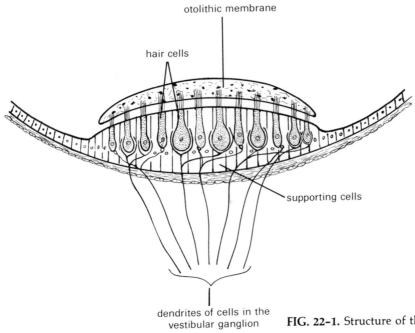

otolithic membrane

hair cells

supporting cells

dendrites of cells in the
vestibular ganglion

FIG. 22-1. Structure of the macula utriculi.

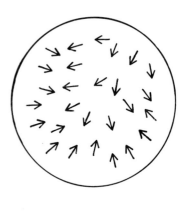

A

B

particular fibers of the vestibular nerve that are conducting impulses to the vestibular nuclei and the cerebellum at any given moment, varies according to the direction in which the head is moving.

VESTIBULAR PATHWAYS

On entering the brain stem at the junction of the medulla and pons, most of the vestibular nerve fibers bifurcate in the usual manner of afferent fibers and end in the vestibular nuclear complex. The remaining fibers enter the cerebellum through the juxtarestiform body of the inferior cerebellar peduncle.

VESTIBULAR NUCLEI

The vestibular nuclei are situated in the rostral part of the medulla, in part beneath the area vestibuli or lateral area of the floor of the fourth ventricle, extending slightly into the pons (Fig. 22–4). Four vestibular nuclei are recognized on the basis of cytoarchitecture and the details of afferent and efferent connections. The **lateral vestibular nucleus,** also known as **Deiters' nucleus,** consists mainly of large multipolar neurons; they have widely branching dendrites, long axons, and prominent Nissl bodies, resembling typi-

cal motor neurons. The **superior, medial,** and **inferior vestibular nuclei** consist of small and medium-sized cells. In transverse sections stained by the Weigert method the inferior vestibular nucleus can be identified by the presence of fine fasciculi consisting of descending branches of vestibular nerve fibers.

CONNECTIONS WITH THE CEREBELLUM

The vestibular portion of the cerebellum or **archicerebellum** consists of the flocculonodular lobe, the adjacent region (uvula) of the inferior vermis, and the fastigial nuclei. The archicerebellum receives fibers from the superior, medial, and inferior vestibular nuclei in addition to a modest number of fibers directly from the vestibular nerve. In the reverse direction fibers from the archicerebellum terminate throughout the vestibular nuclear complex. The role of the archicerebellum in maintaining equilibrium is exerted through pathways from vestibular nuclei to lower motor neurons, and through cerebelloreticular and reticulospinal connections. The cortex of the **paleocerebellum,** which influences muscle tonus in stereotyped movements such as those of postural changes and locomotion, projects to the fastigial nuclei as

---

◀**FIG. 22–2. A.** Simplified sketch of the two types of hair cells in the macula. Excitation occurs when the hairs or microvilli (**a**) bend in the direction of the cilium (**b**), whereas inhibition of the hair cells occurs when the hairs bend in the opposite direction. **B.** Surface of the macula, showing that hair cells in different regions are stimulated and different nerve fibers activated according to the direction of gravitational pull on the otolithic membrane. This pattern results from variations in the position of the cilium relative to the tuft of hairs from one region of the macula to another.

FIG. 22–3. Structure of the crista ampullaris.

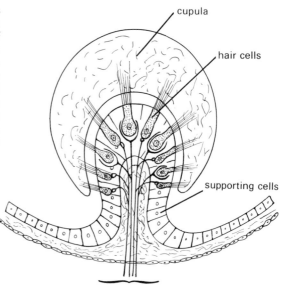

dendrites of cells in the
vestibular ganglion

well as the globose and emboliform nuclei of the cerebellum. The paleocerebellum therefore influences the musculature through pathways thought of as being primarily archicerebellar and through the red nucleus and its projections to lower motor neurons. The afferent and efferent fibers of the archicerebellum compose the juxtarestiform body or medial portion of the inferior cerebellar peduncle.

CONNECTIONS WITH THE SPINAL CORD

The principal connections between the vestibular nuclei and the spinal cord are descending fibers in the vestibulospinal tract and the medial longitudinal fasciculus. (These tracts are sometimes referred to as the lateral and the medial vestibulospinal tracts, respectively.)

The **vestibulospinal tract,** which is uncrossed, originates in the lateral vestibular or Deiters' nucleus exclusively. The fibers descend in the medulla dorsal to the inferior olivary nucleus and continue into the ventral white column of the spinal cord. Vestibulospinal fibers terminate on alpha and gamma motor neurons at all levels of the spinal cord, but most abundantly in the cervical and lumbosacral enlargements. This tract is of prime importance in regulating muscle tonus in such a manner that balance is maintained. A **spinovestibular tract** conveys general sensory data to the vestibular nuclei; the fibers of this minor fasciculus are intermingled with the vestibulospinal tract and confined to the cervical region of the spinal cord.

Fibers from the medial vestibular nucleus, perhaps with some contribution from the inferior vestibular nucleus, project toward the midline and turn caudally in the **medial longitudinal fasciculi** of both sides. This fasciculus is adjacent to the midline, close to the floor of the fourth ventricle, and ventral to the central canal of the medulla more caudally. The fibers continue into the sulcomarginal fasciculus of the ventral white column of the spinal cord, terminating on ventral horn cells throughout the cervical region. Among other possible functions, this vestibulospinal connection may provide for changes in the tonus of neck muscles as required for support of the head in various positions.

CONNECTIONS WITHIN THE BRAIN STEM

The ascending portion of the **medial longitudinal fasciculus** is situated adjacent to the midline in the pons and midbrain, ventral to the floor of the fourth ventricle and the periaqueductal gray matter. The constituent fibers connect the vestibular nuclei with the nuclei of the abducens, trochlear, and oculomotor nerves. More specifically fibers from the superior vestibular nucleus are uncrossed; those from the lateral and inferior vestibular nuclei are crossed, and the medial vestibular nucleus contributes fibers to both fasciculi (Fig. 22-4). This portion of the medial longitudinal fasciculus provides for conjugate movement of the eyes, coordinated with movement of the head, in order to maintain visual fixation. Impulses received by the vestibular nuclei from the cristae ampullares of the kinetic labyrinth are responsible for the ocular adjustments to movement of the head.

The vestibular control of ocular movements needs to be considered in the larger context of multiple neural mechanisms that bear on movements of the eyes. These include the frontal eye field for volitional scanning and the visual association cortex for automatic scanning. There are also connections for reflex turning of the eyes toward the source of visual and acoustic stimuli, and the vestibular coordination of eye and head movements described previously. The precise synchronization of ocular movements as required for binocular vision is controlled in the brain stem, notably through fibers in the medial longitudinal fasciculus. In addition to the vestibular fibers just described, the fasciculus includes axons of internuncial neurons connecting the three cranial nerve nuclei supplying the extraocular muscles. A "center for lateral gaze" is postulated in the pons for specific coordination of the lateral rectus muscle of one eye with the medial rectus muscle of the other eye. The center may consist of a group of neurons in the reticular formation adjacent to the abducens nucleus, and it is therefore called the **parabducens nucleus.** This nucleus is thought to send fibers directly to the abducens nucleus and through the medial longitudinal fasciculus to cells in the contralateral oculomotor nucleus supplying the medial rectus muscle.

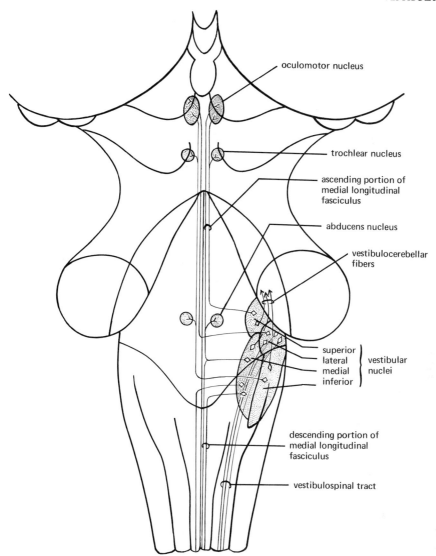

FIG. 22–4. Vestibular pathways to the spinal cord and nuclei of the abducens, trochlear, and oculomotor nerves.

oculomotor nucleus

trochlear nucleus

ascending portion of medial longitudinal fasciculus

abducens nucleus

vestibulocerebellar fibers

superior
lateral   } vestibular
medial   nuclei
inferior

descending portion of medial longitudinal fasciculus

vestibulospinal tract

Excessive or prolonged stimulation of the vestibular system may cause nausea and vomiting. The connections responsible for these effects appear to be collateral branches of efferent fibers from vestibular nuclei, the branches ending in visceral "centers" and parasympathetic nuclei in the brain stem. Excessive input from the labyrinth to the vestibular nuclei is reduced to some extent by a feedback through efferent fibers in the vestibular nerve. These fibers, which are few in number compared with afferent fibers, origi-nate in the vestibular nuclei and possibly the fastigial nucleus. They terminate on hair cells of the maculae and cristae, on which they have an inhibitory effect. The neural mechanisms governing visceral responses to vestibular stimulation are in fact quite complicated because of the important role of psychologic and emotional factors.

CORTICAL REPRESENTATION

Although the vestibular system functions mainly at brain stem, cerebellar, and spinal cord levels, there is a significant projection from the vestibular nuclei to the cerebral cortex. Evoked potentials have been recorded in the parietal lobe of the monkey during electrical stimulation of the vestibular nerve. The vestibular area of cortex thus identified is adjacent to the general sensory area for the head. There are reports of sensations of rotation or body displacement being elicited in man by stimulation of the corresponding area of cortex. The vestibular cortical field probably contributes information for higher motor regulation and conscious spatial orientation. The ascending pathway from the vestibular nuclei is predominantly crossed and runs close to the medial lemniscus. The thalamic relay for the cortical projection is in the ventral posterior nucleus between the region receiving general sensory fibers for the head and the region receiving these fibers for the remainder of the body.

It has been stated that the vestibular area is located in the superior temporal gyrus anterior to the auditory area. This is based on the occasional occurrence of vertigo or of a feeling of dizziness on electrical stimulation of the superior temporal gyrus in conscious patients. The close anatomic relationship between the vestibular and auditory systems in the membranous labyrinth seemed to support the concept of adjoining cortical areas. However, the vestibular system is essentially proprioceptive in function and the presence of a cortical area in the parietal lobe is entirely plausible on physiologic grounds.

TESTS APPLIED TO THE VESTIBULAR SYSTEM

The vestibular projections to nuclei supplying extraocular muscles and motor neurons in the spinal cord can be demonstrated by strong stimulation of the labyrinth. This may be done by rotating a person around a vertical axis about 10 times in 20 sec, then stopping the rotation abruptly. The responses are most pronounced if the head is bent foward 30 degrees to bring the lateral semicircular ducts in a horizontal plane. On stopping rotation, momentum acquired by the endolymph causes it to flow past (and deflect) the cupulae of the lateral semicircular ducts more suddenly and rapidly than for most movements.

The responses of the hair cells in the cristae ampullares produce the following signs immediately after rotation ceases. Impulses conveyed by the ascending fibers of the me-

dial longitudinal fasciculus cause nystagmus, *i.e.*, a slight oscillatory movement of the eyes consisting of fast and slow components. The direction of nystagmus, right or left, is designated by that of the fast component, which is opposite to the direction of rotation. The fast component has been considered as a compensatory reaction mediated by corticobulbar connections. However, both components persist in experimental animals following transection at the rostral end of the midbrain, indicating that the fast component is triggered by a center in the brain stem. The individual serving as a subject deviates in the direction of rotation if asked to walk in a straight line, and the finger deviates in the same direction on pointing to an object. These responses are caused by the effect of vestibulospinal projections on muscle tonus. There is a subjective feeling of turning in a direction opposite to that of rotation, for which the cortical projection is presumably responsible. The spread of impulses to visceral centers may produce sweating and pallor, and even nausea in more susceptible persons.

The **caloric test** is used when there is a reason to suspect a tumor of the vestibulocochlear nerve or a lesion interrupting the vestibular pathway in the brain stem. This procedure has the distinct advantage of testing the pathway from each internal ear separately. The head is positioned so that the lateral semicircular duct is in a vertical plane, and the external acoustic meatus is irrigated with warm or cold water, usually the latter. The ampulla of the duct is near the bone undergoing a change of temperature, and the endolymph "rises" or "falls," depending on whether it is warmed or cooled. The procedure causes nystagmus if the vestibular pathway for the side tested is intact.

Labyrinthine irritation or disease may cause vertigo, sometimes accompanied by nausea and vomiting, pallor, a cold sweat, and nystagmus. Paroxysms of labyrinthine irritation constitute Ménière's disease, the cause of which is usually obscure.

SUGGESTED READING

Brodal A, Pompeiano O, Walberg F: The Vestibular Nuclei and Their Connections, Anatomy and Functional Anatomy. Edinburgh, Oliver & Boyd, 1962

Christoff N, Anderson PJ, Nathanson M, Bender MB: Problems in anatomic analysis of lesions of the medial longitudinal fasciculus. Arch Neurol 2:293–304, 1960

Deeke L, Schwarz DWF, Fredrickson JM: Nucleus ventroposterior inferior (VPI) as the vestibular thalamic relay in the Rhesus monkey. I. Field potential investigation. Exp Brain Res 200:80–100, 1974

Engström H, Wersäll H: The ultrastructural organization of the organ of Corti and of the vestibular sensory epithelia. Exp Cell Res [Suppl] 5:460–492, 1958

Flock A: Structure of the macula utriculi with special reference to directional interplay of sensory responses as revealed by morphological polarization. J Cell Biol 22:413–431, 1964

Fredrickson JM, Figge U, Schied P, Kornhuber HH: Vestibular nerve projection to the cerebral cortex of the rhesus monkey. Exp Brain Res 2:318–327, 1966

Mickle WA, Ades HW: Rostral projection pathway of the vestibular system. Am J Physiol 176:243–246, 1954

Penfield W: Vestibular sensation and the cerebral cortex. Ann Otol Rhinol Laryngol 66:691–698, 1957

Rasmussen GL, Windle WF (eds): Neural Mechanisms of the Auditory and Vestibular Systems. Springfield, IL, Thomas, 1960

23

Motor Systems

Except for certain aspects of visceral function (see Ch. 24, Visceral Afferents and the Autonomic Nervous System), overt expression of activity in the central nervous system depends on the somatic or skeletal musculature. The control of these muscles is vested in the pyramidal and the extrapyramidal motor systems. The pyramidal system, an uninterrupted pathway from the neocortex to the brain stem and spinal cord, is a feature of the mammalian nervous system. The extrapyramidal system is older phylogenetically. It includes several subcortical gray areas, and this polysynaptic system is therefore much more complex than the pyramidal system. Both systems converge on lower motor neurons in motor nuclei of cranial nerves and the ventral gray horns of the spinal cord, these neurons constituting the final common pathway (Sherrington) for determining muscle action.

PYRAMIDAL SYSTEM

The pyramidal system is responsible for certain aspects of voluntary movement. (The contributions of the pyramidal and the extrapyramidal systems to voluntary motor activity are discussed at the conclusion of the chapter.) The corticospinal tract is called the pyramidal tract because it traverses the pyramid of the medulla. But the corticobulbar tract has the same relationship to motor neurons of cranial nerves as the corticospinal tract to motor neurons of the spinal cord, and both tracts are therefore included under the heading of the pyramidal motor system.

CORTICAL AREAS FOR THE PYRAMIDAL MOTOR SYSTEM

The fibers of the pyramidal motor system originate in a rather large expanse of cortex in the frontal and parietal lobes. Within the total area the region with the lowest threshold for eliciting motor responses on electrical stimulation is designated the motor area (or primary motor area). This area in the frontal lobe occupies the precentral gyrus and the anterior part of the paracentral lobule on the lateral and medial surfaces of the hemisphere, respectively (Figs. 15–1 and 15–2). The motor area corresponds with area 4 in Brodmann's cytoarchitectural map, and it is the source of about 40% of the pyramidal motor fibers. The motor area is thicker (4.5 mm) than cortex elsewhere and is classified as agranular heterotypical cortex because it contains a wealth of pyramidal cells which obscure the basic six-layered pattern of neocortex. The presence of giant pyramidal (Betz) cells in layer 5 is a unique feature of the motor area.

Excitation of neurons in area 4 is reflected primarily in the contralateral musculature. This is especially true of muscles of the limbs and the lower facial muscles; there is significant ipsilateral (as well as contralateral) control of many of the muscles of the head and muscles in the neck and trunk. A somatotopic representation has been demonstrated by the electrical stimulation of the cortex required in some neurosurgical procedures. The region for muscles of the head is the ventral one-third of the motor area, a large portion of which is assigned to muscles used in speech. Proceeding dorsally there is a large region for muscles moving the hand, followed by sequential representation of the arm, shoulder, trunk, and thigh. The region for the remainder of the lower limb and the anal and vesical sphincters is in the paracentral lobule. The large portions of area 4 assigned to parts of the body in which movements are delicate and precise reflect the many cortical neurons required for such movements.

The somesthetic cortex in the parietal lobe

(areas 3, 1, and 2), occupying the postcentral gyrus and the posterior part of the paracentral lobule, contributes about 20% of the fibers of the pyramidal system. (Sensory responses can be elicited by stimulating the motor area; because of overlapping functions, the motor and somesthetic areas can usefully be considered as an integrated region of sensorimotor cortex surrounding the central sulcus.) The remaining pyramidal fibers originate in premotor cortex in the frontal lobe (area 6) and cortex of the parietal lobe posterior to the somesthetic area, especially areas 5 and 7 of Brodmann.

CORTICOBULBAR TRACT (Fig. 23-1)

Axons from the ventral one-third of area 4, together with contributions from adjacent areas as already noted, traverse the corona radiata of the medullary center and the internal capsule. These corticobulbar (corticonuclear) fibers pass through the lenticulothalamic portion of the posterior limb of the internal capsule at about the junction of its anterior two-thirds and posterior one-third. They continue into the basis pedunculi of the midbrain, where small bundles separate immediately for the oculomotor and trochlear nuclei. The middle three-fifths of the basis pedunculi consists of corticospinal fibers. Corticobulbar fibers for nuclei of cranial nerves in the pons and medulla run along the medial side of the corticospinal tract, *i.e.*, between the corticospinal and frontopontine tracts. The corticospinal tract continues through the ventral portion of the pons and the pyramid of the medulla, whereas bundles of corticobulbar fibers diverge at intervals to supply motor nuclei of cranial nerves in the pons and medulla. These consist of the motor nucleus of the trigeminal nerve, the abducens nucleus, the motor nucleus of the facial nerve, the nucleus ambiguus for the glossopharyngeal, vagus, and accessory nerves, and the hypoglossal nucleus. With few exceptions intercalated neurons in the reticular formation intervene between the corticobulbar fibers and lower motor neurons in the cranial nerve nuclei.

The majority of corticobulbar fibers cross to the opposite side of the brain stem; cortical control of the musculature of the head through this system is therefore predominantly contralateral. However, significant ipsilateral connections exist, preventing voluntary paralysis of most of the muscles following interruption of corticobulbar connections from one hemisphere. In fact there is exclusive contralateral control only for the motor nucleus of the facial nerve, and even here the cells supplying the frontalis and orbicularis oculi muscles come under bilateral cortical control. A corticobulbar lesion such as may occur in the cortex, corona radiata, or internal capsule, results in paralysis of the contralateral muscles of expression, except that the patient is able to raise the eyebrow and close the eyelids.

The motor nucleus of the trigeminal nerve and the hypoglossal nucleus receive a moderate number of uncrossed cortical fibers. There is nearly always weakness (paresis) rather than paralysis of voluntary contraction of the muscles of mastication and the lingual muscles on the side opposite the lesion, and detection of the deficit may be difficult. The oculomotor, trochlear, and abducens nuclei come under still more substantial bilateral cortical control, and voluntary eye movements are therefore preserved in the presence of a lesion interrupting fibers from one hemisphere. However, fibers from the frontal eye field (lower part of area 8) may be interrupted in such a lesion, resulting in paralysis of contralateral gaze and even transient deviation of the eyes to the side of an acute lesion. Muscles of the soft palate, larynx, and pharynx function satisfactorily following a one-sided corticobulbar type of lesion because the nucleus ambiguus receives a substantial number of fibers from the ipsilateral cortex in addition to a larger number from the opposite side. (As noted later in the chapter, extrapyramidal projections to lower motor neurons must also be taken into consideration when dealing with the physiologic basis of voluntary motor action and voluntary motor paralysis.)

CORTICOSPINAL TRACT (Fig. 23-1)

Emanating from the dorsal two-thirds of the motor area, from premotor cortex, and from cortex of the parietal lobe, corticospinal fibers traverse the corona radiata and the posterior one-third of the lenticulothalamic portion of the posterior limb of the internal capsule. The tract continues through the middle three-fifths of the basis pedunculi of the midbrain and is broken up into many fasciculi on traversing the ventral portion of

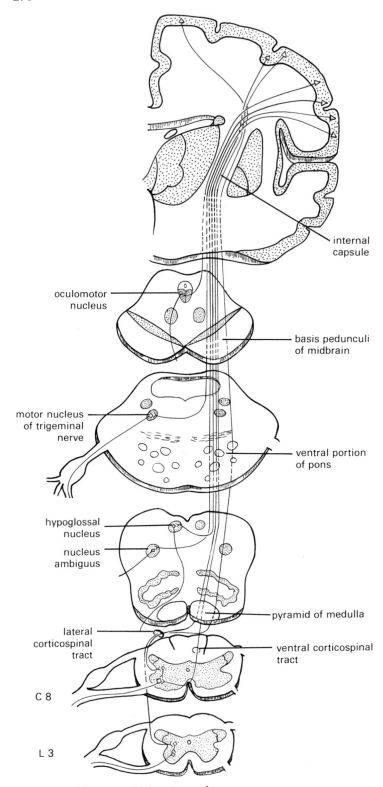

internal
capsule

oculomotor
nucleus

basis pedunculi
of midbrain

motor nucleus
of trigeminal
nerve

ventral portion
of pons

hypoglossal
nucleus

nucleus
ambiguus

pyramid of medulla

lateral
corticospinal
tract

ventral corticospinal
tract

C 8

L 3

FIG. 23–1. The pyramidal motor pathway.

the pons. At the latter site the bundles are separated by the groups of cells comprising the pontine nuclei and by transverse strands of pontocerebellar fibers. The fasciculi coalesce to form the compact corticospinal tract in the pyramid of the medulla. There is considerable intermingling of corticospinal fibers that influence the musculature of different parts of the body. Nevertheless in the internal capsule fibers for the neck and upper limb are concentrated in the anterior part of the region containing corticospinal fibers, followed by fibers for the trunk and then the lower limb. Throughout the brain stem fibers for the upper part of the body tend to be medial and those for the lower part of the body lateral, although the topographical arrangement again lacks precision because of intermingling of fibers concerned with different parts of the body.

A quantitative study of the corticospinal tract in the pyramid of the medulla has shown that there are approximately 1 million fibers of various sizes. About 35,000 fibers (3%) are distinctly larger than the remainder, measuring about 10μ in diameter. The giant pyramidal cells of Betz are best developed in the dorsal two-thirds of area 4, in which the number of Betz cells corresponds closely with the number of large corticospinal fibers. It is assumed, therefore, that the Betz cells are responsible for these large, rapidly conducting fibers in the corticospinal tract. Fibers constituting the bulk of the tract are for the most part axons of pyramidal and fusiform cells in the regions of cortex in which the corticospinal tract originates.

At the caudal end of the medulla, with some variation in the exact level among different individuals, most of the corticospinal fibers cross the midline in the **decussation of the pyramids.** The proportion of crossing fibers also varies from one individual to another, the average being about 85%. The decussation consists of coarse bundles, the bundles from a pyramid alternating with those from the opposite pyramid. Fibers concerned with the upper limbs cross before those for the lower limbs. Having traversed the decussation, the fibers constitute the **lateral corticospinal tract** in the dorsal part of the lateral white column of the spinal cord. The constituent fibers have a segmental topography, those ending in the highest segments being most medial and the longest fibers most lateral. The proportions of fibers

terminating in the major regions of the spinal cord are: cervical, 55%; thoracic, 20%; and lumbosacral, 25%. With few exceptions corticospinal fibers synapse with intercalating neurons, which synapse in turn with alpha motor neurons and some gamma motor neurons; only about 5% of the fibers synapse directly with motor cells.

About 15% of the fibers in a pyramid do not cross over in the decussation. Of these the majority continue into the ventral white column of the spinal cord as the **ventral corticospinal tract,** the fibers terminating in the ventral gray horns of cervical and upper thoracic segments. A few fibers of the pyramid continue into the lateral corticospinal tract of the same side. These, together with fibers of the ventral tract which terminate in the ipsilateral gray matter, account in part for bilateral cortical control of muscles of the neck and trunk. Cortical projections to extrapyramidal centers (described later) also contribute to the bilaterality of voluntary control of the musculature.

The pyramidal tracts contain a small proportion of fibers other than the motor fibers described. These are descending fibers from the sensorimotor cortex surrounding the central sulcus, proceeding with the pyramidal tract to the nucleus of the spinal tract of the trigeminal nerve, the nuclei gracilis and cuneatus, and the dorsal gray horn of the spinal cord. Through this descending pathway, cortical activity facilitates or inhibits transmission of data by second order sensory neurons to the thalamus and the somesthetic cortex.

Fibers of the pyramidal system give off collateral branches as they traverse the internal capsule and the brain stem; these branches terminate in the corpus striatum, red nucleus, pontine nuclei, inferior olivary nucleus, and the reticular formation. Through excitation or inhibition the collateral branches provide connections through which the pyramidal system influences components of the extrapyramidal motor system.

EXTRAPYRAMIDAL SYSTEM

Defining the extrapyramidal motor system presents difficulties, leading to considerable dissatisfaction with a term that is well established in the neurologic literature. As narrowly defined, extrapyramidal pathways consist of those paralleling the direct pyramidal pathways, *i.e.*, corticorubral and corticoreticular fibers, together with projections from the red nucleus and the reticular formation to lower motor neurons. In the comprehensive definition, the extrapyramidal system consists of all components of the central nervous system functioning in the motor sphere, exclusive of the pyramidal system. While acknowledging the conceptual vulnerability of the broad definition, it is followed here as a basis for reviewing the motor components of the central nervous system. This requires that a distinction be made between 1) pathways projecting to motor cortical areas in the frontal lobe and 2) pathways distributed to lower motor neurons.

PATHWAYS TO MOTOR CORTEX

The corpus striatum, substantia nigra, and neocerebellum project to motor areas of the frontal lobe through a relay in the ventral anterior and ventral lateral nuclei of the thalamus, and the subthalamic nucleus is closely related to the corpus striatum (Fig. 23–2).

Corpus Striatum

The corpus striatum receives fibers from the cerebral cortex, the thalamus, and the substantia nigra; they end mainly in the neostriatum (striatum), consisting of the caudate nucleus and the putamen of the lenticular nucleus. Corticostriate fibers originate in

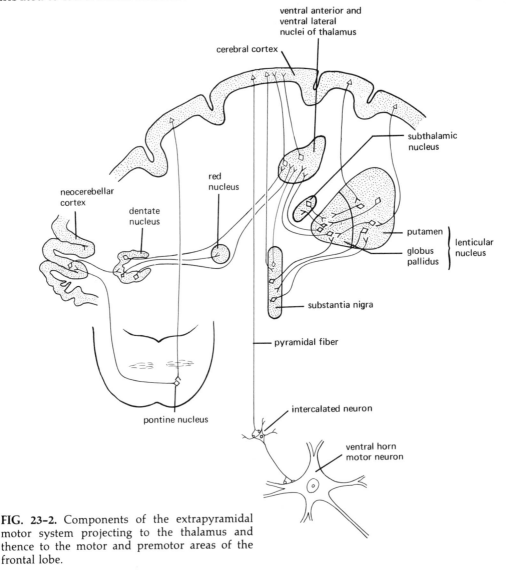

FIG. 23–2. Components of the extrapyramidal motor system projecting to the thalamus and thence to the motor and premotor areas of the frontal lobe.

widespread areas of cortex, but predominantly in cortex of the frontal and parietal lobes. Most of these fibers enter the neostriatum from the internal capsule, although a substantial number reach the putamen by way of the external capsule. Thalamostriate fibers have their origin in the intralaminar, medial, and ventral anterior nuclei of the thalamus. Most of the fibers leaving the neostriatum end in the paleostriatum, i.e., the globus pallidus (pallidum) of the lenticular nucleus, and a few striatal efferents terminate in the substantia nigra.

Efferent fibers of the globus pallidus make up two fasciculi, the lenticular fasciculus and the ansa lenticularis. Almost all of these fibers traverse the subthalamus to reach the ventral anterior and ventral lateral thalamic nuclei, from which fibers project to the motor and premotor cortex of the frontal lobe.

Substantia Nigra

The substantia nigra has reciprocal connections with the corpus striatum, the red nucleus, and the reticular formation of the brain stem. It is also incorporated in a circuit which includes the cerebral cortex. This consists of corticonigral fibers from the frontal, parietal, and occipital lobes, and fibers from the substantia nigra to the ventral anterior and ventral lateral nuclei of the thalamus, relay sites to the motor and premotor cortex in the frontal lobe. The most evident connection of the substantia nigra in the clinical context is the projection to the neostriatum. Degeneration of these neurons, for which dopamine is the neurotransmitter substance, results in paralysis agitans or Parkinson's disease.

Subthalamic Nucleus

This nucleus has a reciprocal connection with the globus pallidus through the subthalamic fasciculus which intersects the intervening internal capsule. Through this connection the subthalamic nucleus has a modifying influence, mainly inhibitory, on the neurons in the globus pallidus.

In summary the corpus striatum, substantia nigra, and subthalamic nucleus constitute a closely integrated group of nuclei. With the intervention of the ventral anterior and ventral lateral nuclei of the thalamus, an important, but poorly understood, influence is exerted on motor areas of the frontal lobe which give rise to fibers of the pyramidal and extrapyramidal motor systems. The importance of these connections is manifest in the dyskinesias resulting from lesions in one or another of the nuclei, lesions which are often referred to as causing extrapyramidal motor disorders.

Neocerebellum

The neocerebellum, consisting of the cortex of the lateral portion of each cerebellar hemisphere and the dentate nuclei, participates in a circuit which ensures efficiency of voluntary muscle action. The circuit connects the cortex of a cerebral hemisphere with the contralateral half of the neocerebellum. It consists of corticopontine and pontocerebellar fibers, dentatothalamic fibers to the ventral lateral nucleus of the thalamus, and thalamocortical fibers to motor areas of cortex in the frontal lobe. Stated generally, the cerebellum is informed concerning volitional movements in progress or about to take place; this and related information is processed by the computerlike circuitry within the cerebellum; neuronal activity in motor areas of the cerebral cortex is influenced in such a way as to produce the intended rate, range, force, and direction of movement.

PATHWAYS TO LOWER MOTOR NEURONS

Lower motor neurons, constituting the final common pathway of the motor system, receive fibers from the red nucleus, the reticular formation, vestibular nuclei, and the superior colliculus, in addition to fibers of the pyramidal system (Fig. 23-3). The extrapyramidal fibers converge on gamma motor neurons as well as alpha motor neurons; in fact the gamma reflex loop involving neuromuscular spindles is used substantially in the control of muscle action by the extrapyramidal motor system.

Red Nucleus and Reticular Formation

The red nucleus of the midbrain and the reticular formation of the brain stem have some connections in common. Corticorubral fibers originate mainly in the motor and premotor areas of the frontal lobe; they traverse the internal capsule in company with fibers of the pyramidal system. The cells of origin of corticoreticular fibers are in various parts of the cortex, including a major contribution from the sensorimotor strip. Corticoreticular fibers reach the brain stem through the internal and external capsules, terminating throughout the reticular formation but preferentially in the magnocellular nuclei of the medial area. The red nucleus and the reticular formation receive fibers from the globose and emboliform nuclei of the cerebellum, and the reticular formation receives fibers

from the fastigial nuclei of the cerebellum. They are therefore included in pathways from the paleocerebellum and the archicerebellum to lower motor neurons. There are also afferents to the red nucleus and the reticular formation from the substantia nigra.

Pallidorubral and pallidoreticular fibers were described on the basis of earlier work, but it now seems unlikely that these connections exist. However, a few fibers from the globus pallidus terminate in the pedunculopontine nucleus, a small group of cells situ-

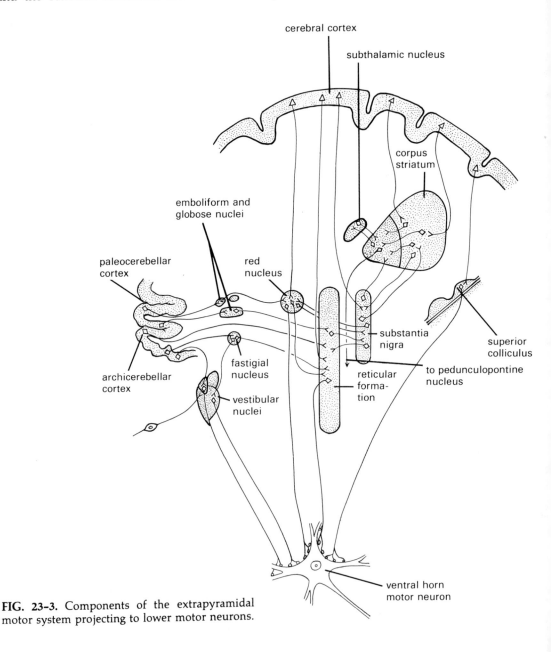

FIG. 23-3. Components of the extrapyramidal motor system projecting to lower motor neurons.

ated in the lateral part of the brain stem at the junction of the cerebral peduncle of the midbrain and the dorsal portion of the pons. The pedunculopontine nucleus sends fibers to the medial area of the reticular formation in which reticulospinal fibers originate. A pathway is thereby provided through which the corpus striatum projects to lower motor neurons, but it must be of minor importance compared with the projection of the corpus striatum, *via* a thalamic relay, to motor areas of the cerebral cortex.

Descending fibers from the red nucleus constitute the crossed **rubrospinal tract** in the lateral white column of the spinal cord; its fibers terminate in all regions of the cord, but mainly in the cervical region. **Reticulospinal fibers** originate in the medial part of the reticular formation, especially the magnocellular region in the medulla and caudal pons. The fibers do not form a discrete fasciculus but are distributed instead in the ventral and lateral white columns of the spinal cord. In addition to reticulospinal conduction by long fibers there is polysynaptic transmission through spinospinalis association fibers. In man rubroreticular and reticulospinal connections probably constitute as important a descending pathway from the red nucleus as the rubrospinal tract. Comparable fibers from the red nucleus and the reticular formation terminate in motor nuclei of cranial nerves innervating striated muscles.

In summary the rubrospinal tract and reticulospinal fibers provide pathways through which the cerebral cortex, the cerebellum, and to some extent the substantia nigra bring their influence to bear on lower motor neurons.

Other Descending Pathways

The cells of origin of the vestibulospinal tract and the medial longitudinal fasciculus are situated in the vestibular nuclear complex. The afferents for these nuclei are fibers of the vestibular nerve and fibers from the archicerebellum. The **vestibulospinal tract** originates in the lateral vestibular (Deiters') nucleus; this uncrossed tract in the ventral white column gives off fibers to the ventral gray horn throughout the spinal cord. Descending fibers of the **medial longitudinal fasciculus** come from the medial and inferior vestibular nuclei; they are included in

the sulcomarginal fasciculus of the ventral white column of the spinal cord and end in the ventral gray horn throughout the cervical region. The ascending fibers of the medial longitudinal fasciculus proceed to the abducens, trochlear, and oculomotor nuclei. The projection from the vestibular nuclei to motor neurons is concerned with maintenance of balance and coordination of head and eye movements.

The **tectospinal tract** in the ventral white column of the spinal cord originates in the contralateral superior colliculus, and its fibers terminate in the ventral gray horn throughout the cervical region. The superior colliculus receives visual data from the retina, acoustic data from the inferior colliculus, and general sensory data by means of the spinotectal tract. The tectospinal tract and tectobulbar fibers for nuclei supplying the extraocular muscles provide for reflex turning of the head and eyes toward the source of visual, acoustic, and cutaneous stimuli. Corticotectal fibers to the superior colliculus from the visual association cortex and the collicular efferents previously mentioned provide for automatic scanning movements.

In addition to impulses received by lower motor neurons through the various descending pathways, impulses received through the dorsal roots of spinal nerves are vital to the normal functioning of these neurons. Following deafferentation by section of dorsal roots for the lower cervical segments, for example, there is severe motor impairment of the upper limb, even to the point of virtual uselessness.

ROLES OF THE PYRAMIDAL AND EXTRAPYRAMIDAL SYSTEMS

A concept of the particular roles of the pyramidal and the extrapyramidal motor systems evolved gradually during the present century and continues to be a subject of investigation. One difficulty stems from differences between experimental results in animals, including subhuman primates, and the traditional clinical interpretation of motor deficits resulting from lesions that involve the pyramidal system. The problem can be appreciated to best advantage by considering the historical development of the concepts of these motor systems.

THE PYRAMIDAL SYSTEM

By the beginning of the present century, cortical stimulation studies on experimental animals were fairly well advanced. A motor area from which movements could be elicited on weak stimulation had been delineated in the cortex of the frontal lobe. At this stage of investigation the assumption was made that the pyramidal tract consisted of fibers that originated primarily, if not exclusively, in the motor cortex in the precentral gyrus. It was known that the pyramidal tract was a relatively recent phylogenetic acquisition, achieving its greatest development in man. It was natural, therefore, that the impairment of voluntary motor function consequent to ablation of the motor cortex in animals or its pathologic involvement in humans led to the concept that the pyramidal system represented the great descending pathway for all voluntary motor activity.

With the greater degree of sophistication in both anatomic and physiologic experimentation, certain presumptions leading to the concept of a strict association between the pyramidal system and voluntary motor function had to be revised. Anatomic studies showed that fibers from the motor area (area 4) constitute about 40% of the fibers of the pyramidal tract, the remainder originating in cortex of the frontal lobe anterior to the motor area and in cortex of the parietal lobe. Physiologic studies on both lower mammals and subhuman primates disclosed that the effects of section of the pyramidal tract are less devastating than one might expect on the basis of traditional views. In addition it was shown that ablation of the motor cortex adds a more severe and complex deficit in motor function to that already present in an animal whose pyramidal tract had been sectioned previously. Thus by 1940 anatomists and physiologists were becoming aware of the shortcomings of equating the pyramidal system strictly with area 4 and of the strict equation of the pyramidal system with voluntary motor function.

THE EXTRAPYRAMIDAL SYSTEM

Many reports appeared in the literature correlating involuntary movement disorders with degenerative changes in subcortical nuclei considered as components of the extrapyramidal motor system. These involuntary movement disorders, now collectively referred to as the dyskinesias, therefore became known as extrapyramidal syndromes, of which the following are the most important.

The variable tremors and rigidity of Wilson's disease are associated with a special type of degenerative change in the lenticular nucleus resulting from a disorder of copper metabolism. Degenerative changes of various kinds in the corpus striatum are associated with involuntary movements of choreiform or athetoid type. Choreiform movements are jerky, rapid, and purposeless, involving particularly the axial and proximal limb musculature. Athetoid movements are slow, sinuous, and aimless, most frequently involving the distal musculature of the limbs. Degenerative changes in these conditions may not be limited to the corpus striatum, but they are less widespread than those seen in dystonia musculorum deformans, the most grotesque of the dyskinesias, which also is associated with striatal pathology. This disorder consists of slow, writhing movements of various parts of the axial and limb musculature. The involuntary movements are more sustained than those of chorea and athetosis, thus accounting in part for its more grotesque nature and the tendency to development of contractures of various parts of the body musculature.

Hemiballismus, consisting of sudden, flailing, gross movements involving the proximal musculature of the limbs, is associated with pathologic changes in the contralateral subthalamic nucleus. The commonest dyskinesia, paralysis agitans or Parkinson's disease, is caused by neuronal degeneration in the substantia nigra and is characterized by muscular rigidity, a fine tremor, and poverty of movement (bradykinesia). Finally lesions of the cerebellum lead to a variety of motor disturbances including a specific type of ataxia, hypotonia, and a characteristic intention tremor. Cerebellar lesions may be said in general to lead to errors in the rate, range, force, and direction of willed movements.

The clinical and pathologic observations just summarized lent support to the concept that the extrapyramidal system is concerned mainly with involuntary and stereotyped movements without being involved directly with voluntary movements.

THE PRESENT POSITION

Naturally occurring lesions in man rarely, if ever, interrupt the pyramidal pathway without simultaneous involvement of extrapyramidal connections. The effects of a pure pyramidal lesion (careful sectioning of the pyramid in the medulla for example) can only be studied in experimental animals. Even when subhuman primates are studied in this way, caution must be exercised in transferring information thus obtained to the human situation. The possibility that the normally functioning pyramidal tract may be responsible for more activities than those which disappear when the tract is sectioned must also be considered. Recognizing these problems, more recent, well-performed studies seem to have made untenable the hypothesis that all voluntary, nonstereotyped movement is mediated by way of the pyramidal system. Many observers now believe that the pyramidal system confers speed and agility on voluntary motor behavior, with the important specific contribution of enabling primates to use the individual digits in an independent and nonstereotyped manner. It follows that much of voluntary movement is mediated by the extrapyramidal motor system. It should also be noted that there is no increase in muscle tonus following a pure pyramidal lesion in the experimental animal and that spasticity is a typical feature of experimental lesions involving extrapyramidal pathways.

The admixture of pyramidal and extrapyramidal involvement is best illustrated by an upper motor neuron type of lesion, which occurs most frequently in the cerebral cortex, the medullary center, or the internal capsule. In addition to affecting neurons of the pyramidal system, such a lesion affects extrapyramidal neurons connecting the cortex with subcortical nuclei. Similarly, a lesion in the brain stem or the spinal cord is most unlikely to interrupt the pyramidal tract without simultaneous involvement of one or more extrapyramidal pathways. For example a lesion in the lateral white column of the spinal cord interrupts not only the lateral corticospinal tract but also some reticulospinal fibers and the rubrospinal tract.

After the effects of the acute lesion wear off the characteristic signs of an upper motor neuron lesion include varying degrees of voluntary paralysis, spasticity with exaggerated tendon reflexes, and the sign of Babinski. According to the concept summarized here the impairment of voluntary movement is partly pyramidal and partly extrapyramidal in origin. The pyramidal deficit is most evident in the voluntary paralysis of the muscles of the arm, in particular muscles which move the digits individually, and perhaps in voluntary paralysis of the muscles of facial expression. The sign of Babinski is also considered to be a pyramidal sign. Interruption of extrapyramidal pathways appears to be responsible for spasticity of the affected muscles and hyperactive tendon reflexes. Even though several types of neuron are involved in an upper motor neuron lesion, the term is useful and appropriate in distinguishing between the neurologic signs previously noted and those of a lower motor neuron lesion, in which there is flaccid paralysis and diminished or absent tendon reflexes.

In view of the overlapping nature of the pyramidal and extrapyramidal motor systems anatomically and functionally, several neuroscientists have strongly advocated that the terms "pyramidal" and "extrapyramidal" be discarded. However, these terms are so firmly entrenched, especially in clinical usage, that their discontinuance could only take place over many years.

SUGGESTED READING

Bertrand G: Stimulation during stereotactic operations for dyskinesias. J Neurosurg 24:419–423, 1966

Bertrand G. Blundell J, Musella R: Electrical exploration of the internal capsule and neighbouring structures during stereotaxic procedures. J Neurosurg 22:333–343, 1965

Brodal A: Some data and perspectives on the anatomy of the so-called "extrapyramidal system." Acta Neurol Scand [Suppl] 39 (4):17–38, 1963

Brooks VB, Stoney SD: Motor mechanisms: the role of the pyramidal system in motor control. Ann Rev Physiol 33:337–392, 1971

Coxe WS, Landau WM: Patterns of Marchi degeneration in the monkey pyramidal tract following small discrete cortical lesions. Neurology (Minneap) 20:89–100, 1970

Denny–Brown D: The Basal Ganglia and Their Relation to Disorders of Movement. London, Oxford University Press, 1962

Denny–Brown D: The Cerebral Control of Movement. Liverpool, Liverpool University Press, 1966

Felix D, Wiesendanger M: Pyramidal and nonpyramidal

motor cortical effects on distal forelimb muscles of monkeys. Exp Brain Res 12:81–91, 1971

Koella WP: Organizational aspects of some subcortical motor areas. Int Rev Neurobiol 4:71–116, 1962

Lassek AM: The Pyramidal Tract. Springfield, IL, Thomas, 1954

Lawrence DG, Kuypers HGJM: The functional organization of the motor system in the monkey. I. The effects of bilateral pyramidal lesions. Brain 91:1–14, 1968

Lawrence DG, Kuypers HGJM: The functional organization of the motor system in the monkey. II. The effects of lesions of the descending brain–stem pathways. Brain 91:15–36, 1968

Martin JP: The Basal Ganglia and Posture. Philadelphia, Lippincott, 1967

Walshe FMR: Critical Studies in Neurology. Edinburgh, Livingstone, 1948

Wiesendanger M: Some aspects of pyramidal tract functions in primates. In Desmedt JE (ed): New Developments in EMG and Clinical Neurophysiology, Vol 3. Basel, Karger, 1973, pp 159–174.

24

Visceral Afferents and the Autonomic Nervous System

The primary role of the afferent and efferent nerve supply of the viscera is to maintain optimal homeostasis in the internal environment (the *"milieu interieur"* of Claude Bernard). This end is attained through regulation of the organs and structures concerned with digestion, circulation, respiration, excretion, and maintenance of normal body temperature. In addition to the regulating role of the visceral reflexes, the activity of smooth muscles, glandular elements, and cardiac muscle is altered by influences from the highest levels of the brain, especially in response to emotional reactions to the external environment.

Afferent impulses of visceral origin reach the central nervous system through primary sensory neurons similar to those for general sensation. Under normal conditions these impulses elicit reflex responses in viscera and a feeling of fullness of hollow organs such as the stomach, the large intestine, and the urinary bladder. Impulses originating in the viscera also contribute to feelings of well being or malaise. In the presence of abnormal function and disease, visceral afferents transmit impulses for pain. The painful sensation is often referred to that part of the body wall which is supplied by the same spinal nerves as those supplying the affected viscus.

The motor or efferent supply of smooth muscle, cardiac muscle, and gland cells differs from that of voluntary muscles in that the connection between the central nervous system and the viscus consists of a succession of two neurons rather than a single motor neuron. The cell body of the first neuron is situated in the brain stem or the spinal cord; its axon terminates on a neuron in an autonomic ganglion, and the axon of the latter neuron ends on effector cells. The two neurons are called preganglionic and postganglionic neurons, respectively. Because of this feature of the visceral efferent system and because of its involuntary nature, Langley (1898) assigned the term "autonomic nervous system" to the visceral efferents exclusively. Although separate consideration of visceral efferents as the autonomic system continues to be the usual practice, this is to some extent unfortunate because the role of visceral reflexes tends to be obscured.

VISCERAL AFFERENTS

Olfactory cells and gustatory neurons transmitting impulses to the brain are classified as **special visceral afferents** because these are special senses eliciting visceral responses. The widely dispersed neurons conveying impulses from the viscera generally constitute the **general visceral afferents,** the main features of which are now discussed.

The cell bodies of general visceral afferent neurons are situated in the sensory ganglia of those cranial and spinal nerves that include the autonomic outflow. (The oculomotor and facial nerves are exceptions; they include autonomic neurons but no general visceral afferent neurons.) The peripheral processes of visceral afferent neurons traverse the various autonomic ganglia and plexuses without interruption to reach the viscera. These neurons are functionally of the following types: 1) physiologic afferents, and 2) afferents for pain resulting from disturbed function or disease. Physiologic afferents accompany both the sympathetic or thoracolumbar division of the autonomic system and the parasympathetic or craniosacral division, although more importantly the latter. The afferents for pain accompany the sympathetic division of the autonomic system almost exclusively.

PHYSIOLOGIC AFFERENTS

The cell bodies of visceral afferent neurons associated with the sympathetic division of the autonomic system are in the dorsal root ganglia of T1 through L2 or L3 spinal nerves. Their peripheral processes reach the sympathetic trunk by way of white communicating rami (Fig. 24–1), then traverse the cardiac, pulmonary, and splanchnic nerves arising from the sympathetic trunk for distribution to thoracic and abdominal viscera. Except for pacinian corpuscles, most of which are in mesenteries, the sensory endings consist of nonencapsulated terminal branches of the nerve fibers in the viscera. The central branches of these neurons enter the spinal cord through dorsal roots and terminate in the gray matter of segments T1 through L2 or L3. Either directly or with the intervention of intercalated neurons, impulses reach the in-

termediolateral cell column in the lateral gray horn, the source of the sympathetic outflow, for visceral reflex action.

Visceral afferents of special physiologic importance are associated with the parasympathetic division of the autonomic system. The following examples will serve to illustrate the reflex arcs of which they form the afferent limb.

Cardiovascular System

Terminal branches of sensory fibers in the aortic arch and the carotid sinus at the bifurcation of the common carotid artery serve as baroreceptors, signaling changes in arterial blood pressure. The cell bodies of neurons supplying the aortic arch are in the inferior ganglion of the vagus nerve, whereas those for the carotid sinuses are in the inferior ganglion of the glossopharyngeal nerve. The central processes terminate in the nucleus of the tractus solitarius in the medulla, from which fibers pass to groups of cells in the reticular formation referred to as cardiovascular "centers." These in turn project to the dorsal nucleus of the vagus nerve and the in-

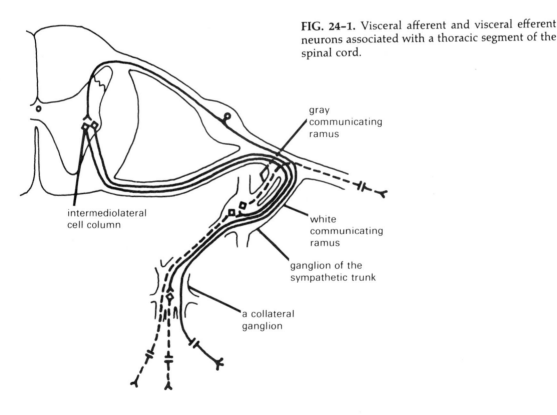

FIG. 24–1. Visceral afferent and visceral efferent neurons associated with a thoracic segment of the spinal cord.

gray communicating ramus

intermediolateral cell column

white communicating ramus

ganglion of the sympathetic trunk

a collateral ganglion

termediolateral cell column of the spinal cord. Through the reflex pathways thereby established, a rapid increase in arterial pressure causes a decrease in heart rate (vagus nerve) and vasodilation through inhibition of the vasoconstrictor action of the sympathetic outflow. A fall in arterial pressure, such as occurs following hemorrhage, initiates reflex responses which are the reverse of those caused by a rise in arterial pressure. Visceral afferents in the glossopharyngeal and vagus nerves are therefore important in the maintenance of normal arterial blood pressure.

Another reflex, the details of which are not fully understood, serves to regulate venous pressure. As originally described by Bainbridge, nerve endings in the wall of the right atrium and adjacent large veins are stimulated by a rise in venous pressure. The impulses are conducted centrally by visceral afferents in the vagus nerve. The response is cardiac acceleration, with lowering of venous pressure, by inhibition of vagal efferents and excitation of sympathetic efferents to the heart. Among other modifications of the concept of the Bainbridge reflex (or effect) that may be necessary, there is the possibility that afferent impulses initiating cardiac acceleration may originate in some part of the pulmonary vascular bed.

Respiratory System

There are respiratory "centers" in the brain stem for automatic control of respiratory movements. Two such groups of neurons are situated in the reticular formation of the medulla, an inspiratory center medially and dorsolateral to it an expiratory center. In addition a pneumotaxic center in the pontine reticular formation regulates the rhythmicity of inspiration and expiration. Inspiration is initiated by stimulation of neurons in the inspiratory center by carbon dioxide of the circulating blood, the impulses reaching lower motor neurons supplying the diaphragm and intercostal muscles by means of reticulospinal connections.

Sensory neurons in the vagus nerve constitute the afferent limb of the Hering–Breuer reflex, through which expiration is initiated. Nerve terminals in the bronchial tree, especially the smaller branches, discharge at an increasing rate as the lungs are inflated. Impulses reach the expiratory center through a relay in the nucleus of the tractus solitarius. The inspiratory phase is terminated by inhibition of neurons of the inspiratory center and neurons supplying the respiratory muscles, expiration normally being a passive (elastic) process.

Respiratory movements are also influenced by nerve impulses conducted centrally from the carotid bodies situated near the bifurcation of the common carotid arteries and from small aortic bodies adjacent to the aortic arch. Nerve terminals in these bodies function as chemoreceptors which are sensitive to a decrease in oxygen tension in the circulating blood. The resulting impulses reach the nucleus of the tractus solitarius through neurons with cell bodies in the inferior ganglia of the glossopharyngeal and vagus nerves. Further connections with respiratory centers in the brain stem bring about an increase in the rate and depth of respiratory movements. This reflex is especially important in vigorous exercise, when a person is exposed to a lowered oxygen tension such as at high altitudes, or in any circumstances that produce asphyxia.

Other Systems

Sensory fibers in the vagus nerve are distributed to the gastrointestinal tract as far as the splenic flexure at the junction of the transverse colon and the descending colon. The nerve terminals are stimulated by distention of the stomach and intestine, contraction of the smooth musculature, and irritation of the mucosa. Although motility and secretion are not dependent on the extrinsic nerves, they are modified by reflex action involving vagal afferent and efferent neurons. The distal colon, the rectum, and the urinary bladder are supplied by splanchnic branches of the second, third, and fourth sacral nerves. Reflexes involving the corresponding segments of the spinal cord and the sacral portion of the parasympathetic system function in emptying the large bowel and the urinary bladder, subject to voluntary control.

There are ascending visceral pathways distinct from the pathway for pain described in the next section. One such pathway originates in the nucleus of the tractus solitarius in the medulla, which receives general visceral afferents from the vagus nerve predominantly. A second pathway originates in the visceral afferent nucleus of the spinal cord, a poorly defined cell column in segments T1 through L2 or L3 and segments S2 through S4. The ascending fibers, supplemented by spinospinalis relays, run in the deeper part of the lateral white column. Through these pathways, impulses of visceral origin reach the reticular formation of the brain stem and the hypothalamus. Impulses also reach the ventral posterior nucleus of the thalamus and are relayed to the cerebral cortex. Through this projection, vagal afferents contribute to a feeling of fullness when the stomach is distended and a feeling of hunger when the stomach is empty. Similarly the ascending visceral pathway from the sacral region of the spinal cord provides for a feeling of fullness in the distal part of the colon and the urinary bladder.

PAIN AFFERENTS

The sensory neurons for pain of visceral origin are associated with the sympathetic division of the autonomic nervous system. The cell bodies of primary sensory neurons are therefore in the dorsal root ganglia of the thoracic and upper two or three lumbar nerves. The peripheral processes of these neurons reach the sympathetic trunk by way of white communicating rami; they run in the sympathetic trunk for variable distances and then continue to the viscera by way of the cardiac, pulmonary, and splanchnic nerves. The termination of the corresponding dorsal root fibers in the spinal gray matter is not known precisely; however, the majority probably enter the dorsolateral fasciculus along with somatic pain fibers and end in the substantia gelatinosa. Synaptic contacts are made in the substantia gelatinosa with dendrites of neurons which transmit impulses for visceral pain to the brain. The ascending pathway for visceral pain may coincide, in part, with the pathway for somatic pain, i.e., through crossed fibers in the lateral spinothalamic tract. There also appears to be crossed and uncrossed conduction by means of fibers deep in the lateral white column, these fibers probably originating in the visceral afferent nucleus. The impulses reach the thalamus through the spinal lemniscus and extralemniscal relays in the reticular formation, along with impulses for pain from somatic structures.

The sensory endings for pain are stimulated in various ways in the presence of abnormal function or disease. Most commonly the pain is caused by distention of a hollow viscus such as the intestine, which may occur when there is localized and forcible contraction of the smooth muscle of the intestine. Similarly distention of a bile duct or the ureter occurs when the lumen is obstructed by a calculus. Visceral pain also results from rapid stretching of the capsule of a solid organ, such as the liver and spleen. Peritoneal irritation contributes to the pain of inflammatory disease. In the case of anginal pain and the pain of coronary thrombosis, the effective stimulus is produced by anoxia of the affected cardiac muscle. The stimulus is probably chemical in nature, perhaps a lowering of pH because of accumulation of acid metabolites.

Referred Pain

Visceral pain has characteristics which distinguish it from pain originating in somatic structures, notably diffuse localization and radiation to somatic areas (referred pain). The zone of reference of the pain for a viscus coincides with the part of the body served by somatic sensory neurons associated with the same segments of the spinal cord as sensory neurons supplying the affected viscus. The principle of referred pain is illustrated by the following examples.

The heart is supplied with sensory fibers for pain by the middle and inferior cervical cardiac branches and the thoracic cardiac branches of the left sympathetic trunk. Central processes of the primary sensory neurons enter segments T1 through T4 or T5 of the spinal cord; pain of cardiac origin is therefore referred to the left side of the chest and the inner aspect of the left arm.

In the case of pain arising from distention of the gallbladder or bile ducts, the impulses pass centrally in the greater splanchnic nerve on the right side, entering the spinal cord through the seventh and eighth thoracic dorsal roots. The pain is referred to the upper quadrant of the abdomen and the infrascapular region on the right side. Disease of the liver or gallbladder may irritate the peritoneum covering the diaphragm. The resulting pain is often referred to the shoulder because the diaphragm is supplied with sensory fibers (as well as motor fibers) by the phrenic nerve, which originates from the third, fourth, and fifth cervical segments of the spinal cord.

Pain of gastric origin is referred to the epigastrium because the stomach is supplied with pain afferents that reach the seventh and eighth thoracic segments of the spinal cord by way of the greater splanchnic branch of the sympathetic trunk. Pain of duodenal origin, as in duodenal ulcer, is referred to the anterior abdominal wall just above the umbilicus, both this area and the duodenum being supplied by the ninth and tenth thoracic nerves. Afferent fibers from the appendix are included in the lesser splanchnic nerve and impulses enter the tenth thoracic segment of the spinal cord. The pain of appendicitis is referred initially to the region of the umbilicus, which lies in the tenth thoracic dermatome, shifting to the lower right quadrant of the abdomen if the parietal peritoneum becomes involved in the inflammatory process. Pain afferents supplying the renal pelvis and the ureter are included in the least splanchnic nerve; nerve impulses enter the first and second lumbar segments of the spinal cord, and the pain is referred to the loin and the inguinal region.

There is no entirely satisfactory explanation for the referral of pain of visceral origin. One proposal implicates a spinal reflex consisting of visceral afferent neurons, intercalated neurons in the spinal gray matter, and the intermediolateral cell column. Such a reflex could cause tonic vasoconstriction in a somatic area supplied by segments of the spinal cord receiving afferents from the affected viscus. A further assumption is required, namely, that metabolic products in the area of vasoconstriction are not carried away and that they stimulate pain receptors. According to another proposal, afferent fibers for visceral and somatic pain synapse with the same tract cells in the spinal cord, these cells being excited by subliminal somatic stimuli when receiving impulses of visceral origin.

A more plausible explanation for referred pain is based on a projection of impulses for both visceral and somatic pain from a specific segment of the spinal cord to the same group of cells in the ventral posterior nucleus of the thalamus. The topographic representation of parts of the body in the thalamus and the cerebral cortex provides a basis for recognizing the site of origin of impulses for the general senses. Localization may be in error when the impulses for pain originate in a viscus, perhaps because pain of somatic origin is a common experience compared with pain due to visceral malfunction or disease. It is of interest that John Hunter, pioneer anatomist and surgeon, called referred pain a "delusion of the mind." Even if this hypothesis proves to have substance, spinal reflexes remain the explanation for the muscle spasm seen in the rigidity of abdominal muscles when there is inflammatory disease of a viscus. The reflex arc consists of visceral afferent neurons, intercalated neurons, and motor neurons in the ventral gray horn.

VISCERAL EFFERENT OR AUTONOMIC SYSTEM

By definition "viscera" refers to the organs of the thoracic, abdominal, and pelvic cavities. The smooth muscle and secretory cells of viscera, as well as cardiac muscle, come under the dual influence of the sympathetic and parasympathetic divisions of the autonomic nervous system. They are functionally antagonistic to one another, and a delicate balance between them maintains a more or less constant level of visceral activity under conditions that usually prevail. However, autonomic innervation extends beyond the viscera of the major body cavities to include the muscles of the iris and the ciliary body in the eye, smooth muscles in the orbit, the lacrimal and salivary glands, sweat glands, arrector pili muscles, and blood vessels.

PARASYMPATHETIC DIVISION

Preganglionic parasympathetic neurons, which have long axons, are located in nuclei of the brain stem and in the sacral portion of the spinal cord. Postganglionic neurons with short axons are located in peripheral ganglia or plexuses near or within the structure being innervated. Examples of these are the ciliary, pterygopalatine, submandibular, and otic ganglia in the head, together with the diffusely arranged peripheral neurons in the heart, in the pulmonary plexus, and in the myenteric and submucosal plexuses of the gastrointestinal tract.

The role of the parasympathetic system is

to bring about changes designed to conserve and restore the energy sources of the body. The responses include a decrease in the rate and force of the heart beat, lowering of the blood pressure, and augmentation of the activity of the digestive system. Acetylcholine is the chemical mediator at the synapses between preganglionic and postganglionic neurons and also at the contacts between postganglionic terminals and effector cells. The parasympathetic system is therefore said to be "cholinergic." The system acts in localized and discrete regions rather than causing a mass reaction throughout the body. The discrete nature of the response is a result of the following factors: 1) each preganglionic neuron synapses with a limited number of postganglionic neurons, and the latter end on a limited number of effector cells; and 2) acetylcholine is rapidly inactivated by cholinesterase, hence each parasympathetic discharge is of short duration.

The preganglionic parasympathetic nuclei and the sites of the corresponding postganglionic neurons are as follows: 1) **Edinger–Westphal nucleus** of the oculomotor complex and ciliary ganglion; 2) **superior salivatory nucleus** of the facial nerve and submandibular ganglion; 3) **lacrimal nucleus** of the facial nerve and pterygopalatine ganglion; 4) **inferior salivatory nucleus** of the glossopharyngeal nerve and otic ganglion; 5) **dorsal nucleus** of the vagus nerve and cardiac ganglia, ganglia in the pulmonary plexus, cells in the myenteric and submucosal plexuses of the gastrointestinal tract, and postganglionic neurons at other sites; and 6) **sacral parasympathetic nucleus** and postganglionic neurons in and near the pelvic viscera.

SYMPATHETIC DIVISION

The sympathetic outflow originates in the **intermediolateral cell column** of all thoracic spinal segments and the upper two or three lumbar segments. The axons of preganglionic neurons reach the sympathetic trunk by way of the corresponding ventral roots and white communicating rami (Fig. 24–1). With respect to the sympathetic supply of structures in the head and thorax, the preganglionic fibers terminate in ganglia of the sympathetic trunk. For smooth muscles and glands in the head, the synapses between pre- and postganglionic neurons are mainly in the superior

cervical ganglion of the sympathetic trunk. In the case of thoracic viscera, the synapses are in the three cervical sympathetic ganglia (superior, middle, and inferior) and the upper five ganglia of the thoracic portion of the sympathetic trunk.

Preganglionic fibers for abdominal and pelvic viscera proceed without interruption through the sympathetic trunk and its splanchnic branches. The fibers terminate on postganglionic neurons located in plexuses surrounding the main branches of the abdominal aorta, notably the celiac plexus and the superior and inferior mesenteric plexuses. The sympathetic supply to the adrenal medulla is exceptional. The secretory cells of the medulla, like postganglionic sympathetic neurons, are derived from the neural crest of the embryo. The adrenal medulla is consequently supplied directly by preganglionic sympathetic neurons.

For the body wall and the limbs, preganglionic fibers terminate in all ganglia of the sympathetic trunk, from which postganglionic fibers are distributed by way of gray communicating rami and spinal nerves to blood vessels, arrector pili muscles, and sweat glands.

The sympathetic system stimulates activities that are accompanied by an expenditure of energy stores. These include acceleration of the heart rate and increase in force of the heart beat, rise of arterial pressure, elevation of the blood sugar level, and direction of blood flow to skeletal muscles at the expense of visceral and cutaneous circulation. Sympathetic responses are most dramatically expressed during stress and emergency situations. However, the "flight or fight" responses to strong sympathetic stimulation are only extreme examples of processes that are going on all the time. One can lead a normal existence in a sheltered environment in the absence of sympathetic function, but reactions to stress are lacking. The neurotransmitter substance between pre- and postganglionic neurons is acetylcholine, as in the parasympathetic system. However, in the case of the sympathetic system, norepinephrine (noradrenalin) is the transmitter substance between postganglionic terminals and effector cells. The sympathetic system is therefore said to be "noradrenergic." The sympathetic supply to sweat glands is cholinergic, constituting an exception to the general rule. Cutaneous areas lack parasympathetic fibers; this may be related to the fact that sudomotor fibers are anatomically sympathetic but functionally parasympathetic.

Strong sympathetic stimulation produces diffuse effects because of the following factors, which are the converse of those present in the parasympathetic system. 1) Each sympathetic preganglionic neuron synapses with as many as 30 or more postganglionic neurons, and each of the latter ends on numerous effector cells. Hence, there is much divergence of stimuli. 2) Norepinephrine liberated at postganglionic terminals, and epinephrine (adrenalin) and norepinephrine secreted by the adrenal medulla on sympathetic stimulation, are deactivated slowly. As expressed by Cannon, "the sympathetics are like the loud and soft pedals, modulating all the tones together, while the parasympathetics are like the separate keys."

EXAMPLES OF AUTONOMIC INNERVATION

The autonomic innervation of certain structures may now be summarized (Figs. 21-2 and 21-3). Descriptive details are omitted; autonomic nuclei within the central nervous system have been referred to in earlier chapters, and detailed accounts of peripheral portions of the autonomic system are included in textbooks of gross anatomy.

SMOOTH MUSCLES OF THE EYE AND THE ORBITAL CAVITY

Parasympathetic

Preganglionic fibers from the Edinger–Westphal nucleus traverse the oculomotor nerve to the orbit, where they terminate in the ciliary ganglion. Postganglionic fibers are distributed to the sphincter pupillae and ciliary muscles of the eye through the short ciliary nerves. *Function:* pupillary constriction; increase in refractive power of the lens.

Sympathetic

Preganglionic neurons are located in the upper two thoracic spinal segments, from where axons travel to the superior cervical ganglion of the sympathetic trunk. Postganglionic fibers reach the orbit through plexuses surrounding the internal carotid and ophthalmic arteries, traverse the ciliary ganglion, and continue to the dilator pupillae muscle through the long ciliary nerves. Other sympathetic fibers supply the smooth muscle component (tarsal muscle) of the levator palpe-

brae superioris muscle and Müller's orbital muscle (the latter being rudimentary in man). *Function:* pupillary dilation; retraction of the upper eyelid; exophthalmos (insignificant in man).

GLANDS IN THE HEAD

Parasympathetic

SUBMANDIBULAR AND SUBLINGUAL SALIVARY GLANDS. The preganglionic neurons make up the superior salivatory nucleus, which is represented by an ill-defined cluster of cells in the pontine tegmentum medial to the motor nucleus of the facial nerve. Fibers from the superior salivatory nucleus end in the submandibular ganglion, which they reach by traversing the sensory root of the facial nerve (nervus intermedius), the facial nerve and its chorda tympani branch, and finally the lingual branch of the mandibular nerve. Short postganglionic fibers then proceed to the submandibular and sublingual glands. *Function:* stimulation of salivary secretion and vasodilation.

LACRIMAL GLAND AND MUCOSAL GLANDS OF THE NOSE AND PALATE. The preganglionic neurons constitute the lacrimal nucleus, which is situated near the superior salivatory nucleus. Fibers from the lacrimal nucleus reach the pterygopalatine ganglion by traversing the sensory root of the facial nerve, the facial nerve, and its greater petrosal branch. Postganglionic fibers proceed to the lacrimal gland either through the zygomatic branch of the maxillary nerve or through direct lacrimal rami from the pterygopalatine ganglion. Other postganglionic fibers are distributed to mucosal glands in the nose and on the palate through the nasopalatine and palatine branches of the maxillary nerve. *Function:* stimulation of secretion and vasodilation.

PAROTID GLAND. The inferior salivatory nucleus, which is situated just caudal to its superior counterpart, contains the cell bodies of preganglionic neurons. The axons leave the brain stem in the glossopharyngeal nerve, then traverse its tympanic branch and the tympanic plexus in the wall of the middle ear, from which they constitute the lesser petrosal nerve and terminate in the otic ganglion. Postganglionic fibers reach the parotid gland by way of the auriculotemporal branch of the mandibular nerve. *Function:* stimulation of salivary secretion and vasodilation.

Sympathetic

The preganglionic neurons for the glands in the head are situated in the upper two thoracic segments of the spinal cord, and their axons terminate in the superior cervical ganglion. Postganglionic fibers are distributed to the glands

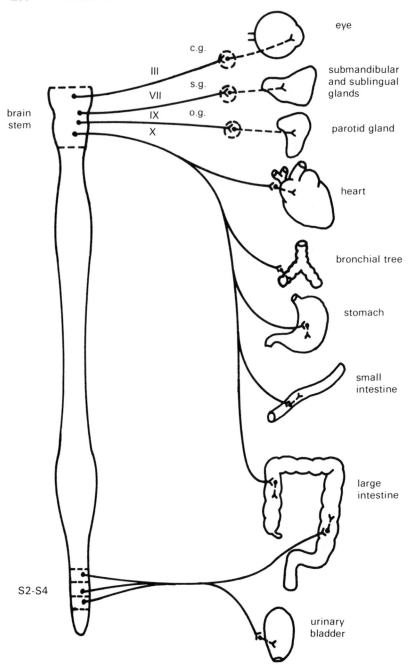

FIG. 24-2. The parasympathetic (craniosacral) division of the autonomic nervous system. **c.g.,** ciliary ganglion; **s.g.,** submandibular ganglion; **o.g.,** otic ganglion.

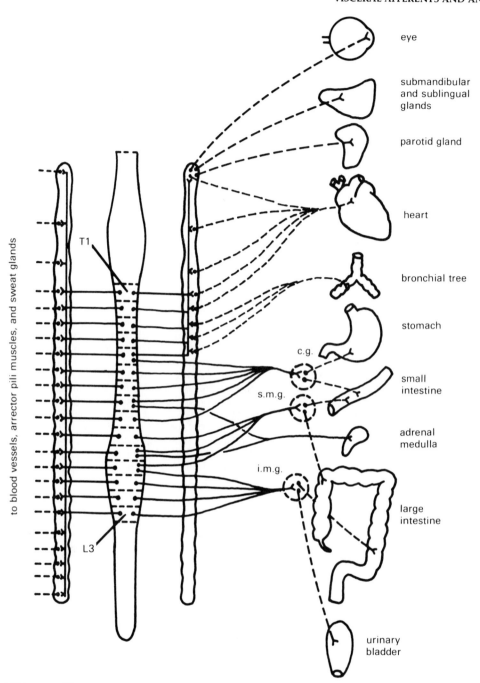

FIG. 24-3. The sympathetic (thoracolumbar) division of the autonomic nervous system. **c.g.,** celiac ganglion; **s.m.g.,** superior mesenteric ganglion; **i.m.g.,** inferior mesenteric ganglion.

through the nerve plexuses surrounding the internal and external carotid arteries. *Function:* vasoconstriction, which decreases secretion.

HEART

Parasympathetic

Preganglionic fibers from the dorsal nucleus of the vagus nerve enter the cardiac branches of the vagus, synapsing with postganglionic neurons in the cardiac plexuses and in scattered cell clusters in the walls of the atria of the heart. Postganglionic fibers supply the sinoatrial and atrioventricular nodes, muscle fibers of the atria and the ventricles, and the coronary arteries. *Function:* cardiac inhibition, *i.e.,* reduction of the rate and force of the heart beat; vasoconstriction.

Sympathetic

Preganglionic fibers originate in the upper five or six thoracic spinal segments; they terminate in the corresponding ganglia of the sympathetic trunk and in the three cervical ganglia. Postganglionic fibers reach the heart by way of the superior, middle, and inferior cardiac branches of the cervical portion of the sympathetic trunk, and through varying numbers of thoracic cardiac nerves. The fibers terminate in the sinoatrial and atrioventricular nodes, on cardiac muscle fibers, and in coronary vessels. *Function:* cardiac acceleration and vasodilation.

LUNGS

Parasympathetic

Preganglionic fibers from the dorsal nucleus of the vagus nerve reach the pulmonary plexus through pulmonary branches of the nerve and end in tracheal and bronchial ganglia embedded in the plexus. Postganglionic fibers supply the smooth muscle and mucosal glands of the trachea and the bronchial tree and also the blood vessels of the lung. *Function:* bronchoconstriction and stimulation of secretion.

Sympathetic

Preganglionic fibers from spinal segments T3 through T5 synapse with neurons in the inferior cervical ganglion of the sympathetic trunk and the upper four or five thoracic ganglia. Postganglionic fibers traverse pulmonary branches of the sympathetic trunk and the pulmonary plexus to supply the smooth muscle and glands of the trachea and the bronchial tree, together with blood vessels. *Function:* bronchodilation and inhibition of secretion. (Although autonomic fibers have been shown to supply pulmonary and bronchial blood vessels, the functional significance of this innervation is debated.)

STOMACH AND INTESTINE

Parasympathetic

Vagal preganglionic fibers traverse the esophageal plexus and enter the abdomen in the anterior and posterior vagal trunks. The fibers achieve a wide distribution to abdominal viscera, including the stomach and the intestine as far as the splenic flexure of the colon. Those fibers supplying the gastrointestinal tract terminate on postganglionic neurons in the myenteric (Auerbach's) and submucosal (Meissner's) plexuses. The short postganglionic fibers end on smooth muscle and gland cells. *Function:* increase in peristaltic rate and tonus of smooth muscle; relaxation of sphincters; stimulation of secretion.

Sympathetic

Preganglionic fibers from spinal segments T5 through T12 traverse the sympathetic trunk and its greater and lesser splanchnic branches, terminating on postganglionic neurons in the celiac and superior mesenteric ganglia. Axons of these neurons are distributed to the stomach with the celiac artery, and to the intestine as far as the splenic flexure with the superior mesenteric artery. Blood vessels for the stomach and intestine are also supplied with sympathetic fibers. *Function:* inhibition of peristalsis and contraction of sphincters; inhibition of secretion; vasoconstriction.

DESCENDING COLON AND PELVIC VISCERA

Parasympathetic

Preganglionic fibers originate in the parasympathetic nucleus in the ventral gray horn of spinal segments S2 through S4. The fibers traverse the pelvic splanchnic branches (nervi erigentes) of the corresponding spinal nerves and terminate on postganglionic neurons in and near the organs innervated. These visceral structures include the descending colon, sigmoid colon, rectum, urinary bladder, prostate, seminal vesicles, testes, uterus and tubes, ovaries, erectile tissue, and blood vessels supplying pelvic organs. *Function:* contraction of the smooth muscle of the lower bowel and the detrusor muscle of the bladder; stimulation of glands; vasodilation; erection.

Sympathetic

Preganglionic fibers originate in spinal segments T12 through L2 or L3, traverse the lumbar splanchnic branches of the sympathetic trunk, and synapse with postganglionic neurons in the inferior mesenteric ganglion. From the latter site, fibers are distributed to the pelvic organs already noted. *Function:* inhibition of peristalsis in the lower bowel; contraction of muscles in the trigone of the bladder; ejaculation of semen; vasoconstriction.

KIDNEY

Nerve fibers assumed to be efferent have been described ending in relation to the renal tubules and the renal glomeruli. However, true secretory fibers appear to be of little importance because the denervated kidney can carry on approximately normal function.

The activity of the renal tubules is influenced by vasomotor fibers. The vasodilator supply is parasympathetic and consists of preganglionic vagal fibers and postganglionic neurons in the renal plexus surrounding the renal artery and the renal vein. The vasoconstrictor sympathetic supply consists of preganglionic fibers from spinal cord segments T11 through L1 and postganglionic fibers traversing the renal plexus from the celiac ganglion.

ADRENAL GLAND

The adrenal medulla is supplied directly by preganglionic sympathetic neurons, since postganglionic sympathetic neurons as well as parasympathetic innervation are lacking. The fibers come from spinal cord segments T8 through T11 and reach the gland by way of the lesser splanchnic branch of the sympathetic trunk. The absence of postganglionic sympathetic neurons stems from the fact that the secretory cells of the adrenal medulla arise from neural crest cells and are comparable in their origin to postganglionic neurons. The transmitter substance between the nerve terminals and the secretory cells is acetylcholine, as at synapses between pre- and postganglionic neurons. Sympathetic stimulation increases the output of epinephrine and norepinephrine.

Convincing evidence of innervation of secretory cells of the adrenal cortex is lacking. However, the blood vessels of both parts of the gland are supplied by postganglionic sympathetic fibers. The preganglionic neurons correspond to those ending on parenchymatous cells of the medulla. The postganglionic neurons are mainly in the aorticorenal plexus, which is an extension of the celiac plexus.

PERIPHERAL BLOOD VESSELS

Preganglionic neurons for blood vessels in the body wall and the limbs are located throughout the intermediolateral cell column; their axons reach the sympathetic trunk through the ventral roots and white communicating rami from T1 through L2 or L3 segments. Many of the fibers run rostrally and caudally, so that preganglionic fibers terminate in all ganglia of the sympathetic trunk. Postganglionic fibers enter all spinal nerves through the gray communicating rami and are distributed to blood vessels of the skin and deep structures, especially the muscles. Although blood vessels supplying some visceral structures (*e.g.,* salivary glands, heart, and kidney) receive parasympathetic as well as sympathetic efferents, peripheral blood vessels have only a sympathetic innervation. Sympathetic stimulation causes vasoconstriction in the skin and vasodilation in skeletal muscle.

BLOOD VESSELS OF THE HEAD

In addition to having a sympathetic innervation for vasoconstriction, a parasympathetic supply which is vasodilator in function has been demonstrated for arteries supplying some structures in the head. The preganglionic sympathetic fibers are from T1 and T2 spinal segments, and most of them synapse with postganglionic neurons in the superior cervical ganglion. Fibers from this ganglion are distributed along the various branches of the internal and external carotid arteries. In addition, postganglionic fibers from the inferior cervical ganglion accompany the vertebral and basilar arteries and their branches. With respect to cerebral arteries, sympathetic fibers supplying the branches on the surface of the brain and arterioles in the pia mater are more numerous than fibers supplying blood vessels in the brain substance.

Most of the preganglionic parasympathetic fibers are included in the facial nerve; those supplying the arterial branches to the lacrimal, submandibular, and sublingual glands have already been noted. Other preganglionic fibers in the facial nerve enter the greater petrosal nerve and join the internal carotid plexus in the region of the middle cranial fossa. Postganglionic neurons are in small clusters of cells in the periarterial plexuses of cerebral arteries. Parasympathetic vasodilator fibers to the parotid gland are included in the glossopharyngeal nerve and accompany the secretomotor fibers.

ARRECTOR PILI MUSCLES AND SWEAT GLANDS

The sympathetic supply of the smooth muscles attached to hair follicles and of the sweat glands corresponds to that of cutaneous blood vessels. The postganglionic terminals in sweat glands are cholinergic; they are therefore parasympathetic with respect to the chemical transmitter, although sympathetic anatomically.

CENTRAL CONTROL OF THE AUTONOMIC SYSTEM

The cells of origin of the autonomic outflow come under the influence of various levels of the nervous system. The main controlling and integrating center is the hypothalamus, but visceral afferent nuclei and visceral "centers" in the reticular formation of the brain stem are also very important. Impulses from the brain stem reach the intermediolateral cell column of the spinal cord and the sacral parasympathetic nucleus by way of reticulospinal connections (descending autonomic fibers).

Of visceral afferent neurons, those in the vagus nerve are among the more important; impulses thus conveyed centrally are relayed to autonomic preganglionic neurons through the nucleus of the tractus solitarius and the reticular formation. The special visceral sense of taste has similar connections. Fibers from the olfactory and limbic systems reach brain stem nuclei of autonomic significance through the olfactotegmental component of the medial forebrain bundle. These systems also project to the brain stem through a complex pathway which includes the habenular nucleus, midbrain nuclei, and the dorsal longitudinal fasciculus. Through the foregoing connections and through projections of the olfactory and limbic systems to the hypothalamus, visceral functions are influenced by the sense of smell (a special visceral sense) and by the emotions. Visceral centers in the reticular formation of the brain stem include those influencing the cardiovascular system through connections with the dorsal nucleus of the vagus nerve and the intermediolateral cell column of the spinal cord.

Impulses from the hypothalamus reach autonomic efferent neurons through the dorsal longitudinal fasciculus and the mammillotegmental tract, with relays in the reticular formation. The hypothalamic control of the endocrine system, however, is based primarily on mechanisms which do not involve the autonomic outflow. Hormones released into the blood stream in the neurohypophysis are produced in the hypothalamus and reach the neurohypophysis by axoplasmic flow in fibers of the hypothalamohypophysial tract. The hypothalamus controls hormone production in the adenohypophysis by means of releasing factors, which reach the adenohypophysis through the pituitary portal system of blood vessels.

The neurons in the hypothalamus receive nerve impulses from several sources. These include visceral afferent impulses, both general and for taste, by way of ascending fibers in the brain stem, and impulses from the olfactory cortex and the limbic system through the medial forebrain bundle. Other important afferents to the hypothalamus come from the medial and anterior thalamic nuclei, the amygdala, and the hippocampus; these parts of the brain are of special significance with respect to the emotions. Corticohypothalamic fibers, most of them originating in the orbital cortex of the frontal lobe, bring the hypothalamus under the influence of the neocortex. Hypothalamic neurons are also sensitive to slight changes in the temperature, the osmolarity, and the level of various chemical substances (including hormones) in the circulating blood. By the various means outlined previously, the autonomic system comes under a wide range of influences, extending from primitive visceral afferents to psychic processes at the cortical level.

SUGGESTED READING

Appenzeller O: The Autonomic Nervous System: An Introduction to Basic and Clinical Concepts. New York, American Elsevier, 1970

Cannon WB, Rosenbleuth A: Autonomic Neuro-effector Systems. New York, Macmillan, 1937

Crosby EC, Humphrey T, Lauer EW: Correlative Anatomy of the Nervous System. New York, Macmillan, 1962

Kuntz A: The Autonomic Nervous System, 4th ed. Philadelphia, Lea & Febiger, 1953

Mitchell GAG: Anatomy of the Autonomic Nervous System. Edinburgh, Livingstone, 1953

Pick J: The Autonomic Nervous System: Morphological, Comparative, Clinical and Surgical Aspects. Philadelphia, Lippincott, 1970

Romanes GJ (ed): Cunningham's Textbook of Anatomy, 10th ed. London, Oxford University Press, 1964

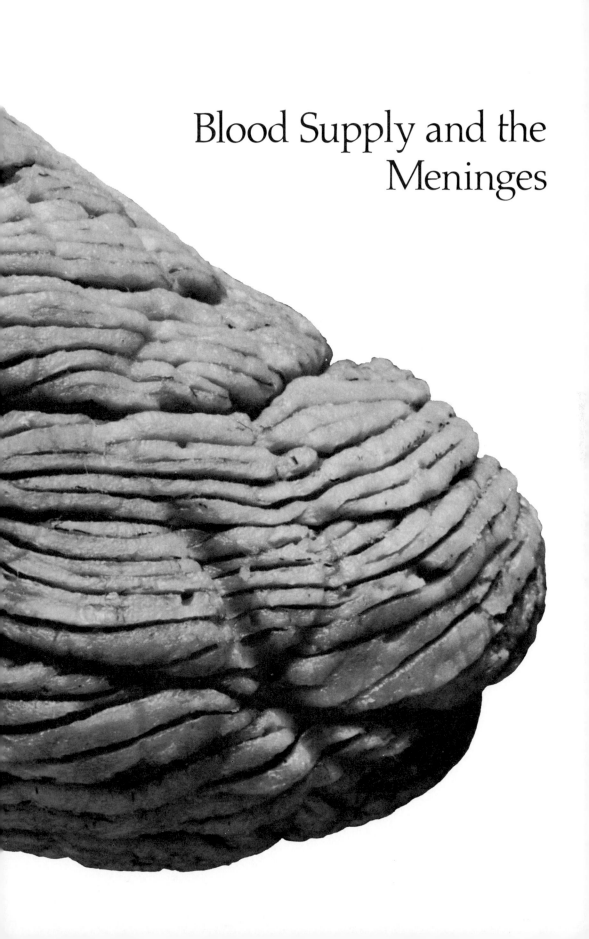

Blood Supply and the Meninges

25

Blood Supply of the Central Nervous System

Lesions of vascular origin are responsible for more neurologic disorders than any other category of disease process. Arterial occlusion by a thrombus, which is usually followed by infarction of a portion of the region supplied by the affected artery, is the most common type of cerebral vascular accident. This type of arterial occlusion occurs most frequently in persons past middle life because the thrombus usually develops at the site of atheromatous changes in the intima. An embolus originating at some other site in the vascular system is another cause of cerebral arterial occlusion. In addition to intracranial occlusions, impairment of the cerebral circulation is often the result of stenosis of a carotid or vertebral artery extracranially.

The slender, thin-walled arteries which penetrate the ventral surface of the brain to supply the internal capsule and adjacent gray masses are especially prone to rupture. Hypertension and degenerative changes in these arteries are important factors leading to cerebral hemorrhage. Aneurysms usually occur at the site of branching of one of the larger arteries at the base of the brain. An aneurysm may leak or rupture, in which case the bleeding is typically into the subarachnoid space; however, the hemorrhage may be intracerebral.

There are anastomotic channels between branches of the major arteries on the surface of the brain. There are also communications at the arteriolar level, and the capillary bed is continuous throughout the brain. These anastomoses, however, are usually inadequate to sustain the circulation in the region supplied normally by a major artery. The size of an infarction depends on the caliber of the occluded artery, existing anastomoses,

and the time elapsing before complete occlusion.

Because of the practical importance of cerebral vascular disease and because the neurologic signs depend on the site of the lesion, an understanding of the distribution of the arteries supplying the brain is essential.

The blood supply of the central nervous system has a special interest because of the metabolic demands of nervous tissue. The brain depends on aerobic metabolism of glucose and is one of the most metabolically active organs of the body. Although composing only 2% of the body weight, the brain receives approximately 17% of the cardiac output and consumes about 20% of the oxygen utilized by the entire body. Unconsciousness follows cessation of cerebral circulation in about 10 sec.

ARTERIAL SUPPLY OF THE BRAIN

The brain is supplied by the paired internal carotid and vertebral arteries through an extensive system of branches.

INTERNAL CAROTID SYSTEM

The **internal carotid artery,** a terminal branch of the common carotid artery, traverses the carotid canal in the base of the skull and enters the middle cranial fossa beside the dorsum sellae of the sphenoid bone. Beyond this point the artery undergoes the following sequence of bends which constitute the "carotid siphon" in a cerebral angiogram. The internal carotid artery first runs forward in the cavernous venous sinus, then turns upward on the medial side of the anterior clinoid process. At this point the artery enters the subarachnoid space by piercing the dura mater and the arachnoid, courses backward below the optic nerve, and finally turns upward immediately lateral to the optic chiasma. This brings the artery under the anterior perforated substance, where it divides into the middle and anterior cerebral arteries (Fig. 25–1).

Collateral Branches

The following branches arise from the internal carotid artery before its terminal bifurcation.

HYPOPHYSIAL ARTERIES. These arteries originate from the cavernous and postclinoid portions of the internal carotid artery. In addition to supplying the infundibular process of the neurohypophysis, hypophysial arteries enter the median eminence of the hypothalamus. The latter blood vessels break up into capillary loops, into which hypothalamic releasing factors gain access, and the capillary loops drain through small veins into the sinusoids of the adenohypophysis. This constitutes the important pituitary portal system through which the hypothalamus influences the output of pituitary hormones.

OPHTHALMIC ARTERY. This branch comes off immediately after the internal carotid artery enters the subarachnoid space. The ophthalmic artery passes forward into the orbit, supplying the eye and other orbital contents, the frontal area of the scalp, the frontal and ethmoid paranasal sinuses, and parts of the nose.

POSTERIOR COMMUNICATING ARTERY. This slender artery arises from the internal carotid artery close to its terminal bifurcation. The posterior communicating artery runs backward to join the proximal part of the posterior cerebral artery, thereby forming part of the arterial circle (circle of Willis).

ANTERIOR CHOROIDAL ARTERY. This branch comes off the distal part of the internal carotid artery or the beginning of the middle cerebral artery and has a wider distribution than its name suggests. The artery passes back along the optic tract and the choroid fissure at the medial edge of the temporal lobe. In addition to supplying the choroid plexus in the inferior horn of the lateral ventricle, the anterior choroidal artery gives off branches to the optic tract, uncus, amygdala, hippocampus, globus pallidus, lateral geniculate nucleus, and ventral part of the internal capsule. The further distribution of this artery varies considerably, but additional branches have been traced into the subthalamus, the ventral portion of the thalamus, and the rostral part of the midbrain (including the red nucleus). The anterior choroidal artery is said to be prone to thrombosis because of its small caliber and rather long subarachnoid course. The globus pallidus and the hippocampus, both of which are supplied in part by the anterior choroidal artery, are considered to be favored sites of neuronal degeneration as a result of circulatory deficiency.

Middle Cerebral Artery

Of the terminal branches of the internal carotid artery, the middle cerebral artery is the larger and the more direct continuation of the parent vessel (Fig. 25–1). This artery runs deep in the lateral fissure between the frontal and temporal lobes. **Frontal, parietal,** and **temporal branches** emerge from the lateral fissure and ramify over the lateral surface of the cerebral hemisphere (Fig. 25–2).

The area of distribution of the middle cerebral artery includes the sensorimotor strip surrounding the central sulcus, except for the dorsal part of the strip for the lower limb. Occlusion of the artery therefore results in contralateral paralysis most noticeable in the lower part of the face and the arm, together with general sensory deficits of the cortical type. The auditory cortex is included in the area of distribution; however, a unilateral lesion causes little impairment of hearing because of the bilateral cortical projection from the organ of Corti. Occlusion of a branch of the middle cerebral artery in the dominant hemisphere is the principal cause of aphasia (Chapter 15). The cortical areas concerned are the sensory language area in the temporal and parietal lobes, especially Wernicke's area in the temporal lobe, and Broca's area in the inferior frontal gyrus (Fig. 25–2).

Anterior Cerebral Artery

The smaller terminal branch of the internal carotid artery is the anterior cerebral artery,

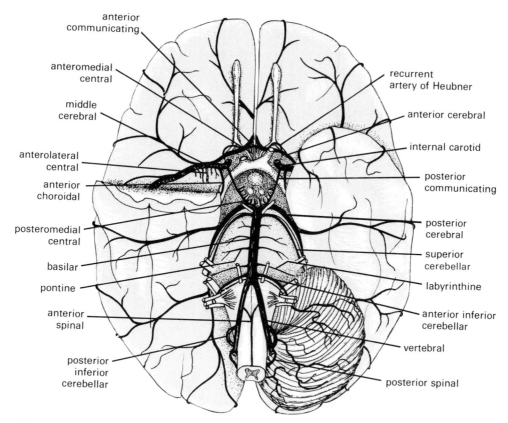

anterior
communicating

anteromedial
central

middle
cerebral

anterolateral
central

anterior
choroidal

posteromedial
central

basilar

pontine

anterior
spinal

posterior
inferior
cerebellar

recurrent
artery of Heubner

anterior cerebral

internal carotid

posterior
communicating

posterior
cerebral

superior
cerebellar

labyrinthine

anterior inferior
cerebellar

vertebral

posterior spinal

FIG. 25-1. The blood supply of the brain as seen on the ventral surface.

FIG. 25-2. Distribution of the middle cerebral artery on the lateral surface of the cerebral hemisphere.

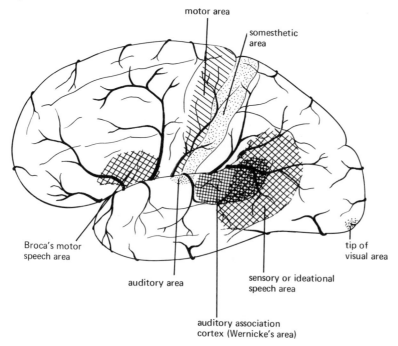

motor area

somesthetic
area

Broca's motor
speech area

tip of
visual area

auditory area

sensory or ideational
speech area

auditory association
cortex (Wernicke's area)

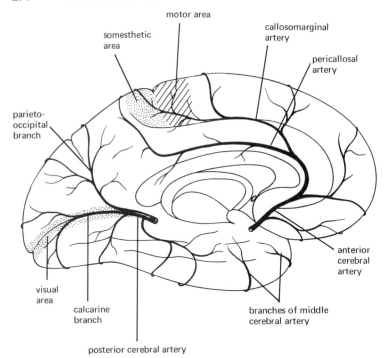

FIG. 25–3. Distribution of the anterior and posterior cerebral arteries on the medial surface of the cerebral hemisphere.

which is first directed medially above the optic nerve (Fig. 25-1). The two anterior cerebral arteries almost meet at the midline where they are joined together by the **anterior communicating artery.** The anterior cerebral artery then ascends in the longitudinal fissure and bends backward around the genu of the corpus callosum (Fig. 25-3). Branches given off just distal to the anterior communicating artery supply the medial portion of the orbital surface of the frontal lobe, including the olfactory bulb and the olfactory tract.

The artery continues along the upper surface of the corpus callosum as the **pericallosal artery,** and a large branch, the **callosomarginal artery,** follows the cingulate sulcus. The anterior cerebral artery supplies the medial portions of the frontal and parietal lobes and the corpus callosum. In addition, branches extend over the dorsomedial border of the hemisphere and supply a strip on the lateral surface (Fig. 25-2). The dorsal part of the sensorimotor strip is included in the area of distribution; occlusion of the anterior cerebral artery therefore causes paralysis and sensory deficits in the contralateral leg.

A special branch of the anterior cerebral artery is given off just proximal to the anterior communicating artery. This is the **recurrent artery of Heubner,** which penetrates the anterior perforated substance to supply the ventral part of the head of the caudate nucleus, the adjacent portion of the putamen, and the anterior limb and genu of the internal capsule. The recurrent artery of Heubner is sometimes called the **medial striate artery** because of its contribution to the blood supply of the corpus striatum.

VERTEBRAL SYSTEM

The **vertebral artery,** a branch of the subclavian artery, ascends in the foramina of the transverse processes of the upper six cervical vertebrae. On reaching the base of the skull, the artery winds around the lateral mass of the atlas, pierces the posterior atlantooccipital membrane, and enters the subarachnoid space at the level of the foramen magnum by piercing the dura mater and the arachnoid. The vertebral artery runs forward with a medial inclination beneath the medulla, joining its fellow of the opposite side at the caudal border of the pons to form the **basilar artery.** The latter artery runs forward in the midline of the pons and divides into the **posterior cerebral arteries** (Fig. 25-1).

Branches of the Vertebral Artery

SPINAL ARTERIES. The upper portion of the cervical cord receives blood through spinal branches of the vertebral arteries. A single **anterior spinal artery** is formed by a contribution from each vertebral artery. A **posterior spinal artery** arises on each side as a branch of either the vertebral or the posterior inferior cerebellar artery (Fig. 25–1). The anterior and posterior spinal arteries continue throughout the length of the spinal cord. However, except for their proximal portions, the blood comes from reinforcements by the anterior and posterior radicular arteries, as described later.

POSTERIOR INFERIOR CEREBELLAR ARTERY. This artery, the largest branch of the vertebral artery, pursues an irregular course between the medulla and the cerebellum. Branches are distributed to the posterior part of the cerebellar hemisphere, the inferior vermis, the central nuclei of the cerebellum, and the choroid plexus of the fourth ventricle. There are also medullary branches to the dorsolateral region of the medulla. Occlusion of the posterior inferior cerebellar artery therefore results in the lateral medullary or Wallenberg's syndrome (see Chapter 7). In addition to branches from the posterior inferior cerebellar artery, fine branches arising directly from the vertebral artery supply the medulla.

Branches of the Basilar Artery

The basilar artery gives off the following branches before dividing into the posterior cerebral arteries at the rostral border of the pons.

ANTERIOR INFERIOR CEREBELLAR ARTERY. Arising from the caudal end of the basilar artery, the anterior inferior cerebellar artery supplies the cortex of the inferior surface of the cerebellum anteriorly and the underlying white matter; it assists in the supply of the central cerebellar nuclei. In addition slender twigs from the artery penetrate the upper medulla and lower pons.

LABYRINTHINE ARTERY. This artery, a branch of either the basilar artery or the anterior inferior cerebellar artery, traverses the internal acoustic meatus and ramifies throughout the membranous labyrinth of the internal ear.

Although of rare occurrence, occlusion of the labyrinthine artery results in the expected deafness in the corresponding ear and signs of vestibular dysfunction.

PONTINE ARTERIES. These are slender branches arising from the basilar artery along its length. They penetrate the pons and ramify in both the ventral portion of the pons and the pontine tegmentum.

SUPERIOR CEREBELLAR ARTERY. This branch arises close to the terminal bifurcation of the basilar artery, ramifies over the dorsal surface of the cerebellum, and supplies the cortex, medullary center, and central nuclei. Branches from the proximal part of the superior cerebellar artery are distributed to the pons, the superior cerebellar peduncle, and the inferior colliculus of the midbrain.

Posterior Cerebral Artery

Each posterior cerebral artery curves around the midbrain and reaches the medial surface of the cerebral hemisphere beneath the splenium of the corpus callosum (Fig. 25–3). The artery gives off **temporal branches,** which ramify over the inferior surface of the temporal lobe, and **calcarine** and **parietooccipital branches,** which run along the corresponding sulci. All these arteries send branches around the border of the cerebral hemisphere to supply a peripheral strip on the lateral surface (Fig. 25–2). The calcarine branch is of special significance because it supplies the visual area of cortex, and occlusion causes blindness in the contralateral field of vision. Central or macular vision is usually spared, perhaps because the large portion of the visual area at the occipital pole for macular vision is partially sustained by collateral circulation from the middle cerebral artery. However, the possibility exists that "macular sparing" is an artifact of testing due to the person being tested shifting his fixation point slightly during examination of the visual field.

The **posterior choroidal artery** comes off the posterior cerebral artery in the region of the splenium and runs forward in the transverse fissure beneath the corpus callosum. The posterior choroidal artery supplies the choroid plexus of the central part of the lateral ventricle, the choroid plexus of the third ventricle, the posterior part of the thalamus, the fornix, and the tectum of the midbrain.

CORTICAL BRANCHES OF THE CEREBRAL ARTERIES

Anastomoses between branches of the anterior, middle, and posterior cerebral arteries are concealed in the sulci. The caliber of an anastomotic vessel may be sufficient to sustain a portion of the territory of another artery if the latter is occluded. The cerebral arteries are also interconnected through an arteriolar network in the pia mater. Short cortical branches from the pial plexus supply the rich capillary network of the cortex, whereas longer branches of arteries in the subarachnoid space penetrate into the white matter and form a more open capillary network.

Sympathetic fibers from cervical ganglia of the sympathetic trunk form perivascular plexuses around the internal carotid and vertebral arteries. Some fibers can be followed to the finer ramifications of the blood vessels. Parasympathetic fibers, most of them coming from the facial nerve, have also been described in the perivascular plexuses. The functional significance of the autonomic supply of cerebral vessels is still obscure. The cerebral circulation changes according to fluctuations in local requirements; this is probably a response to alterations in carbon dioxide and hydrogen ion concentrations. Circulatory changes of autonomic origin are probably superimposed on those caused by local chemical factors. More recent studies using histochemical stains for nerve fibers have shown that more fibers are associated with blood vessels of various calibers than could be identified with the silver and methylene blue techniques used previously. The influence of autonomic innervation on cerebral blood flow seems, therefore, to be of physiologic and clinical significance.

ARTERIAL CIRCLE (CIRCLE OF WILLIS)

The major arteries supplying the cerebrum are joined to one another at the base of the brain in the form of an arterial circle or the circle of Willis (Fig. 25-1). Starting from the midline in front, the circle consists of the anterior communicating, anterior cerebral, internal carotid (a short segment), posterior communicating, and posterior cerebral arteries; then it continues to the starting point in reverse order. There is normally little exchange of blood between the main arteries through the slender anterior and posterior communicating arteries. However, the arterial circle provides alternative routes when one of the major arteries leading into it is occluded. These anastomoses are frequently inadequate, especially in elderly persons, in whom the communicating arteries may be narrowed because of vascular disease.

There are frequent variants of the conventional configuration of the arterial circle. The posterior cerebral artery is a branch of the internal carotid artery embryologically. In the course of development the posterior cerebral artery becomes a terminal branch of the basilar artery, the vestige of the embryologic condition being seen in the posterior communicating artery. The embryologic condition persists in about a third of all individuals, in whom one of the posterior cerebral arteries is a major branch of the internal carotid artery. The embryologic type of connection of the posterior cerebral artery occurs bilaterally very rarely. One of the anterior cerebral arteries may be unusually small in the first part of its course, in which case the anterior communicating artery has a larger than usual caliber.

CENTRAL BRANCHES

Numerous central branches arise from arteries in the region of the arterial circle (Fig. 25-1). These slender, thin-walled blood vessels, also known as ganglionic or nuclear arteries, supply portions of the corpus striatum, internal capsule, diencephalon, and midbrain. There are four groups of central branches in the region of the arterial circle. (The recurrent artery of Heubner is similar to the central arteries with respect to its distribution, as are the anterior and posterior choroidal arteries with respect to portions of their distribution.)

Anteromedial Group

These central branches arise from the anterior cerebral arteries and the anterior communicating artery. They penetrate the medial part of the anterior perforated substance and are distributed mainly to the preoptic and suprachiasmatic regions of the hypothalamus.

Anterolateral Group

This group of central arteries consists mainly of branches of the middle cerebral artery. They enter the anterior perforated substance and are also called **striate arteries** (or lateral striate arteries) because they supply a major portion of the corpus striatum. The region of distribution of the anterolateral central arteries includes the head of the caudate nucleus, putamen, lateral part of the globus pallidus, much of the internal capsule (anterior limb, genu, and dorsal portion of the posterior limb), external capsule, and claustrum. Several of these arteries also send twigs into the lateral area of the hypothalamus.

Posteromedial Group

The posteromedial central arteries are branches of the posterior cerebral and posterior communicating arteries. After penetrating the posterior perforated substance between the cerebral peduncles, they are distributed to the anterior and medial portions of the thalamus, the subthalamus, the middle and posterior regions of the hypothalamus, and the medial parts of the cerebral peduncles of the midbrain.

Posterolateral Group

These central arteries come off the posterior cerebral artery as it curves around the midbrain. They are distributed to the posterior portion of the thalamus (including the medial and lateral geniculate bodies), the tectum of the midbrain, and the lateral part of the cerebral peduncle.

Distribution of Central Arteries

The following summary identifies the blood supply of structures situated within the region of the brain that is nourished by the central arteries.

Head of caudate nucleus and putamen (striatum): anterolateral central arteries; recurrent artery of Heubner

Globus pallidus (pallidum): anterolateral central arteries; anterior choroidal artery

Thalamus: posteromedial and posterolateral central arteries; anterior and posterior choroidal arteries

Subthalamus: posteromedial central arteries; anterior choroidal artery

Hypothalamus: anteromedial, posteromedial, and anterolateral central arteries

Pineal gland: posterolateral central arteries

Internal capsule: anterolateral and posterolateral central arteries; anterior choroidal artery; recurrent artery of Heubner

Amygdala, uncus, and hippocampal formation: anterior choroidal artery; temporal branches of posterior cerebral artery

External capsule and claustrum: anterolateral central arteries

Tectum of midbrain: posterolateral central arteries; posterior choroidal artery; superior cerebellar artery

Cerebral peduncle: posteromedial and posterolateral central arteries; anterior choroidal artery

VENOUS DRAINAGE OF THE BRAIN

The capillary bed of the brain stem and the cerebellum is drained by unnamed veins which empty into dural venous sinuses situated adjacent to the posterior cranial fossa. The cerebrum has an external and an internal venous system. The external cerebral veins lie in the subarachnoid space on all surfaces of the hemispheres, whereas the central core of the cerebrum is drained by internal cerebral veins situated beneath the corpus callosum in the transverse fissure. Both sets of cerebral veins empty into dural venous sinuses, which are identified in the following chapter.

EXTERNAL CEREBRAL VEINS

The **superior cerebral veins,** 8–12 in number, course upward over the lateral surface of the hemisphere. On nearing the midline, they pierce the arachnoid, run between the arachnoid and the dura mater for 1–2 cm, and empty into the superior sagittal sinus or into venous lacunae adjacent to the sinus. Trauma to the head may tear a superior cerebral vein as it lies between the arachnoid and the dura mater, resulting in a subdural hemorrhage.

The **superficial middle cerebral vein** runs downward and forward along the lateral fissure and empties into the cavernous sinus. However, anastomotic channels allow for drainage in other directions. These are the superior anastomotic vein (of Trolard), which opens into the superior sagittal sinus, and the inferior anastomotic vein (of Labbé), which opens into the transverse sinus.

The **deep middle cerebral vein** runs downward and forward in the depths of the lateral fissure to the ventral surface of the brain; the **anterior cerebral vein** corresponds with the anterior cerebral artery. These veins unite in the region of the anterior perforated substance to form the **basal vein** (of Rosenthal), which runs backward at the base of the brain, curves around the midbrain, and empties into the great cerebral vein (see Internal Cerebral Veins). The basal vein receives tributaries from the optic tract, hypothalamus, temporal lobe, and midbrain.

In addition to the named veins just noted, there are numerous small veins which drain limited areas. These have no consistent pattern and empty into adjacent dural sinuses.

INTERNAL CEREBRAL VEINS

The internal venous system forms in the floor of each lateral ventricle and continues through the transverse cerebral fissure beneath the corpus callosum (Fig. 25–4). The **vena terminalis** or **thalamostriate vein** begins in the region of the amygdaloid nucleus in the temporal lobe and follows the curve of the tail of the caudate nucleus on its medial side. The vena terminalis receives tributaries from the corpus striatum, internal capsule, thalamus, fornix, and septum pellucidum. The **choroidal vein,** which is rather tortuous, runs along the choroid plexus of the lateral ventricle. In addition to draining the plexus, the choroidal vein receives tributaries from the hippocampus, fornix, and corpus callosum. The vena terminalis and the choroidal vein unite immediately behind the interventricular foramen to form the **internal cerebral vein.** The paired internal cerebral veins run posteriorly in the transverse fissure, uniting beneath the splenium of the corpus callosum to form the **great cerebral vein** (of Galen). The latter vein, which is about 2 cm in length, receives the basal veins and tributaries from the cerebellum. The great cerebral vein empties into the straight

sinus, situated in the midline of the tentorium cerebelli.

BLOOD SUPPLY OF THE SPINAL CORD

SPINAL ARTERIES

Three arterial channels, the **anterior spinal artery** and the paired **posterior spinal arteries,** run longitudinally throughout the length of the spinal cord. The anterior spinal artery originates in a Y-shaped configuration from the vertebral arteries, as already described, and runs caudally along the ventral median fissure. Each posterior spinal artery is a branch of either the vertebral artery or the posterior inferior cerebellar artery and consists of plexiform channels along the line of attachment of the dorsal roots of the spinal nerves.

The blood received by the spinal arteries from the vertebral arteries is sufficient for only the upper cervical segments of the spinal cord. The arteries are therefore reinforced at intervals in the following manner. The vertebral artery in the cervical region, the posterior intercostal branches of the thoracic aorta, and the lumbar branches of the abdominal aorta give off segmental **spinal arteries,** which enter the vertebral canal through the intervertebral foramina. In addition to supplying the vertebrae, these segmental spinal arteries give rise to **anterior** and **posterior radicular arteries,** which run along the ventral and dorsal roots of the spinal nerves. Most of the radicular arteries are of small caliber, sufficient only to supply the nerve roots and contribute to a vascular plexus in the pia mater covering the spinal cord. A variable number of anterior radicular arteries, approximately 12 including both sides, join the anterior spinal artery. Similarly a variable number of posterior radicular arteries, approximately 14 including both sides, join the plexiform channels composing the posterior spinal arteries. These radicular arteries are of substantial size and are situated mainly in the lower cervical, lower thoracic, and upper lumbar regions; the largest, an anterior radicular artery known as the spinal artery of Adamkiewicz, is usually in the upper lumbar region. The spinal cord is vulnerable to circulatory impairment if the important contribution by a radicular artery is compromised by injury or the placing of a

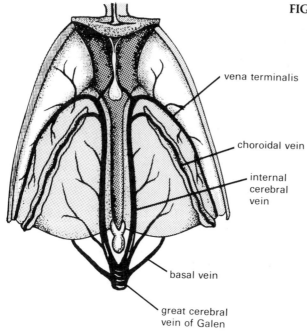

FIG. 25-4. The internal cerebral system of veins.

vena terminalis

choroidal vein

internal
cerebral
vein

basal vein

great cerebral
vein of Galen

ligature. The upper thoracic and upper lumbar regions of the spinal cord are considered to be especially vulnerable to degenerative changes caused by a deficiency in blood supply.

Sulcal branches arise in succession from the anterior spinal artery and enter the right and left sides of the spinal cord alternately from the ventral median fissure. The sulcal arteries are least frequent in the thoracic part of the spinal cord. The anterior spinal artery supplies the ventral gray horns, part of the dorsal gray horns, and the ventral and lateral white columns, including the lateral corticospinal tracts. Penetrating branches from the posterior spinal arteries supply the remainder of the dorsal gray horns and the dorsal columns of white matter. A fine plexus (the vasocorona) derived from the spinal arteries is present in the pia mater on the lateral and ventral surfaces of the cord. Penetrating branches from the vasocorona supply a narrow zone of white matter beneath the pia mater.

SPINAL VEINS

Although the pattern of spinal veins is irregular, there are essentially six of them. **Anterior spinal veins** run along the midline and each ventrolateral sulcus; **posterior spinal veins** are situated in the midline and along the dorsolateral sulci. The spinal veins are drained at intervals by up to 12 **anterior radicular veins** and a similar number of **posterior radicular veins.** The radicular veins empty into an epidural venous plexus, which in turn drains into an external vertebral plexus through channels in the intervertebral foramina. Blood from the external vertebral plexus empties into the vertebral, intercostal, and lumbar veins.

THE BLOOD-BRAIN BARRIER

Certain substances fail to pass from capillary blood into the central nervous system, although the same substances gain access to nonnervous tissues. They include dye substances used in animal experimentation and, more importantly, some agents that would otherwise be of therapeutic value. The lumen of a capillary and the parenchyma of the brain and spinal cord are separated by endothelium, a basement membrane in which pericytes are embedded, and perivascular foot plates of astrocytic processes. Much research has been directed toward the identification of the blood–brain barrier in an

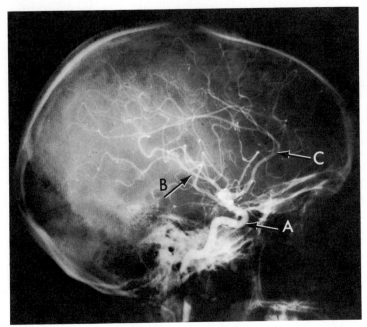

FIG. 25-5. Carotid angiogram, lateral view. **A.** carotid siphon; **B.** branches of the middle cerebral artery; **C.** anterior cerebral artery. (Courtesy of Dr. J. M. Allcock)

FIG. 25-6. Carotid angiogram, anteroposterior view. **A.** carotid siphon; **B.** branches of the middle cerebral artery; **C.** anterior cerebral artery. (Courtesy of Dr. J. M. Allcock)

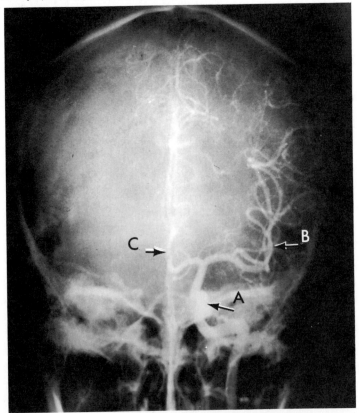

anatomic or physical sense. The best evidence points to the tight junctions between endothelial cells and special properties of the internal plasma membrane of these cells. In a few small regions, *e.g.,* the area postrema in the medulla, the classical blood–brain barrier is lacking.

CEREBRAL ANGIOGRAPHY

In 1927 de Egas Moniz introduced the technique of cerebral angiography, which developed into a valuable diagnostic aid in the hands of neuroradiologists. Briefly stated the method consists of injecting a radiopaque solution into the artery, followed by serial x-ray photography at approximately 1-sec intervals. The roentgenograms show the contrast medium in progressive stages of its passage through the arterial tree and the venous return. Injection into the common carotid artery or the internal carotid artery shows the distribution of the middle and anterior cerebral arteries (Figs. 25–5 and 25–6). Similarly injection of the vertebral artery permits visualization of the vertebral, basilar, and posterior cerebral arteries, together with their larger branches. The cerebral veins are seen in later roentgenograms of a series.

The technique of cerebral angiography is especially useful in identifying vascular malformations and aneurysms. The method often provides valuable information concerning occlusive vascular disease and space-occupying lesions.

SUGGESTED READING

Aird RB: Barriers in the brain. Sc Am 194/2:101–106, 1956

Bull JWD: Use and limitations of angiography in the diagnosis of vascular lesions of the brain. Neurology (Minneap) 11[2]:80–85, 1961

Carpenter MB: Human Neuroanatomy, 7th ed. Baltimore, Williams & Wilkins, 1976

Gillilan LA: The arterial blood supply of the human spinal cord. J Comp Neurol 110:75–103, 1958

Harper AM, Deshmukh VD, Rowan JO, Jennett WB: The influence of sympathetic nervous activity on cerebral blood flow. Arch Neurol 27:1–6, 1972

Long DM: Capillary ultrastructure and the blood-brain barrier in human malignant brain tumors. J Neurosurg 32:127–144, 1970

Nelson E, Rennels M: Innervation of cranial arteries. Brain 93:475–490, 1970

Pappas GD: Some morphological considerations of the blood-brain barrier. J Neurol Sci 10:241–246, 1970

Shaw Dunn J, Wyburn GM: The anatomy of the blood brain barrier: a review. Scottish Med J 17:21–36, 1972

Stephens RB, Stilwell DL: Arteries and Veins of the Human Brain. Springfield, IL, Thomas, 1969

Taveras JM: Angiographic observation in occlusive cerebrovascular disease. Neurology (Minneap) 11[2]:86–90, 1961

26

Meninges and Cerebrospinal Fluid

The consistency of the brain is soft and gelatinous, although the spinal cord is slightly firmer. The meninges provide protection for the central nervous system in addition to the protection provided by the skull and the vertebral column and its ligaments. They consist of the thick dura mater externally, the delicate arachnoid lining the dura, and the thin pia mater adhering to the brain and spinal cord. The latter two layers, which may be combined under the heading of the pia-arachnoid, bound the subarachnoid space filled with cerebrospinal fluid. The main support and protection provided by the meninges come from the dura mater and the cushion of cerebrospinal fluid in the subarachnoid space.

DURA MATER AND ASSOCIATED STRUCTURES

The internal surfaces of the bones enclosing the cranial cavity are clothed by periosteum, such as covers bones elsewhere. This periosteum is continuous with the periosteum on the external surface of the cranium at the margins of the foramen magnum and smaller foramina for nerves and blood vessels. The cranial dura mater is attached intimately to the periosteum, which is sometimes referred to incorrectly as the external layer of the dura mater.

PERIOSTEUM AND MENINGEAL BLOOD VESSELS

The periosteum consists of collagenous connective tissue and contains arteries, somewhat inappropriately called meningeal ar-

teries, which mainly supply the underlying bone. Of these the largest is the **middle meningeal artery,** a branch of the maxillary artery entering the cranial cavity through the foramen spinosum in the floor of the middle cranial fossa. The artery divides into anterior and posterior branches soon after entering the middle cranial fossa; these branches ramify over the lateral surface of the cranium, producing grooves on the underlying bones. A fracture in the temporal region of the skull may tear a branch of the middle meningeal artery. The extravasated blood accumulates between the bone and the periosteum, forming an epidural hematoma. As in the case of any space-occupying lesion in the nonexpansile cranial cavity, intracranial pressure rises and surgical intervention is usually necessary. Less extensive areas are supplied by several small arteries. These include meningeal branches of the ophthalmic artery, branches of the occipital artery traversing the jugular foramen and the hypoglossal canal, and small twigs arising from the vertebral artery at the foramen magnum.

The meningeal arteries are accompanied by **meningeal veins,** which are also subject to tearing in fractures of the skull. The largest meningeal veins accompany the middle meningeal artery, leave the cranial cavity through the foramen spinosum or the foramen ovale, and drain into the pterygoid venous plexus.

DURA MATER

The dura mater or pachymeninx (thick membrane) is a dense, firm layer consisting of collagenous connective tissue. The **spinal dura mater** takes the form of a tube, pierced by the roots of spinal nerves, extending from the foramen magnum to the second segment of the sacrum. The spinal dura mater is separated from the wall of the spinal canal by an epidural space containing adipose tissue and a venous plexus. The **cranial dura mater** is firmly attached to the periosteum, as previously described, from which it receives small blood vessels. The smooth inner surface of the dura mater consists of simple squamous epithelium, and a thin film of fluid occupies the potential subdural space between the dura and the arachnoid. The cranial dura mater has several features of importance, notably the dural reflections and the dural venous sinuses.

DURAL REFLECTIONS

The dura mater is reflected along certain lines to form the dural reflections or dural septa. The intervals between the periosteum and the dura along the lines of attachment of the septa accommodate dural venous sinuses (Fig. 26–1). The largest septa, the falx cerebri and the tentorium cerebelli, form incomplete partitions dividing the cranial cavity into three compartments (Fig. 26–2).

The **falx cerebri,** so named because of its

FIG. 26–1. Coronal section at the vertex of the skull, including the superior sagittal sinus and the attachment of the falx cerebri.

sickle shape, is a vertical partition in the longitudinal fissure between the cerebral hemispheres. This dural reflection is attached to the crista galli of the ethmoid bone in front, to the midline of the vault as far back as the internal occipital protuberance, and to the tentorium cerebelli. The free edge is close to the splenium of the corpus callosum, but some distance from the corpus callosum further forward. The anterior portion of the falx cerebri is often fenestrated.

The **tentorium cerebelli** intervenes between the occipital lobes of the cerebral hemispheres and the cerebellum. The attachment of the falx cerebri along the midline draws the tentorium upward, giving it a shallow tentlike configuration. The peripheral border of the tentorium is attached to the upper edges of the petrous portion of the temporal bones and to the margins of the sulci on the occipital bone for the transverse sinuses. The free border bounds the **incisura of the tentorium** (tentorial notch); the incisura is completed by the sphenoid bone and accommodates the midbrain.

The narrow interval between the midbrain and the boundary of the tentorial incisura is the only communication between the subtentorial and supratentorial regions of the subarachnoid space. The cerebrospinal fluid produced in the ventricles enters the subarachnoid space of the posterior cranial fossa, then moves slowly upward around the

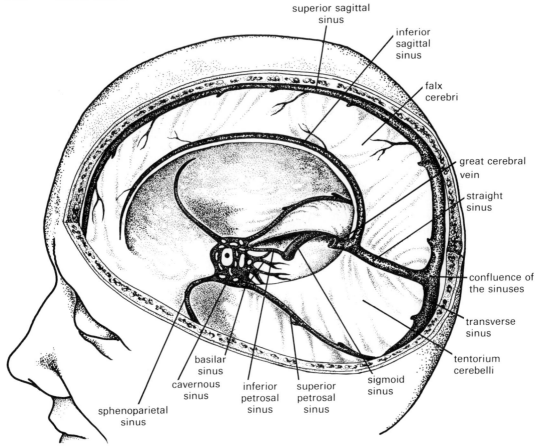

FIG. 26-2. Dural reflections and dural venous sinuses.

midbrain to be absorbed into venous blood along the attached border of the falx cerebri. Obstruction of the subarachnoid space around the midbrain results in dilation of the ventricles and the subarachnoid space in the posterior cranial fossa (communicating hydrocephalus). Also of clinical interest, an expanding lesion in a cerebral hemisphere may cause the medial part of the temporal lobe to herniate into the incisura of the tentorium. The midbrain is displaced toward the opposite side, and the pressure of the firm edge of the tentorium on the basis pedunculi may result in the unusual finding of voluntary motor paresis on the same side of the body as the cerebral lesion.

The **falx cerebelli** is a small dural fold in the posterior cranial fossa, extending vertically for a short distance between the cerebellar hemispheres. The **diaphragma sellae**

roofs over the pituitary fossa or sella turcica of the sphenoid bone and has an opening for passage of the infundibular stem of the neurohypophysis.

NERVE SUPPLY OF THE DURA MATER

The cranial dura mater has a plentiful supply of sensory nerve fibers, mainly from the trigeminal nerve. The fibers terminate as nonencapsulated endings, for the most part, and are of significance in certain types of headache.

The dura lining the anterior cranial fossa is supplied by ethmoid branches of the ophthalmic nerve. The mandibular nerve supplies a large area through the nervus spinosum, which enters the middle cranial fossa with the middle meningeal artery and ramifies with the arterial branches. A meningeal branch comes off the maxillary nerve while it is still in the cranial cavity and joins the fibers of the nervus spinosum which accompany the anterior branch of the middle meningeal artery. The tentorium cerebelli and the dura mater lining the vault above it are supplied by several large branches coming off the first part of the ophthalmic nerve. These nerves run backward in the tentorium, spreading out over the vault and in the falx cerebri. The dura lining the floor of the posterior cranial fossa is supplied by the vagus nerve and upper cervical nerves. The meningeal branch of the vagus nerve arises from the superior ganglion at the level of the jugular foramen, through which it enters the posterior fossa. Sensory twigs from the first three cervical spinal nerves enter the posterior fossa through the hypoglossal canal. (The first cervical nerve lacks a sensory component in about half of individuals.) Recurrent branches of all spinal nerves enter the vertebral canal through the intervertebral foramina and give off meningeal branches to the spinal dura mater.

DURAL VENOUS SINUSES

The veins draining the brain empty into the venous sinuses of the dura mater, from which blood flows into the internal jugular veins. The walls of the sinuses consist of dura mater and periosteum, lined by endothelium. The location of most of the dural venous sinuses is shown in Figure 26–2.

The **superior sagittal sinus** lies along the attached border of the falx cerebri. It begins in front of the crista galli of the ethmoid bone, where there may be a narrow communication with nasal veins. Venous lacunae lie alongside the superior sagittal sinus and open into it. The superior cerebral veins drain into the sinus or into the lacunae. The superior sagittal sinus is usually continuous with the right transverse sinus.

The **inferior sagittal sinus** is smaller than the one just described; it runs along the free border of the falx cerebri and receives veins from the medial aspects of the cerebral hemispheres. The inferior sagittal sinus opens into the **straight sinus,** which lies in the attachment of the falx cerebri to the tentorium cerebelli. The straight sinus receives the great cerebral vein; it therefore drains the system of internal cerebral veins and the territories of the cerebral hemispheres drained by the basal vein, formed by the union of the deep

middle cerebral and anterior cerebral veins. The straight sinus is usually continuous with the left transverse sinus. Venous channels connect the transverse sinuses at the internal occipital protuberance; the configuration of sinuses in this location is called the **confluence of the sinuses** (torcular Herophili).

Each **transverse sinus** lies in a groove on the occipital bone along the attached margin of the tentorium cerebelli. On reaching the petrous portion of the temporal bone, the transverse sinus continues as the **sigmoid sinus;** the latter follows a curved course in the posterior fossa on the mastoid portion of the petrous bone and becomes continuous with the internal jugular vein at the jugular foramen.

The **cavernous sinuses** are situated one on each side of the body of the sphenoid bone; each sinus receives the ophthalmic vein and the superficial middle cerebral vein. Venous channels in the anterior and posterior margins of the diaphragma sellae connect the cavernous sinuses; these channels and the cavernous sinuses constitute the **circular sinus.** The cavernous sinus drains into the transverse sinus through the **superior petrosal sinus,** running along the attachment of the tentorium cerebelli to the petrous portion of the temporal bone. The **inferior petrosal sinus** lies in the groove between the petrous portion of the temporal bone and the basilar portion of the occipital bone, providing a communication between the cavernous sinus and the internal jugular vein. Small venous channels posterior to the circular sinus constitute the **basilar sinus,** which is connected with the cavernous and inferior petrosal sinuses. Finally the **sphenoparietal sinus** is a small venous channel under the lesser wing of the sphenoid bone draining into the cavernous sinus, and the small **occipital sinus** in the falx cerebelli drains into the confluence of the sinuses. The sinuses at the base of the cranium receive veins from adjacent parts of the brain.

Emissary veins connect dural venous sinuses with veins outside the cranial cavity. Blood may flow in either direction, depending on venous pressure relationships. The parietal and mastoid emissary veins are the largest of these connecting channels. The parietal emissary vein traverses the parietal foramen, joining the superior sagittal sinus with tributaries of the occipital veins. The mastoid emissary vein traverses the mastoid foramen and joins the sigmoid sinus with the occipital and posterior auricular veins.

PIA-ARACHNOID

The **pia mater** and the **arachnoid** develop initially as a single layer from the mesodermal tissue surrounding the embryonic brain and spinal cord. Fluid-filled spaces appear within the layer; these become the subarachnoid space, and the origin of the membranes from a single layer is reflected in the numerous trabeculae passing between them. Histologically the pia and the arachnoid consist of collagenous fibers and some elastic fibers. Both surfaces of the arachnoid and the external surface of the pia mater are covered by simple squamous epithelium. The trabeculae crossing the subarachnoid space consist of delicate strands of connective tissue with squamous epithelial cells on their surfaces. The pia mater and the arachnoid together constitute the leptomeninges (slender membranes).

The avascular arachnoid is separated from the dura mater by a film of fluid in the potential subdural space. The pia mater, which contains a network of fine blood vessels, adheres to the surface of the brain and spinal cord, following all their contours. The connective tissue fibers of the spinal pia mater tend to run in a longitudinal direction. This is accentuated along the ventromedian line of the spinal cord, where a thickened strand of fibers superficial to the anterior spinal artery is known as the **linea splendens.** The **denticulate ligament,** described in Chapter 5, is derived from the pia mater.

The larger arteries and veins entering and leaving the substance of the brain are surrounded by a sleeve of pia mater. There are thus formed **perivascular spaces** (Virchow-Robin spaces), continuous with the subarachnoid space and extending in increasingly attenuated form as far as arterioles and venules in the brain.

SUBARACHNOID CISTERNS

The width of the subarachnoid space varies because the arachnoid rests on the dura

mater, whereas the pia mater adheres to the irregular contours of the brain. The space is narrow over the summits of gyri, wider in the regions of major sulci, and wider yet at the base of the brain and in the lumbosacral region of the spinal canal. Regions of the subarachnoid space containing more substantial amounts of cerebrospinal fluid are called **subarachnoid cisterns** (Fig. 26–3).

The **cerebellomedullary cistern** (cisterna magna) occupies the interval between the cerebellum and the medulla and receives cerebrospinal fluid through the median aperture of the fourth ventricle. The basal cisterns beneath the brain stem and the diencephalon include the **pontine** and **interpeduncular cisterns** and the **cistern of the optic chiasma.** The last-named cistern is continuous with the **cistern of the lamina terminalis,** which in turn continues into the **cistern of the corpus callosum** above this commissure. The subarachnoid space dorsal to the midbrain is called the **superior cistern** or, alternatively, the **cistern of the great cerebral vein.** This cistern and the subarachnoid space on the sides of the midbrain constitute the **cisterna ambiens.** The **cistern of the lateral fissure** corresponds with that fissure. The **lumbar cistern** of the spinal subarachnoid space is especially large, extending from the second lumbar vertebra to the second segment of the sacrum. It contains the cauda equina, formed by lumbosacral spinal nerve roots.

The meningeal layers and the subarachnoid space extend around cranial nerves and spinal nerve roots for a short distance, approximately to the level of sensory ganglia when these are present. For example, an extension of the subarachnoid space, enclosed by dura mater, around the proximal part of the trigeminal ganglion in the middle cranial fossa at the tip of the petrous portion of the temporal bone constitutes the trigeminal cave (Meckel's cave). The most important meningeal extension clinically surrounds the optic nerve to its attachment to the eyeball. The central artery and the central vein of the retina run within the anterior part of the optic nerve and cross the extension of the subarachnoid space to join the ophthalmic artery and the ophthalmic vein. An increase of cerebrospinal fluid pressure slows the return of venous blood, causing edema of the retina. This is most apparent on ophthalmoscopic examination as swelling of the optic

cistern of the
corpus callosum

interventricular foramen

third ventricle

cerebral
aqueduct

superior
cistern

cistern
of the
lamina
terminalis

cistern of
the optic
chiasma

(a)

(b)

fourth
ventricle

interpeduncular cistern

pontine cistern

median aperture of the
fourth ventricle

cerebellomedullary
cistern

FIG. 26–3. Subarachnoid cisterns. **(a)** cerebrospinal fluid entering the third ventricle from the right lateral ventricle though an interventricular foramen; **(b)** cerebrospinal fluid entering the cerebellomedullary cistern from the fourth ventricle through the median aperture.

papilla or disk (papilledema). Inspection of the ocular fundi is an important part of the neurologic examination.

CEREBROSPINAL FLUID

The cerebrospinal fluid is produced mainly by the choroid plexuses of the lateral, third, and fourth ventricles, those in the lateral ventricles being the largest and most important.

The **choroid plexus** of each lateral ventricle is formed by an invagination of vascular pia mater (the tela choroidea) on the medial surface of the cerebral hemisphere. The vascular connective tissue picks up a covering layer of epithelium from the ependymal lining of the ventricle. The choroid plexuses of the third and fourth ventricles are similarly formed by invaginations of the tela choroidea attached to the roofs of these ventricles. The choroid plexuses, which have a minutely folded surface, therefore consist of a core of connective tissue containing many wide capillaries and a surface layer of simple cuboidal or low columnar epithelium (the choroid epithelium) (Fig. 26–4). The surface area of the choroid plexuses of the two lateral ventricles combined is about 40 sq cm.

Several features of the choroid epithelium as seen in electron micrographs are of functional interest (Fig. 26–5). The large spherical nucleus, abundant cytoplasm, and numerous mitochondria indicate that the production of cerebrospinal fluid is at least partly an active process requiring expenditure of energy on the part of these cells. The plasma membrane at the free surface is greatly increased in area by irregular microvilli. The membranes of

FIG. 26–4. A fragment of choroid plexus showing the large capillaries and the choroid epithelium (Hematoxylin and eosin stain, × 400)

adjoining cells are thrown into complicated folds at the base of the cells. The choroid epithelial cells bear motile cilia in the embryo, and patches of ciliated epithelium persist for varying periods postnatally. A basement membrane separates the epithelium from the subjacent stroma with its rich vascular network. The capillaries are unlike those supplying nervous tissue generally in that the junctions between endothelial cells are more permeable and the cells have fenestrations or pores closed by thin diaphragms.

Production of cerebrospinal fluid is a complex process, the details of which are still being studied. Some components of the blood plasma negotiate the capillary wall and the choroid epithelium with difficulty, others enter the cerebrospinal fluid readily by diffusion, and still others reach the fluid with the assistance of metabolic activity on the part of choroid epithelial cells. An important factor appears to be active transport of certain ions (notably sodium ions) through the epithelial cells, followed by passive movement of water to maintain the osmotic equilibrium between cerebrospinal fluid and blood plasma.

The flow of cerebrospinal fluid is from the lateral ventricles into the third ventricle through the interventricular foramina, and then into the fourth ventricle by way of the cerebral aqueduct. Cerebrospinal fluid leaves the ventricular system through the median and lateral apertures of the fourth ventricle, the former opening into the cerebellomedullary cistern and the latter into the pontine cistern. From these sites there is a sluggish movement of fluid through the spinal subarachnoid space, determined in part by movements of the vertebral column. More importantly the cerebrospinal fluid flows slowly forward through the basal cisterns and then upward over the medial and lateral surfaces of the cerebral hemispheres. Movement of cerebrospinal fluid is assisted by the pulsation of arteries in the subarachnoid space, especially in the subarachnoid space around the spinal cord.

The main site of absorption of the cerebrospinal fluid into venous blood is through the **arachnoid villi** projecting into dural venous sinuses, especially the superior sagittal sinus and adjacent venous lacunae (Fig. 26–1). The arachnoid villi consist of a thin cellular layer, derived from the epithelium of the arachnoid and the endothelium of the sinus, which encloses an extension of the subarachnoid space containing trabeculae. The absorptive mechanism depends on the higher hydrostatic pressure of the cerebrospinal fluid compared with venous blood in the dural sinuses, the difference of colloidal osmotic pressure between the virtually protein-free cerebrospinal fluid and the blood, and active transport by cells forming the walls of the arachnoid villi. The arachnoid villi become hypertrophied with age, when they are called **arachnoid granulations** or **pacchionian bodies;** these may be sufficiently large to produce erosion or pitting of the cranial bones.

Although the choroid plexuses are the main source of cerebrospinal fluid and the arachnoid villi of its absorption, there are exchanges between blood plasma and cerebrospinal fluid elsewhere. Studies using radioactive isotopes in experimental animals show that the chemical composition of cerebrospinal fluid is determined in part by passive, two-way transfer of solutes across the ependymal lining of the ventricles and the walls of small blood vessels in the pia mater. Some cerebrospinal fluid is probably ab-

FIG. 26–5. Electron micrograph of a choroid epithelial cell. **ER,** endoplasmic reticulum; **M,** mitochondria; **MV,** microvilli; **N,** nucleus; **PM,** folds of plasma membrane. (× 8,800) (Courtesy of Dr. D. H. Dickson)

sorbed into lymphatic vessels adjacent to the extensions of the subarachnoid space around cerebrospinal nerves.

The volume of the cerebrospinal fluid varies from 80–200 ml, with an average of about 130 ml; these figures include the fluid in both the ventricles and the subarachnoid space. The ventricular system alone contains from 15–40 ml fluid. The rate of production of fluid is thought to be sufficient to effect a total replacement in 24 hours. The pressure of cerebrospinal fluid is from 80–180 ml water when a person is recumbent; the pressure in the lumbar cistern is approximately twice these values when measured in a sitting position. Venous congestion in the closed space of the cranial cavity and the spinal canal, as produced by straining or coughing, is reflected in a prompt rise of cerebrospinal fluid pressure.

Cerebrospinal fluid is clear and colorless,

with a specific gravity of 1.003–1.008. The few cells present are mainly lymphocytes. These vary in number from one to eight in each cubic millimeter; a count of over ten cells is indicative of disease. The glucose level is about half that of blood, and the protein content is very low (15–45 mg/100 ml).

When there is an excess of cerebrospinal fluid, the condition is known as **hydrocephalus,** of which there are several types. **External hydrocephalus,** in which the excess fluid is mainly in the subarachnoid space, is found in senile atrophy of the brain. **Internal hydrocephalus** refers to dilation of the ventricles. All the ventricles are enlarged if the apertures of the fourth ventricle are occluded, the third and lateral ventricles if the obstruction is in the cerebral aqueduct, and one lateral ventricle only in the rare occurrence of occlusion of an interventricular foramen. The term **communicating hydrocephalus** refers to a combination of internal hydrocephalus and subtentorial external hydrocephalus. In this instance, the flow of cerebrospinal fluid through the incisura of the tentorium around the midbrain is obstructed.

SUGGESTED READING

Alksne, JF, Lovings ET: Functional ultrastructure of the arachnoid villus. Arch Neurol 27:371–377, 1972

Bowsher D: Cerebrospinal Fluid Dynamics in Health and Disease. Springfield, IL, Thomas, 1960

Bull JWD: The volume of the cerebral ventricles. Neurology (Minneap) 11:1–9, 1961

Crosby EC, Humphrey T, Lauer EN: Correlative Anatomy of the Nervous System. New York, Macmillan, 1962

Davson, H: Physiology of the Cerebrospinal Fluid. London, Churchill, 1967

Davson H, Hollingsworth G, Segal MB: The mechanism of drainage of the cerebrospinal fluid. Brain 93:665–678, 1970

Dohrmann, GJ: The choroid plexus: a historical review. Brain Res 18:197–218, 1970

Dohrmann GJ, Bucy PC: Human choroid plexus: a light and electron microscopic study. J Neurosurg 33:506–516, 1970

Jones EG: On the mode of entry of blood vessels into the cerebral cortex. J Anat 106:507–520, 1970

Kimmel DL: Innervation of spinal dura mater and dura mater of the posterior cranial fossa. Neurology (Minneap) 11:800–809, 1961

Millen JW, Woollam DHM: On the nature of the pia mater. Brain 84:514–520, 1961

Millen JW, Woollam DHM: The Anatomy of the Cerebrospinal Fluid. London, Oxford University Press, 1962

Penfield W, McNaughton F: Dural headache and innervation of the dura mater. Arch Neurol Psychiatry 44:43–75, 1940

Wolstenholme GEW, O'Connor CM (eds): Ciba Foundation Symposium on the Cerebrospinal Fluid: Production, Circulation and Absorption. London, Churchill, 1958

Woollam DHM, Millen JW: The perivascular spaces of the mammalian central nervous system and their relation to the perineuronal and subarachnoid spaces. J Anat 89:193–200, 1955

Appendix

Investigators Mentioned in the Text

ADAMKIEWICZ, ALBERT (1850–1921) Polish pathologist. Described the blood supply of the spinal cord of man (an anterior radicular artery supplying the lumbar region of the spinal cord is known as the artery of Adamkiewicz).

ANGSTRÖM, ANDERS JONAS (1814–1874) Swedish physicist. Angström unit (Å) equals one-ten-thousandth of a micron.

ARGYLL ROBERTSON, DOUGLAS MORAY COOPER LAMB (1837–1909) Scottish ophthalmologist. The Argyll Robertson pupil includes, among other signs, pupillary constriction in accommodation, but not in response to light.

AUERBACH, LEOPOLD (1828–1897) German anatomist. Auerbach's plexus (myenteric plexus) in the gastrointestinal tract; end bulbs of Held–Auerbach (synaptic end bulbs or boutons terminaux).

BABINSKI, JOSEPH FRANÇOIS FÉLIX (1857–1932) French neurologist of Polish origin. The Babinski sign, which consists of up-turning of the great toe and spreading of the toes on stroking the sole, is characteristic of an upper motor neuron lesion.

BAILLARGER, JULES GABRIEL FRANÇOIS (1806–1891) French psychiatrist. The lines of Baillarger consist of two transverse strata of nerve fibers in the cerebral cortex.

BAINBRIDGE, FRANCIS ARTHUR (1874–1921) British physiologist. Found that an increase of pressure on the venous side of the heart accelerates the heart rate.

BEEVOR, CHARLES EDWARD (1854–1908) English neurologist. Contributed to our knowledge of neurology, especially with respect to localization of function in the cerebral cortex.

BELL, SIR CHARLES (1774–1842) Scottish anatomist, neurologist, and surgeon. Bell's palsy is a form of facial paralysis caused by interruption of conduction by the facial nerve. The Bell–Magendie law states that dorsal spinal roots are sensory, whereas ventral roots are motor.

BERNARD, CLAUDE (1813–1878) French physiologist and one of the great investigators of the nineteenth century. One of his outstanding contributions was the demonstration of vasomotor mechanisms.

BETZ, VLADIMIR A. (1834–1894) Russian anatomist. Discovered and described the giant pyramidal cells (Betz cells) in the motor area of the cerebral cortex.

BIELSCHOWSKY, MAX (1869–1940) German neuropathologist and neurologist. Bielschowsky's silver staining method for nerve cells and fibers.

BODIAN, DAVID Contemporary American anatomist who has made important contributions to neurology. Bodian's stain for nerve cells and fibers, using the organic silver compound protargol.

BOWMAN, SIR WILLIAM (1816–1892) English anatomist and ophthamologist. His name is associated with glands in the olfactory mucosa, the capsule of the renal glomerulus, and a layer in the cornea.

BREUER, JOSEF (1842–1925) Austrian physician and psychologist. Contributed to our knowledge of reflexes controlling respiratory movements.

BROCA, PIERRE PAUL (1824–1880) French pathologist and anthropologist. Localized the cortical motor speech area in the inferior frontal gyrus; also described a band of nerve fibers (the diagonal band of Broca) in the anterior perforated substance on the ventral surface of the cerebral hemisphere.

BRODMANN, KORBINIAN (1868–1918) German neuropsychiatrist. Brodmann's cytoarchitectural map of the cerebral cortex is used frequently when referring to specific regions of the cortex.

BROWN–SÉQUARD, CHARLES EDOUARD (1817–1894) British physiologist and neurologist. The Brown–Séquard syndrome consists of the sensory and motor abnormalities that follow hemisection of the spinal cord.

BRUCH, KARL WILHELM LUDWIG (1819–1884) German anatomist. Bruch's membrane is the innermost layer of the choroid of the eye, separating the capillary layer of the choroid from the retina.

BUCY, PAUL C. Contemporary American neurosurgeon. The Klüver–Bucy syndrome is caused by extensive bilateral lesions of the temporal lobes.

BÜNGNER, OTTO VON (1858–1905) German neurologist. Described the endoneurial tubes containing modified Schwann cells in the distal portion of a sectioned peripheral nerve (bands of von Büngner).

CAJAL, See Ramón y Cajal.

CANNON, WALTER BRADFORD (1871–1945) Outstanding American physiologist who contributed much to our understanding of autonomic regulation of visceral functions. Among other contributions he developed the concept of homeostasis of the internal environment and demonstrated the "fight or flight" reactions of the body to stress.

CLARKE, JACOB AUGUSTUS LOCKHARD (1817–1880) English anatomist and neurologist. Among numerous contributions, described the nucleus dorsalis (thoracicus) of the spinal cord, which is also known as Clarke's column.

CORTI, MARCHESE ALFONSO (1822–1888) Italian histologist. Described the sensory epithelium of the cochlea (organ of Corti).

CUSHING, HARVEY (1869–1939) Pioneer American neurosurgeon. Contributed to many basic aspects of neurology, including the function of the pituitary gland, pituitary tumors, tumors of the eighth cranial nerve, and classification of brain tumors.

DARKSCHEWITSCH, LIVERIJ OSIPOVICH (1858–1925) Russian neurologist. Nucleus of Darkschewitsch in the central gray matter of the midbrain.

DE EGAS MONIZ, ANTÔNIO CAETANO DE ABREAU FRIERE (1874–1955) Portuguese physician. Awarded the Nobel Prize in 1949 for demonstration of the therapeutic value of prefrontal leukotomy; introduced the technique of cerebral angiography in 1927.

DEITERS, OTTO FRIEDRICH KARL (1834–1863) German anatomist. The lateral vestibular nucleus, the origin of the vestibulospinal tract, is known as Deiters' nucleus.

DUSSER DE BARENNE, JOHANNES GREGORIUS (1885–1940) Dutch neurophysiologist. Studied cortical function and introduced the technique of physiologic neuronography.

EDINGER, LUDWIG (1855–1918) German neuroanatomist and neurologist. An outstanding teacher of functional neuroanatomy and a pioneer in comparative neuroanatomy. The Edinger–Westphal nucleus is the parasympathetic component of the oculomotor nucleus.

FERRIER, SIR DAVID (1843–1928) Scottish neuropathologist, neurophysiologist, and neurologist. Best known for his studies of the motor and sensory areas of the cerebral cortex.

FLECHSIG, PAUL EMIL (1847–1929) German psychiatrist and neurologist. Flechsig's method of tracing fiber tracts in the immature brain and spinal cord is based on differing times of myelination for different tracts.

FOERSTER, OTFRID (1873–1941) German neurologist and neurosurgeon. Made important contributions to the study of epilepsy, pain, the dermatomes, brain tumors, and the cytoarchitecture and functional localization of the cerebral cortex; introduced the chordotomy (tractotomy) operation for intractable pain.

FOREL, AUGUSTE H. (1843–1931) Swiss neuropsychiatrist. Described certain fiber bundles in the subthalamus, which are known as the fields of Forel. The ventral tegmental decussation of Forel in the midbrain consists of crossing rubrospinal and rubroreticular fibers. Forel proposed the Neuron Theory on the basis of the response of nerve cells to injury.

FRIEDREICH, NIKOLAUS (1826–1882) German physician. Best known for his studies of neuromuscular disorders; hereditary spinal ataxia is known as Friedreich's ataxia.

FRITSCH, GUSTAV THEODOR (1838–1927) German anthropologist and anatomist. With Hitzig, he studied localization of motor function in the dog's cerebral cortex by electrical stimulation.

FRÖLICH, ALFRED (1871–1953) Austrian pharmacologist and neurologist. Described the adiposogenital syndrome, which is caused by a lesion involving the hypothalamus.

GALEN, CLAUDIUS (131–201) Roman physician. Galen was the leading medical authority of the Christian world for 1400 years. His name is attached to the great cerebral vein.

GASSER, JOHANN LAURENTIUS Eighteenth century Austrian anatomist. The sensory ganglion of the trigeminal nerve was named for him by one of his students, A.B.R. Hirsch, in 1765.

GENNARI, FRANCESCO (1750–1796?) Italian physician. Described the white line in the visual cortex, now known as the line of Gennari, while still a medical student in Parma, Italy.

GOLGI, CAMILLO (1843–1926) Italian histologist. Introduced a silver staining method which provided the basis of numerous advances in neurohistology. Awarded the Nobel Prize in Physiology and Medicine in 1906 (with Santiago Ramón y Cajal). Golgi staining method, type I and type II neurons, tendon spindles, and so on.

GRÜNBAUM, ALBERT S.F. (later Leyton, A.S.F.) (1869–1921) British bacteriologist and physiologist. Worked with Sir Charles Sherrington on functional localization of the cerebral cortex.

GUDDEN, BERNHARD ALOYS VON (1824–1886) German neuropsychiatrist. Described the partial crossing of optic nerve fibers in the optic chiasma together with certain small commissural bundles adjacent to the chiasma. Gudden also studied connections in the brain by observing changes subsequent to lesions made in the brains of young animals.

HEAD, SIR HENRY (1861–1940) English neurologist. Studied the dermatomes, cutaneous sensory physiology, and especially sensory disturbances and aphasia following cerebral lesions.

HELD, HANS (1866–1942) German anatomist. Made extensive studies of interneuronal relationships (axonal synaptic terminals or end bulbs of Held–Auerbach).

HENLE, FRIEDRICH GUSTAV JACOB (1809–1885) German anatomist and a pioneer in histology. The endoneurial sheath surrounding individual fibers of a peripheral nerve is known as the sheath of Henle.

HENSEN, VICTOR (1835–1924) German embryologist and physiologist. Studied the anatomy and physiology of the sense organs (cells of Hensen in the organ of Corti).

HERING, HEINRICH EWALD (1866–1948) German

physiologist. Best known for his study of the reflex that initiates expiration.

HEROPHILUS (*ca.* 300-250 B.C.) Greek physician in Alexandria. Made early observations on the anatomy of the brain and other organs. The confluence of the dural venous sinuses at the internal occipital protuberance is known as the torcular Herophili.

HESCHL, RICHARD (1824-1881) Austrian anatomist and pathologist. Described the anterior transverse temporal gyri (Heschl's convolutions), which serve as a landmark for the auditory area of the cerebral cortex.

HEUBNER, JOHANN OTTO LEONHARD (1843-1926) German pediatrician. Described the recurrent branch of the anterior cerebral artery.

HIS, WILHELM (1831-1904) Swiss anatomist and a founder of human embryology. Proposed the Neuron Theory on the basis of his embryologic studies of the development of nerve cells.

HITZIG, EDUARD (1838-1907) German physiologist and neurologist. Studied localization of motor function in the cerebral cortex of dogs and monkeys by electrical stimulation.

HORNER, JOHANN FRIEDRICH (1831-1886) Swiss ophthalmologist. Horner's syndrome, caused by interruption of the sympathetic innervation of the eye, includes pupillary constriction and ptosis of the upper eyelid.

HORSLEY, SIR VICTOR ALEXANDER HADEN (1857-1916) A founder of neurosurgery in England. Studied the motor cortex and other parts of the brain by electrical stimulation; introduced the Horsley–Clarke stereotaxic apparatus.

HUNTER, JOHN (1728-1793) Outstanding British anatomist and pioneer surgeon of the eighteenth century. His collection of anatomic and pathologic specimens formed the basis of the Hunterian Museum of the Royal College of Surgeons.

HUNTINGTON, GEORGE SUMNER (1850-1916) American general medical practitioner. Described a hereditary form of chorea resulting from neuronal degeneration in the corpus striatum and the cerebral cortex.

JACKSON, JOHN HUGHLINGS (1835-1911) English neurologist and pioneer of modern neurology. Gave a thorough description of focal epilepsy (jacksonian seizures) resulting from local irritation of the motor cortex.

KLÜVER, HEINRICH Contemporary American psychologist. The Klüver–Bucy syndrome is caused by bilateral lesions of the temporal lobes.

KORSAKOFF, SERGEI SERGEIEVICH (1854-1900) Russian psychiatrist. Korsakoff's psychosis or syndrome, which is usually a sequel of chronic alcoholism, includes a memory defect, fabrication of ideas, and polyneuritis.

KRAUSE, WILHELM JOHANN FRIEDRICH (1833-1910) German anatomist. Described sensory endings in the skin, including the end bulbs of Krause.

LABBÉ LÉON (1832-1916) French surgeon. Studied the veins of the brain (lesser anastomotic vein of Labbé).

LANGLEY, JOHN NEWPORT (1852-1925) English physiologist. Best known for his studies of the autonomic nervous system, a term which he introduced in 1898.

LANTERMAN, A. J. Nineteenth century American anatomist. Described the incisures of Schmidt–Lanterman in myelin sheaths of peripheral nerve fibers.

LISSAUER, HEINRICH (1861-1891) German neurologist. Described the dorsolateral fasciculus of the spinal cord (Lissauer's tract or zone).

LUSCHKA, HUBERT VON (1820-1875) German anatomist. Among other contributions to anatomy, described the lateral apertures of the fourth ventricle (foramina of Luschka).

LUYS, JULES BERNARD (1828-1895) French neurologist. Described the subthalamic nucleus (nucleus of Luys), whose degeneration causes hemiballismus.

MAGENDIE, FRANÇOIS (1783-1855) French physiologist and pioneer of experimental physiology. The sensory function of dorsal spinal nerve roots and motor function of ventral roots constitutes the Bell–Magendie law. Also described the median aperture of the fourth ventricle (foramen of Magendie).

MARCHI, VITTORIO (1851-1908) Italian physician and histologist. The Marchi staining method for tracing the course of degenerating myelinated fibers is a valuable neuroanatomic technique.

MARIE, PIERRE (1853-1940) French neurologist. Described a number of disorders, including aphasia and hereditary cerebellar ataxia. The fasciculus sulcomarginalis of Marie is situated in the ventral white column of the spinal cord.

MARTINOTTI, GIOVANNI (1857-1928) Italian physician and student of Golgi. Described a type of neuron known as the cell of Martinotti in the cerebral cortex.

MECKEL, JOHANN FRIEDRICH (1714-1774) German anatomist. Especially known for his careful description of the trigeminal nerve. The trigeminal ganglion is situated in an extension of the meninges called Meckel's cave.

MEISSNER, GEORG (1829-1905) German anatomist and physiologist. His name is associated with touch corpuscles in the dermis and the submucous nerve plexus of the gastrointestinal tract.

MÉNIÈRE, PROSPER (1801-1862) French otologist. Described the syndrome characterized by episodes of vertigo, nausea, and vomiting, occurring in some diseases of the internal ear.

MERKEL, FRIEDRICH SIEGMUND (1845-1919) German anatomist. Described tactile endings in the epidermis, known as Merkel's disks.

MEYER, ADOLPH (1866-1950) A prominent American psychiatrist. The fibers of the geniculocalcarine tract which loop forward in the temporal lobe constitute Meyer's loop.

MEYNERT, THEODOR HERMANN (1833-1892) Austrian neuropsychiatrist and neurologist. The habenulointerpeduncular fasciculus is also called the fasciculus retroflexus of Meynert. The dorsal tegmental decussation of Meynert in the midbrain consists of crossing tectobulbar and tectospinal fibers.

MONAKOW, CONSTATIN VON (1853–1930) Neurologist of Russian birth who lived in Switzerland. Made fundamental contributions to knowledge of the thalamus, red nucleus, rubrospinal tract, and so on. The dorsolateral region of the medulla is known as Monakow's area.

MONIZ, See de Egas Moniz.

MONRO, ALEXANDER (1733–1817) Scottish anatomist, also known as Alexander Monro (Secundus). Including tenure by his father (Primus) and son (Tertius), the Chair of Anatomy in the University of Edinburgh was occupied by Alexander Monros for over a century. The interventricular foramen between the lateral and third ventricles is known as the foramen of Monro.

MÜLLER, HEINRICH (1820–1864) German anatomist. Müller's orbital muscle and cells of Müller in the retina.

NAUTA, WALLE JETZE HARINX Contemporary American neuroanatomist. Has made numerous contributions to knowledge of the functional anatomy of the central nervous system. The Nauta silver staining method is used widely for tracing the course of nerve fibers.

NISSL, FRANZ (1860–1919) German neuropsychiatrist. Made important contributions to neurohistology and neuropathology. Introduced a method of staining gray matter with basic aniline dyes to show the basophil material (Nissl bodies) of nerve cells.

PACCHIONI, ANTONIO (1665–1726) Italian anatomist. The arachnoid villi become hypertrophied with age and are then known as arachnoid granulations or pacchionian bodies.

PACINI, FILIPPO (1812–1883) Italian anatomist and histologist. Described the sensory endings known as the corpuscles of Vater-Pacini.

PARKINSON, JAMES (1775–1824) English physician, surgeon, and paleontologist. Described "shaking palsy" or paralysis agitans, which is frequently referred to as Parkinson's disease.

PENFIELD, WILDER GRAVES (1891–1976) Canadian neurosurgeon. Made fundamental contributions to neurocytology and neurophysiology, including functions of the cerebral cortex, speech mechanisms, and factors underlying epilepsy.

PERRONCITO, A. (1882–1929) Italian histologist. Described the whorls of regenerating fibers (spirals of Perroncito) in the central stump of a sectioned peripheral nerve.

PURKINJE, JOHANNES (JAN) EVANGELISTA (1787–1869) Bohemian physiologist, pioneer in histologic techniques, and accomplished histologist. Described the Purkinje cells of the cerebellar cortex and Purkinje fibers in the heart, among others.

RAMÓN Y CAJAL, SANTIAGO (1852–1934) Spanish histologist who is acknowledged as the foremost among neurohistologists. Awarded the Nobel Prize in Physiology and Medicine (with Camillo Golgi) in 1906. Among innumerable contributions Cajal vigorously championed the Neuron Theory on the basis of his observations with silver staining methods.

RANVIER, LOUIS-ANTOINE (1835–1922) French histologist and a founder of experimental histology. Described the nodes of Ranvier in the myelin sheaths of nerve fibers.

RASMUSSEN, GRANT LITSTER Contemporary American neuroanatomist. Has made numerous contributions to neuroanatomy, including a description of the olivocochlear bundle.

REIL, JOHANN CHRISTIAN (1759–1813) German physician. The insula, lying in the depths of the lateral fissure of the cerebral hemisphere, is known as the island of Reil.

REISSNER, ERNST (1824–1878) German anatomist. The vestibular membrane of the cochlea is known as Reissner's membrane.

RENSHAW, BIRDSEY (1911–1948) American neurophysiologist. Certain intercalated neurons in the ventral gray horn of the spinal cord are called Renshaw cells.

REXED, BROR Contemporary Swedish neuroanatomist. Divided the gray matter of the spinal cord into regions (laminae of Rexed) on the basis of differences in cytoarchitecture.

RIO HORTEGA, PIO DEL (1882–1945) Spanish histologist who worked in his later years in England and Argentina. Best known for his studies of neuroglial cells, especially the microglia.

ROBIN, CHARLES PHILIPPE (1821–1885) French anatomist. The perivascular spaces of the brain are known as Virchow–Robin spaces.

ROLANDO, LUIGI (1773–1831) Italian anatomist. Among various contributions to neurology, described the central sulcus of the cerebral hemisphere and the substantia gelatinosa of the spinal cord.

ROMBERG, MORITZ HEINRICH (1795–1873) German neurologist. Romberg's sign of impaired conduction in the dorsal white columns of the spinal cord consists of abnormal unsteadiness when standing with the feet together and the eyes closed.

ROSENTHAL, FRIEDRICH CHRISTIAN (1779–1829) German anatomist. Studied the veins of the brain (basal vein of Rosenthal).

RUFFINI, ANGELO (1864–1929) Italian anatomist. Described sensory endings, especially those known as the end bulbs of Ruffini.

RUSSELL, JAMES SAMUEL RISIEN (1863–1939) British physician and neurologist. Published on diseases of the nervous system and described the uncinate fasciculus of efferent cerebellar fibers.

SCARPA, ANTONIO (1747–1832) Italian anatomist and surgeon. Made numerous contributions to anatomy, including a description of the vestibular ganglion.

SCHMIDT, HENRY D. (1823–1888) American anatomist and pathologist. Described the incisures of Schmidt–Lanterman in myelin sheaths of peripheral nerve fibers.

SCHÜTZ, H. German anatomist. Described the dorsal longitudinal fasciculus of the brain stem in 1891.

SCHWANN, THEODOR (1810–1882) German anatomist. Formulated the Cell Theory (with M. J. Schleiden) and described the neurolemmal cells (Schwann cells) of peripheral nerve fibers.

SHERRINGTON, SIR CHARLES SCOTT (1856–1952) English neurophysiologist. A foremost contributor to basic knowledge of the function of the nervous system. His researches included studies of reflexes, decerebrate rigidity, reciprocal innervation, the synapse, and the concept of the integrative action of the nervous system.

SYDENHAM, THOMAS (1624–1689) English physician, known as the English Hippocrates. Described the form of chorea to which his name is attached.

SYLVIUS, FRANCIS DE LA BOE (1614–1672) French anatomist. Gave the first description of the lateral fissure of the cerebral hemisphere.

SYLVIUS, JACOBUS (also known as Jacques Dubois) (1478–1555) French anatomist. Described the cerebral aqueduct of the midbrain.

TROLARD, PAULIN (1842–1910) French anatomist. Described the venous drainage of the brain (greater anastomotic vein of Trolard).

VATER, ABRAHAM (1684–1751) German anatomist. Among other contributions to anatomy, described the sensory endings known as the corpuscles of Vater–Pacini.

VICQ D'AZYR, FELIX (1748–1794) French anatomist and a leading comparative anatomist. The mammillothalamic fasciculus bears his name.

VIRCHOW, RUDOLPH LUDWIG KARL (1821–1902) German pathologist. Founder of cellular pathology, or modern pathology. The perivascular spaces of the brain are known as Virchow–Robin spaces.

WALDEYER, HEINRICH WILHELM GOTTFRIED (1836–1921) German anatomist. Popularized the Neuron Theory on the basis of studies by Cajal, Forel, His, and others.

WALLENBERG, ADOLF (1862–1949) German physician. Described the lateral medullary syndrome.

WALLER, AUGUSTUS VOLNEY (1816–1870) English physician and physiologist. Described the degenerative changes in the distal portion of a sectioned peripheral nerve, known as wallerian degeneration.

WARWICK, ROGER Contemporary British anatomist. Among other contributions, described the organization of the oculomotor nucleus with respect to the ocular muscles which it supplies.

WEBER, SIR HERMANN DAVID (1823–1918) English physician. Described the midbrain lesion causing hemiparesis and ocular paralysis.

WEIGERT, KARL (1843–1905) German pathologist. Introduced several staining methods, including a stain for myelin and therefore for white matter in sections of nervous tissue.

WERNICKE, CARL (1848–1905) German neuropsychiatrist. Made a special study of disorders in the use of language. Wernicke's sensory language area, Wernicke's aphasia.

WESTPHAL, KARL FRIEDRICH OTTO (1883–1890) German neurologist. Among other contributions to neurology, described the Edinger–Westphal nucleus in the oculomotor complex

WILLIS, THOMAS (1621–1675) English physician. One of the dominant figures in English medicine of the seventeenth century and one of the founders of the Royal Society. Among numerous contributions to the anatomy of the brain, described the arterial circle that bears his name.

WILSON, SAMUEL ALEXANDER KINNIER (1878–1937) British neurologist. Described hepatolenticular degeneration, known as Wilson's disease.

WRISBERG, HEINRICH AUGUST (1739–1808) German anatomist. Among other contributions to anatomy, described the sensory root of the facial nerve (nervus intermedius of Wrisberg).

Glossary of Neuroanatomic Terms

Adiadochokinesia. *a*, neg. + Gr. *diadochos*, succeeding + *kinēsis*, movement. Inability to perform rapidly alternating movements. Also called dysdiadochokinesia.

Agnosia. *a*, neg. + Gr. *gnōsis*, knowledge. Lack of ability to recognize the significance of sensory stimuli (auditory, visual, tactile, etc. agnosia).

Agraphia. *a*, neg. + Gr. *graphō*, to write. Inability to express thoughts in writing owing to a central lesion.

Ala cinerea. L. wing + *cinereus*, ashen-hued. Vagal triangle in floor of fourth ventricle.

Alexia. *a*, neg. + Gr. *lexis*, word. Loss of the power to grasp the meaning of written or printed words and sentences.

Allocortex. Gr. *allos*, other + L. *cortex*, bark. The phylogenetically older cerebral cortex, consisting of three layers. Includes paleocortex and archicortex.

Alveus. L. trough. The thin layer of white matter covering the ventricular surface of the hippocampus.

Amacrine. *a*, neg. + Gr. *makros*, long + *is, inos*, fiber. Amacrine nerve cell of the retina.

Ammon's horn. The hippocampus, which has an outline in cross section suggestive of a ram's horn. Also known as the cornu Ammonis. Ammon: an Egyptian diety with a ram's head.

Amygdala. L. from Gr. *amygdalē*, almond. Amygdala or amygdaloid nucleus in the temporal lobe of the cerebral hemisphere.

Anopsia. *an*, neg. + Gr. *opsis*, vision. A defect of vision.

Aphasia. *a*, neg. + Gr. *phasis*, speech. A defect of the power of expression by speech or of comprehending spoken or written language.

Apraxia. *a*, neg. + Gr. *pratto*, to do. Inability to carry out purposeful movements in the absence of paralysis.

Arachnoid. Gr. *arachnē*, spider's web + *eidos*, resemblance. The delicate meningeal layer forming the outer boundary of the subarachnoid space.

Archicerebellum. Gr. *archē*, beginning + diminutive of cerebrum. A phylogenetically old part of the cerebellum, functioning in the maintenance of equilibrium.

Archicortex. Gr. *archē*, beginning + L. *cortex*, bark. Three-layered cortex included in the limbic system; located mainly in the hippocampus and dentate gyrus of the temporal lobe.

Area postrema. An area in the lowest part of the floor of the fourth ventricle.

Astereognosis. *a*, neg. + *stereos*, solid + *gnōsis*, knowledge. Loss of ability to recognize objects or to appreciate their form by touching or feeling them.

Astrocyte. Gr. *astron*, star + *kytos*, hollow (cell). A type of neuroglial cell of ectodermal origin.

Asynergy. *a*, neg. + Gr. *syn*, with + *ergon*, work. Disturbance of that proper association in the contraction of muscles which assures that the different components of an act follow in proper sequence, at the proper moment, and of the proper degree, so that the act is executed accurately.

Ataxia, *a*, neg. + Gr. *taxis*, order. A loss of power of muscle coordination, with irregularity of muscle action.

Athetosis. Gr. *athetos*, without position or place. An affection of the nervous system, caused by degenerative changes in the corpus striatum and cerebral cortex, and characterized by bizarre, writhing movements of the fingers and toes, especially.

Autonomic. Gr. *autos*, self + *nomos*, law. Autonomic system: the efferent or motor innervation of viscera.

Autoradiography. Gr. *autos*, self + L. *radius*, ray + Gr. *graphō*, to write. A technique that uses a photographic emulsion to detect the location of radioactive isotopes in tissue sections. Also called radioautography.

Axolemma. Gr. *axōn*, axis + *lemma*, husk. The plasma membrane of an axon.

Axon. Gr. *axōn*, axis. Efferent process of a neuron conducting impulses to other neurons or to muscle fibers (striated and smooth) and gland cells.

Axon hillock. The region of the nerve cell body from which the axon arises; it contains no Nissl material.

Axon reaction. Changes in the cell body of a neuron following damage to its axon.

Axoplasm. Gr. *axōn*, axis + *plasm*, anything formed or molded. The cytoplasm of the axon.

Baroreceptor. Gr. *baros*, weight + *receptor*, receiver. A sensory nerve terminal that is stimulated by changes in pressure.

Basis pedunculi. The ventral part of the cerebral peduncle of the midbrain on each side, separated from the dorsal part by the substantia nigra. Also called the crus cerebri.

Brachium. L. from Gr. *brachiōn*, arm. As used in the central nervous system, denotes a large bundle of fibers connecting one part with another (*e.g.*, brachia associated with the cerebellum and the colliculi of the midbrain).

Bradykinesia. Gr. *brady*, slow + *kinēsis*, movement. Abnormal slowness of movements.

Brain stem. In the mature human brain, usually denotes the medulla, pons, and midbrain. In descriptions of the embryonic brain the diencephalon is included as well.

Bulb. Referred at one time to the medulla oblongata; but in the context of "corticobulbar tract," refers to the brain stem, in which motor nuclei of cranial nerves are located.

Calamus scriptorius. L. *calamus*, a reed, therefore a reed pen. Refers to an area in the caudal part of the floor of the fourth ventricle, which is shaped somewhat like a pen point.

Calcar. L. spur, used to denote any spur-shaped structure. Calcar avis, an elevation on the medial aspect of the lateral ventricles at the junction of posterior and inferior horns. Also calcarine sulcus of occipital lobe, which is responsible for the calcar avis.

Cauda equina. L. horse's tail. The lumbar and sacral spinal nerve roots in the lower part of the spinal canal.

Caudate nucleus. Part of the corpus striatum, so named because it has a long extension or tail.

Cerebellum. L. diminutive of *cerebrum*, brain. A large part of the brain with motor functions, situated in the posterior cranial fossa.

Cerebrum. L. brain. The principal portion of the brain, including the diencephalon and cerebral hemispheres, but not the brain stem and cerebellum.

Chordotomy. Gr. *chordē*, cord + *tomē*, a cutting. Division of the lateral spinothalamic tract for intractable pain. Also spelled cordotomy.

Chorea. L. from Gr. *choros*, a dance. A disorder characterized by irregular, spasmodic, involuntary movements of the limbs or facial muscles. Attributed to degenerative changes in the neostriatum.

Choroid. Gr. *chorion*, a delicate membrane + *eidos*, form. Choroid or vascular coat of the eye; choroid plexuses in the ventricles of the brain. Also spelled chorioid.

Chromatolysis. Gr. *chrōma*, color + *lysis*, dissolution. Dispersal of the Nissl material of neurons following axon section or in viral infections of the nervous system.

Cinerea. L. *cinereus*, ashen hued, from *cinis*, ashes. Refers to gray matter, but limited in usage. Tuber cinereum (ventral portion of the hypothalamus, from which the infundibular stem of the neurohypophysis arises); tuberculum cinereum (slight elevation on medulla formed by spinal tract and nucleus of trigeminal nerve); ala cinerea (vagal triangle in floor of fourth ventricle).

Cingulum. L. girdle. A bundle of association fibers in the white matter of the cingulate gyrus on the medial surface of the cerebral hemisphere.

Claustrum. L. a barrier. A thin sheet of gray matter, of unknown function, situated between the lenticular nucleus and the insula.

Clava. L. club. A slight swelling on the dorsal surface of the medulla, produced by the nucleus gracilis.

Colliculus. L. a small elevation or mound. Superior and inferior colliculi comprising the tectum of the midbrain; facial colliculus in the floor of the fourth ventricle.

Conjunctivum. L. *conjungo*, to bind together. Brachium conjunctivum: efferent fibers in the superior cerebellar peduncle, originating in central nuclei of the cerebellum.

Corona. L. from Gr. *korōnē*, a crown. Corona radiata (fibers radiating from the internal capsule to various parts of the cerebral cortex).

Corpus callosum. L. body + *callosus*, hard. The main neocortical commissure of the cerebral hemispheres.

Corpus striatum. L. body + *striatus*, furrowed or striped. A mass of gray matter, with motor functions, at the base of each cerebral hemipshere.

Cortex. L. bark. Outer layer of gray matter of the cerebral hemispheres and cerebellum.

Crus. L. leg. The crus cerebri is the ventral part of the cerebral peduncle of the midbrain on each side, separated from the dorsal part by the substantia nigra (also called the basis pedunculi). Crus of the fornix.

Cuneus. L. wedge. A gyrus on the medial surface of the cerebral hemisphere. Fasciculus cuneatus in the spinal cord and medulla; nucleus cuneatus in the medulla.

Dendrite. Gr. *dendrītēs*, related to a tree. A process of a nerve cell, on which axons of other neurons terminate. Also peripheral process of a primary sensory neuron.

Dentate. L. *dentatus*, toothed. Dentate nucleus of the cerebellum; dentate gyrus in the temporal lobe.

Diencephalon. Gr. *dia*, through + *enkephalos*, brain. Part of the cerebrum, consisting of the thalamus, epithalamus, subthalamus, and hypothalamus. The posterior of the two brain vesicles formed from the prosencephalon of the developing embryo.

Dura. L. *durus*, hard. Dura mater (the thick external layer of the meninges).

Dyskinesia. Gr. *dys*, difficult or disordered + *kinēsis*, movement. Abnormality of motor function, characterized by involuntary, purposeless movements.

Dysmetria. Gr. *dys*, difficult or disordered + *metron*, measure. Disturbance of the power to control the range of movement in muscular action.

Emboliform. Gr. *embolos*, plug + L. *forma*, form. Emboliform nucleus of the cerebellum.

Endoneurium. Gr. *endon*, within + *neuron*, nerve. The delicate connective tissue sheath surrounding an individual nerve fiber of a peripheral nerve. Also called the sheath of Henle.

Engram. Gr. *en*, in + *gramma*, mark. Used in psychology to mean the lasting trace left in the psyche by previous experience; a latent memory picture.

Entorhinal. Gr. *entos,* within + *rhis (rhin-),* nose. The entorhinal area is the anterior part of the parahippocampal gyrus of the temporal lobe adjacent to the uncus. Functions as olfactory association cortex.

Ependyma. Gr. *ependyma,* an upper garment. Lining epithelium of the ventricles of the brain and central canal of the spinal cord.

Epineurium. Gr. *epi,* upon + *neuron,* nerve. The connective tissue sheath surrounding a peripheral nerve.

Epithalamus. Gr. *epi,* upon + *thalamos,* inner chamber. A region of the diencephalon above the thalamus; includes the pineal gland.

Exteroceptor. L. *exterus,* external + *receptor,* receiver. A sensory receptor which serves to acquaint the individual with his environment (exteroception).

Extrapyramidal system. In broadest terms, consists of all motor parts of the central nervous system except the pyramidal motor system. "Extrapyramidal system" is subject to various interpretations.

Falx. L. sickle. Two of the dural partitions in the cranial cavity are the falx cerebri and the small falx cerebelli.

Fasciculus. L. diminutive of *fascis,* bundle. A bundle of nerve fibers.

Fastigial. L. *fastigium,* the top of a gabled roof. Fastigial nucleus of the cerebellum.

Fimbria. L. *fimbriae,* fringe. A band of nerve fibers along the medial edge of the hippocampus, continuing as the fornix.

Forceps. L. a pair of tongs. Used in neurologic anatomy for the U-shaped configuration of fibers constituting the anterior and posterior portions of the corpus callosum (forceps minor and forceps major).

Fornix. L. arch. The efferent tract of the hippocampus, arching over the thalamus and terminating mainly in the mammillary body of the hypothalamus.

Fovea. L. a pit or depression. Fovea centralis (the depression in the center of the macula lutea of the retina).

Funiculus. L. diminutive of *funis,* cord. An area of white matter which may consist of several functionally different fasciculi, as in the lateral funiculus (column) of white matter of the spinal cord.

Ganglion. Gr. knot or subcutaneous tumor. A swelling composed of nerve cells, as in cerebrospinal and sympathetic ganglia. Also used inappropriately for certain regions of gray matter in the brain, *e.g.,* basal ganglia of the cerebral hemisphere.

Gemmule. L. *gemmula,* diminutive of *gemma,* bud. Minute projections on dendrites of certain neurons, especially pyramidal cells and Purkinje cells, for synaptic contact with other neurons.

Genu. L. *genus,* knee. Anterior end of corpus callosum; genu of facial nerve. Also geniculate ganglion of facial nerve and geniculate nuclei of thalamus.

Glia. Gr. glue. Neuroglia, the interstitial or accessory cells of the central nervous system.

Gliosome. Gr. *glia,* glue + *soma,* body. Granules in neuroglial cells, in particular astrocytes.

Globus pallidus. L. a ball + pale. Medial part of lentic-

ular nucleus of corpus striatum. Also globose nuclei of cerebellum.

Gracilis. L. slender. Fasciculus gracilis of the spinal cord and medulla; nucleus gracilis of the medulla.

Granule. L. *granulum,* diminutive of *granum,* grain. Used to denote small neurons, such as granule cells of cerebellar cortex and stellate cells of cerebral cortex. Hence granular cell layers of both cortices.

Habenula. L. diminutive of *habena,* strap or rein. A small swelling in the epithalamus, adjacent to the posterior end of the roof of the third ventricle.

Hemiballismus. Gr. *hēmi,* half + *ballismos,* jumping. A violent form of motor restlessness involving one side of the body, caused by a destructive lesion involving the subthalamic nucleus.

Hemiplegia. Gr. *hēmi,* half + *plēgē,* a stroke. Paralysis of one side of the body.

Hippocampus. Gr. *hippocampus,* sea horse. A gyrus which constitutes an important part of the limbic system; produces an elevation on the floor of the inferior (temporal) horn of the lateral ventricle.

Homeostasis. Gr. *homois,* like + *stasis,* standing. A tendency toward stability in the internal environment of the organism.

Hydrocephalus. Gr. *hydrōr,* water + *kephalē,* head. Excessive accumulation of cerebrospinal fluid.

Hypothalamus. Gr. *hypo,* under + *thalamos,* inner chamber. A region of the diencephalon which serves as the main controlling center of the autonomic nervous system.

Indusium. L. a garment, from *induo,* to put on. Indusium griseum, a thin layer of gray matter on the dorsal surface of the corpus callosum (gray tunic).

Infundibulum. L. funnel. Infundibular stem of the neurohypophysis.

Insula. L. island. Cerebral cortex concealed from surface view and lying at the bottom of the lateral fissure. Also called the island of Reil.

Interoceptor. L. *inter,* between + *receptor,* receiver. One of the sensory end organs within viscera.

Isocortex. Gr. *isos,* equal + L. *cortex,* bark. Cerebral cortex having six layers (neocortex).

Kinesthesia. Gr. *kinēsis,* movement + *aisthēsis,* sensation. The sense of perception of movement.

Koniocortex. Gr. *konis,* dust + L. *cortex,* bark. Areas of cerebral cortex containing large numbers of small neurons; typical of sensory areas.

Lemniscus. Gr. *lēmniskos,* fillet (a ribbon or band). Used to designate a bundle of nerve fibers in the central nervous system, *e.g.,* medial lemniscus and lateral lemniscus.

Lenticular. L. *lenticula,* a lentil (of the shape of a lentil or a lens). Lenticular nucleus, a component of the corpus striatum. Also called lentiform nucleus.

Leptomeninges. Gr. *leptos,* slender + *mēninx,* membrane. The arachnoid and pia mater.

Limbus. L. a border. Limbic lobe: a C-shaped configuration of cortex on the medial surface of the cerebral hemisphere, consisting of the cingulate and parahippocampal gyri. Limbic system: Limbic lobe, hippocampal formation, and portions of the diencephalon, especially the mammillary body and anterior thalamic nucleus.

Limen. L. threshold. Limen insulae: the ventral part of the insula (island of Reil); included in the lateral olfactory area.

Locus ceruleus. L. place + *caeruleus*, dark blue. A small dark spot on each side of the floor of the fourth ventricle; marks the position of a group of nerve cells that contain melanin pigment.

Macroglia. Gr. *makros*, large + *glia*, glue. The larger types of neuroglial cells, namely, astrocytes, oligodendrocytes, and ependymal cells; of ectodermal origin.

Macrosmatic. Gr. *makros*, large + *osmē*, smell. Having the sense of smell strongly or acutely developed.

Macula. L. a spot. Macula lutea: a spot at the posterior pole of the eye, having a yellow color when viewed with red-free light. Maculae sacculi and utriculi: sensory areas in the vestibular portion of the membranous labyrinth.

Mammillary. L. *mammilla*, diminutive of *mamma*, breast (shaped like a nipple). Mammillary bodies: small swellings on the ventral surface of the hypothalamus. Also spelled mamillary.

Massa intermedia. A bridge of gray matter connecting the thalami of the two sides across the third ventricle; present in 70% of brains. Also called the interthalamic adhesion.

Medulla. L. marrow, from *medius*, middle. Medulla spinalis: spinal cord. Medulla oblongata: caudal portion of the brain stem. In current usage, "medulla" refers to the medulla oblongata.

Mesencephalon. *Gr. mesos*, middle + *enkephalos*, brain. The midbrain; the second of the three primary brain vesicles.

Mesocortex. Gr. *mesos*, middle + L. *cortex*, bark. Cerebral cortex that is intermediate between three-layered and six-layered cortex (present in the cingulate gyrus).

Mesoglia. Gr. *mesos*, middle + *glia*, glue. Microglial cells, of mesodermal origin.

Metathalamus. Gr. *meta*, after + *thalamos*, inner chamber. The medial and lateral geniculate bodies (nuclei).

Metencephalon. Gr. *meta*, after + *enkephalos*, brain. Pons and cerebellum; the anterior of the two divisions of the rhombencephalon or posterior primary brain vesicle.

Microglia. Gr. *mikros*, small + *glia*, glue. Neuroglial cells of mesodermal origin, belonging to the reticuloendothelial system of cells of the body.

Microsmatic. Gr. *mikros*, small + *osmē*, smell. Having a sense of smell, but relatively poor development.

Mitral. L. *mitra*, a coif or turban (bishop's miter). Mitral cell of the olfactory bulb.

Mnenomic. Gr. *mnēmē*, memory. Pertaining to memory.

Molecular. L. *molecula*, diminutive of *moles*, mass. Used in neurohistology to denote tissue containing large numbers of fine nerve fibers, and which therefore has a punctate appearance in silver-stained sections. Molecular layers of cerebral and cerebellar cortices.

Myelencephalon. Gr. *myelos*, marrow + *enkephalos*, brain. Medulla oblongata; the posterior of the two divisions of the rhombencephalon or posterior primary brain vesicle.

Myelin. Gr. *myelos*, marrow. The layers of lipid and protein substances composing a sheath around nerve fibers.

Neocerebellum. Gr. *neos*, new + diminutive of cerebrum. The phylogenetically newest part of the cerebellum, present in mammals and especially well developed in man. Ensures smooth muscle action in the finer voluntary movements.

Neocortex. Gr. *neos*, new + L. *cortex*, bark. Six-layered cortex, characteristic of mammals and constituting most of the cerebral cortex in man.

Neostriatum. Gr. *neos*, new + L. *striatus*, striped or grooved. The phylogenetically newer part of the corpus striatum consisting of the caudate nucleus and putamen; the striatum.

Neurobiotaxis. Gr. *neuron*, nerve + *bios*, life + *taxis*, arrangement. The tendency of nerve cells to move during embryologic development toward the area from which they receive the most stimuli.

Neurofibril. Gr. *neuron*, nerve + L. *fibrilla*, diminutive of *fibra*, a fiber. Delicate filaments in the cytoplasm of neurons.

Neuroglia. Gr. *neuron*, nerve + *glia*, glue. Accessory or interstitial cells of the central nervous system; includes astrocytes, oligodendrocytes, microglial cells, and ependymal cells.

Neurolemma. Gr. *neuron*, nerve + *lemma*, husk. The delicate sheath surrounding a peripheral nerve fiber consisting of a series of neurolemma cells or Schwann cells. Also spelled neurilemma.

Neuron. Gr. a nerve. The morphologic unit of the nervous system, consisting of the nerve cell body and its processes (dendrites and axon).

Neuropil. Gr. *neuron*, nerve + *pilos*, felt. A complex net of nerve cell processes occupying the intervals between cell bodies in gray matter.

Nociceptive. L. *noceo*, to injure + *capio*, to take. Responsive to injurious stimuli.

Nystagmus. Gr. *nystagmos*, a nodding, from *nystazō*, to be sleepy. An involuntary oscillation of the eyes.

Obex. L. barrier. A small transverse fold overhanging the opening of the fourth ventricle into the central canal of the closed portion of the medulla.

Oligodendrocyte. Gr. *oligos*, few + *dendron*, tree + *kytos*, hollow (cell). A neuroglial cell of ectodermal origin; forms the myelin sheath in the central nervous system in the same manner as the Schwann cell in peripheral nerves.

Olive. L. *oliva*. Oval bulging of the lateral area of the medulla. Inferior, accessory, and superior olivary nuclei.

Operculum. L. a cover or lid, from *opertus*, to cover. Frontal, parietal, and temporal opercula bound the lateral fissure of the cerebral hemisphere and conceal the insula.

Pachymeninx. Gr. *pachys*, thick + *mēninx*, membrane. The dura mater.

Paleocerebellum. Gr. *palaios*, ancient + diminutive of cerebrum. A phylogenetically old part of the cerebellum functioning in postural changes and locomotion.

Paleocortex. Gr. *palaios*, ancient + L. *cortex*, bark. Three-layered olfactory cortex.

Paleostriatum. Gr. *palaios*, ancient + L. *striatus*, striped or grooved. The phylogenetically older and efferent part of the corpus striatum; the globus pallidus or pallidum.

Pallidum. L. *pallidus*, pale. The globus pallidus of the corpus striatum; medial portion of the lenticular nucleus comprising the paleostriatum.

Pallium. L. cloak. The cerebral cortex with subjacent white matter, but usually used synonymously with cortex.

Paraplegia. Gr. *para*, beside + *plēgē*, a stroke. Paralysis of both legs and lower part of trunk.

Perikaryon. Gr. *peri*, around + *karyon*, nut, kernel. The cytoplasm surrounding the nucleus. Sometimes refers to the cell body of a neuron.

Perineurium. Gr. *peri*, around + *neuron*, nerve. The connective tissue sheath surrounding a bundle of nerve fibers in a peripheral nerve.

Pes. L. foot. Pes hippocampi: the anterior thickened end of the hippocampus.

Pia mater. L. tender mother. The thin innermost layer of the meninges, attached to the surface of the brain and spinal cord; forms the inner boundary of the subarachnoid space.

Pineal. L. *pineus*, relating to the pine. Shaped like a pine cone (pertaining to the pineal gland, also called the pineal body).

Pneumoencephalography. Gr. *pneuma*, air + *enkephalos*, brain + *graphō*, to write. The replacement of cerebrospinal fluid by air, followed by x-ray examination (pneumoencephalogram); permits visualization of the ventricles and subarachnoid space. This technique has been replaced by computerized tomography (CT scan).

Pons. L. bridge. That part of the brain stem which lies between the medulla and the midbrain; appears to constitute a bridge between the right and left halves of the cerebellum.

Proprioceptor. L. *proprius*, one's own + *receptor*, receiver. One of the sensory endings in muscles, tendons, and joints; provides information concerning movement and position of body parts (proprioception).

Prosencephalon. Gr. *pros*, before + *enkephalos*, brain. The forebrain, consisting of the telencephalon (cerebral hemispheres) and diencephalon; the anterior primary brain vesicle.

Pulvinar. L. a cushioned seat. The posterior projection of the thalamus beneath which the medial and lateral geniculate bodies are situated.

Putamen. L. shell. The larger and lateral part of the lenticular nucleus of the corpus striatum.

Pyramidal system. Corticospinal and corticobulbar tracts. So called because the corticospinal tracts occupy pyramid-shaped areas on the ventral surface of the medulla. The term pyramidal tract refers specifically to the corticospinal tract.

Pyriform. L. *pyrum*, pear + *forma*, form. Pyriform area is a region of olfactory cortex consisting of the uncus, limen insulae, and entorhinal area; has a pear-shaped outline in animals with a well-developed olfactory system.

Quadriplegia. L. *quadri*, four + Gr. *plēgē*, stroke. Paralysis affecting the four limbs. Also called tetraplegia.

Restiform. L. *restis*, rope + *forma*, form. Restiform body: the main mass of the inferior cerebellar peduncle, containing afferent fibers to the cerebellum.

Reticular. L. *reticularis*, pertaining to or resembling a net. Reticular formation of the brain stem.

Rhinal. Gr. *rhis*, nose, therefore related to the nose. Rhinal sulcus in the temporal lobe indicates the margin of the lateral olfactory area and its association cortex.

Rhinencephalon. Gr. *rhis* (rhin-), nose + *enkephalos*, brain. Refers in man to components of the olfactory system. In comparative neurology structures incorporated in the limbic system (especially the hippocampus and dentate gyrus) are included.

Rhombencephalon. Gr. *rhombos*, a lozenge-shaped figure + *enkephalos*, brain. The pons and cerebellum (metencephalon) and medulla (myelencephalon); the posterior primary brain vesicle.

Rostrum. L. beak. Recurved portion of the corpus callosum, passing backward from the genu to the lamina terminalis.

Satellite. L. *satteles*, attendant. Satellite cells: flattened cells of ectodermal origin forming a capsule for nerve cell bodies in dorsal root ganglia and sympathetic ganglia. Also satellite oligodendrocytes adjacent to nerve cell bodies in the central nervous system.

Septal area. Cortex and underlying septal nuclei, the latter extending into the septum pellucidum, ventral to the genu and rostrum of the corpus callosum on the medial aspect of the frontal lobe. Also called the medial olfactory area.

Septum pellucidum. L. partition + transparent. A triangular double membrane separating the anterior horns of the lateral ventricles. Situated in the median plane, it fills in the interval between the corpus callosum and the fornix.

Somatic. Gr. *somatikos*, bodily. Used in neurology to denote the body, exclusive of the viscera (as in somatic efferent neurons supplying the skeletal musculature).

Somesthetic. Gr. *soma*, body + *aisthēsis*, perception. The consciousness of having a body. Somesthetic senses are the general senses of pain, temperature, touch, pressure, position, movement, and vibration. Also spelled somatesthetic.

Splenium. Gr. *splēnion*, bandage. The thickened posterior extremity of the corpus callosum.

Stratum zonale. A layer of myelinated nerve fibers on the dorsal surface of the thalamus.

Stria terminalis. L. a furrow, groove + boundary, limit. A slender strand of fibers running along the medial side of the tail of the caudate nucleus. Originating in the amygdaloid nucleus, most of the fibers end in the septal area and hypothalamus.

Striatum. L. *striatus*, furrowed. The phylogenetically

more recent part of the corpus striatum (neostriatum) consisting of the caudate nucleus and the putamen or lateral portion of the lenticular nucleus.

Subiculum. L. diminutive of *subex* (*subic-*), a layer. Transitional cortex between that of the parahippocampal gyrus and the hippocampus.

Substantia gelatinosa. A column of small neurons at the apex of the dorsal gray horn throughout the spinal cord.

Substantia nigra. A large nucleus with motor functions in the midbrain; many of the constituent cells contain dark melanin pigment.

Subthalamus. L. under + Gr. *thalamos*, inner chamber. Region of the diencephalon beneath the thalamus, containing fiber tracts and the subthalamic nucleus.

Synapse. Gr. *synaptō*, to join. The word was introduced by Sherrington in 1897 for the site of contact between neurons, at which site one neuron is excited or inhibited by another neuron.

Syringomyelia. Gr. *syrinx*, pipe, tube + *myelos*, marrow. A condition characterized by central cavitation of the spinal cord and gliosis around the cavity.

Tapetum. L. *tapete*, a carpet. Fibers of the corpus callosum sweeping over the lateral ventricle and forming the lateral wall of its posterior and inferior horns.

Tectum. L. roof. Roof of the midbrain consisting of the paired superior and inferior colliculi.

Tegmentum. L. cover, from *tego*, to cover. The dorsal portion of the pons; also the major portion of the cerebral peduncle of the midbrain, lying between the substantia nigra and the tectum.

Tela choroidea. L. a web + Gr. *chorioeidēs*, like a membrane. The vascular connective tissue continuous with that of the pia mater which continues into the core of the choroid plexuses.

Telencephalon. Gr. *telos*, end + *enkephalos*, brain. Cerebral hemispheres; the anterior of the two divisions of the prosencephalon or anterior primary brain vesicle.

Telodendria. Gr. *telos*, end + *dendrion*, tree. The terminal branches of axons.

Tentorium. L. tent. The tentorium cerebelli is a dural partition between the occipital lobes of the cerebral hemispheres and the cerebellum.

Thalamus. Gr. *thalamos*, inner chamber. A major portion of the diencephalon with sensory and integrative functions.

Torcular. L. wine press, from *torquere*, to twist. The confluence of the dural venous sinuses at the internal occipital protuberance was formerly known as the torcular Herophili.

Transducer. L. *transducere*, to lead across. A structure or mechanism for converting one form of energy into another; applied to sensory receptors.

Trapezoid body. Transverse fibers of the auditory pathway situated at the junction of the dorsal and ventral portions of the pons.

Uncinate. L. hook-shaped. Uncinate fasciculus: association fibers connecting cortex of the ventral surface of the frontal lobe with that of the temporal pole. Also a bundle of fastigiobulbar fibers (uncinate fasciculus of Russell) which curves over the superior cerebellar peduncle in its passage to the inferior cerebellar peduncle.

Uncus. L. a hook. The hooked-back portion of the rostral end of the parahippocampal gyrus of the temporal lobe, constituting a landmark for the lateral olfactory area.

Uvula. L. little grape. A portion of the inferior vermis of the cerebellum.

Vallecula. L. diminutive of *vallis*, valley. The midline depression on the inferior aspect of the cerebellum.

Ventricle. L. *ventriculus*, diminutive of *venter*, belly. Lateral, third, and fourth ventricles of the brain.

Vermis. L. worm. The midline portion of the cerebellum.

Zona incerta. Gray matter in the subthalamus representing a rostal extension of the reticular formation of the brain stem.

INDEX